D1358575

RECENT DEVELOPMENTS IN
ALCOHOLISM

VOLUME 8
COMBINED ALCOHOL AND
OTHER DRUG DEPENDENCE

RECENT DEVELOPMENTS IN

Edited by

MARC GALANTER

New York University School of Medicine
New York, New York

Associate Editors

HENRI BEGLEITER, RICHARD DEITRICH,
DONALD GALLANT, DONALD GOODWIN,
EDWARD GOTTHEIL, ALFONSO PAREDES,
MARCUS ROTHSCHILD, and DAVID VAN THIEL

Assistant Editor

DENISE CANCELLARE

An Official Publication of the American Society of Addiction Medicine
and the Research Society on Alcoholism.
This series was founded by the National Council on Alcoholism.

ALCOHOLISM

VOLUME 8
COMBINED ALCOHOL AND OTHER DRUG DEPENDENCE

The Syndrome
Social Deviancy
Biological Issues
Clinical Issues

PLENUM PRESS • NEW YORK AND LONDON

The Library of Congress has cataloged this work as follows:

Recent developments in alcoholism: an official publication of the American Medical Soci-
ety on Alcoholism, and the Research Society on Alcoholism, and the National Council on
Alcoholism—Vol. 1– —New York: Plenum Press, c1983–
   v.: ill.; 25 cm.
   Cataloging in publication.
   Editor: Marc Galanter.
   ISSN 0738-422X = Recent developments in alcoholism.

   1. Alcoholism—Periodicals. I. Galanter, Marc. II. American Medical Society on Alcoholism. III. Research Society on Alcohol (U.S.) IV. National Council on Alcoholism. [DNLM:
1. Alcoholism—periodicals. W1 RE106AH(P)]

| HV5001.R4 | 616.86′1′05—dc19 | 83-643791 |
| Library of Congress | [8311] | AACR 2 MARC-S |

ISBN 0-306-43349-4

© 1990 Plenum Press, New York
A Division of Plenum Publishing Corporation
233 Spring Street, New York, N.Y. 10013

All rights reserved

No part of this book may be reproduced, stored in a retrieval system, or transmitted
in any form or by any means, electronic, mechanical, photocopying, microfilming,
recording, or otherwise, without written permission from the Publisher

Printed in the United States of America

Editorial Board

Chairman:
 Charles S. Lieber, M.D.
James Beard, Ph.D.
Henri Begleiter, Ph.D.
William F. Bosron, Ph.D.
Richard A. Deitrich, Ph.D.
Carlton K. Erickson, Ph.D.
V. Gene Erwin, Ph.D.
Daniel Flavin, M.D.
Dora B. Goldstein, M.D.
R. Adron Harris, Ph.D.
Maria A. Leo, M.D.
Lawrence Lumeng, M.D.
Roger Meyer, M.D.
Esteban Mezey, M.D.
Larissa A. Pohorecky, M.D.
Carrie L. Randall, Ph.D.
Edward Riley, Ph.D.
Percy E. Ryberg, M.D.
Herman H. Samson, Ph.D.
Boris Tabakoff, Ph.D.
Don W. Walker, Ph.D.
Sharon C. Wilsnack, Ph.D.

Research Society on Alcoholism

President:
 Henri Begleiter, Ph.D.
Vice President:
 David Van Thiel, M.D.
Secretary:
 Lawrence Lumeng, M.D.
Treasurer:
 Carlton K. Erickson, Ph.D.
Immediate Past President:
 Ting-Kai Li, M.D.

Board of Directors:
James Beard, Ph.D.
C. Robert Cloninger, M.D.
Marc Galanter, M.D.
Charles S. Lieber, M.D.
Roger Meyer, M.D.

**American Society of
Addiction Medicine**

President:
 Margaret Bean-Bayog, M.D.
President-Elect:
 Jasper G. Chen See, M.D.
Secretary:
 Jess W. Bromley, M.D.
Treasurer:
 William B. Hawthorne, M.D.
Immediate Past President:
 Max A. Schneider, M.D.

Board of Directors

Directors-at-Large:

Sheila B. Blume, M.D.
Marc Galanter, M.D.
Ann Geller, M.D.
Stanley E. Gitlow, M.D.
David E. Smith, M.D.
G. Douglas Talbott, M.D.
Charles L. Whitfield, M.D.

Regional Directors:
Charles S. Lieber, M.D.
Anthony B. Radcliffe, M.D.
David Mee-Lee, M.D.
Jean L. Forest, M.D.
Al J. Mooney, III, M.D.
Roland E. Herrington, M.D.
Donald M. Gallant, M.D.
Sandra Jo Counts, M.D.
Joseph C. MacMillan, M.D.

Contributors

M. Douglas Anglin, UCLA Drug Abuse Research Group, Neuropsychiatric Institute, University of California–Los Angeles, Los Angeles, California 90024

Thomas F. Babor, Department of Psychiatry, University of Connecticut School of Medicine, Farmington, Connecticut 06032

Ann M. Begin, Butler Hospital, and Department of Psychiatry and Human Behavior, Brown University, Providence, Rhode Island 02906

Joseph Brown, Department of Psychiatry, University of Connecticut School of Medicine, Farmington, Connecticut 06032

Kathleen K. Bucholz, Department of Psychiatry, The Jewish Hospital at Washington University School of Medicine, St. Louis, Missouri 63110

Marilyn E. Carroll, Department of Psychiatry, University of Minnesota Medical School, Minneapolis, Minnesota 55455

Allan C. Collins, School of Pharmacy, and Institute for Behavioral Genetics, University of Colorado, Boulder, Colorado 80309

Linda B. Cottler, Department of Psychiatry, Washington University School of Medicine, St. Louis, Missouri 63110

Richard A. Deitrich, Alcohol Research Center, and Department of Pharmacology, University of Colorado School of Medicine, Denver, Colorado 80262

Edward Gottheil, Division of Substance Abuse, Department of Psychiatry and Human Behavior, Thomas Jefferson University, Philadelphia, Pennsylvania 19107

Dwight B. Heath, Department of Anthropology, Brown University, Providence, Rhode Island 02912

Reid K. Hester, Behavior Therapy Associates, Albuquerque, New Mexico 87110

Leo E. Hollister, Department of Psychiatry and Pharmacology, University of Texas Medical School at Houston, Houston, Texas 77025-0249

Yih-Ing Hser, UCLA Drug Abuse Research Group, Neuropsychiatric Institute, University of California–Los Angeles, Los Angeles, California 90024

Robert L. Hubbard, Alcohol and Drug Abuse Research, Research Triangle Institute, Research Triangle Park, North Carolina 27709

Susan K. Keating, Department of Psychiatry, Washington University School of Medicine, St. Louis, Missouri 63110

E. J. Khantzian, Department of Psychiatry, Harvard Medical School at The Cambridge Hospital, Cambridge, Massachusetts 02139

Therese A. Kosten, Substance Abuse Treatment Unit, Department of Psychiatry, Yale University School of Medicine, New Haven, Connecticut 06519

Thomas R. Kosten, Substance Abuse Treatment Unit, Department of Psychiatry, Yale University School of Medicine, New Haven, Connecticut 06519

Neil Liebowitz, Department of Psychiatry, University of Connecticut School of Medicine, Farmington, Connecticut 06032

Richard A. Meisch, University of Texas Health Science Center at Houston, Houston, Texas 77030

Ted D. Nirenberg, Department of Psychiatry and Human Behavior, Brown University, Providence, Rhode Island 02906; and Substance Abuse Treatment Center, Roger Williams General Hospital, Providence, Rhode Island 02908

Barbara Orrok, Department of Psychiatry, University of Connecticut School of Medicine, Farmington, Connecticut 06032

Alfonso Paredes, Brentwood Division, West Los Angeles VA Medical Center, and Department of Psychiatry, School of Medicine, University of California–Los Angeles, Los Angeles, California 90073

Keiko Powers, UCLA Drug Abuse Research Group, Neuropsychiatric Institute, University of California–Los Angeles, Los Angeles, California 90024

Stanley W. Sadava, Department of Psychology, Brock University, St. Catharines, Ontario L2S 3A1, Canada

Ronald Salomon, Department of Psychiatry, University of Connecticut School of Medicine, Farmington, Connecticut 06032

Maxine L. Stitzer, Department of Psychiatry and Behavioral Sciences, Johns Hopkins University School of Medicine/Key Medical Center, Baltimore, Maryland 21224

Eric Strain, Department of Psychiatry and Behavioral Sciences, Johns Hopkins University School of Medicine/Key Medical Center, Baltimore, Maryland 21224

Arnold M. Washton, The Washton Institute on Addictions, New York, New York 10016

Kazuo Yamaguchi, Department of Sociology, University of California–Los Angeles, Los Angeles, California 90024

James P. Zacny, Drug Abuse Research Center, Department of Psychiatry, University of Chicago, Chicago, Illinois 60637

Preface

From the President of the Research Society on Alcoholism

In the last decade research concerning the causes and consequences of alcohol abuse and alcoholism has come of age. We have witnessed a plethora of scientific findings that have shed light on some of the actions of alcohol at the molecular level. Interesting new data have been forthcoming on the complexities of the development of tolerance to alcohol. It is becoming increasingly appropriate to consider that tolerance to alcohol involves biological as well as psychological factors.

New scientific insights have been gained concerning the treatment of withdrawal as well as the presence of persistent withdrawal signs that may possibly be involved with relapse. More recently, new and compelling data indicating that alcoholism is a common familial disorder have appeared. Clinical studies indicate that alcoholism is a heterogeneous disorder with multiformity in clinical symptomatology and genetic heterogeneity. The heterogeneity of the clinical features and the heritability of the predisposing factors of alcoholism are currently under vigorous scientific investigation.

In the past several years sophisticated psychosocial studies have provided fundamental information on subjects at high risk for alcoholism. Psychosocial and biological studies of families including alcoholics and subjects at high risk are likely to bring new insights to our understanding of etiological factors. Moreover, as a result of these studies we stand to develop better prevention initiatives and treatment approaches.

Much of the aforementioned research has appeared in two publications sponsored and supported by the Research Society on Alcoholism (RSA), namely *Recent Developments in Alcoholism* and the journal *Alcoholism: Clinical and Experimental Research*. The present volume of *Recent Developments in Alcoholism* deals with the topic of combined alcohol and other drug dependencies; it includes chapters on definition of the dependence syndrome, social deviancy and alcohol dependence, and biological and clinical issues of combined alcohol and other drug dependencies. While the wide range of topics typically reflects the broad range of interest among members of RSA, the high quality of the papers is a tribute to Dr. Marc Galanter, the editor of this fine publication. The Research Society on Alcoholism is pleased to once again sponsor the publication of *Recent Developments in Alcoholism*.

Henri Begleiter, Ph.D.
President, Research Society on Alcoholism

From the President of the American Society of Addiction Medicine

The eighth volume of *Recent Developments in Alcoholism* brings up to date several areas important to physicians who care for people with addictive disorders. The first section increases the specificity and reproducibility of definitions and concepts in alcohol and drug abuse, in order to allow clinical work to be more coherent and rational. The second section describes a variety of contextual and social correlates of alcoholism.

The section on biological issues explores recent exciting findings and interactions between alcohol and nicotine, clinically vital because of the high risk of nicotine dependence and lower rates of stopping nicotine use in alcoholics; it also examines the controversial issue of benzodiazepines and alcohol. The final section includes diverse topics important to understanding treatment and recovery: cultural, psychological, and behavioral concerns, and the controversy about treating drug and alcohol abuse together in single programs.

This volume, like its predecessors, provides a wonderful tool to medical practitioners who care for addicted people, helping them to integrate recent findings from both clinical and basic science research into a higher standard of clinical practice. The members of ASAM are grateful for the contribution of this volume toward this goal.

Margaret Bean-Bayog, M.D.
President, American Society of Addiction Medicine

Editor's Note

The contents of this volume are subject to peer review, but do not necessarily represent either the views or policies of the sponsoring societies. On many issues, particularly those involving diagnostic and therapeutic techniques, other perspectives, particularly those drawn from the preponderance of clinical observations, may be most pertinent to the issues raised.

Marc Galanter, M.D.

Contents

I. The Nature of the Syndrome 1

Thomas F. Babor, Section Editor

Chapter 1

The Behavioral Pharmacology of Alcohol and Other Drugs:
Emerging Issues
    Marilyn E. Carroll, Maxine L. Stitzer, Eric Strain, and Richard A. Meisch

1. Introduction 5
2. Factors Related to the Establishment of Alcohol and Other Drugs
   as Reinforcers 7
   2.1. Acquisition Techniques 7
   2.2. Schedule of Access: Limited vs. Unlimited 11
   2.3. Route of Self-Administration 12
   2.4. Organism Factors 14
3. Factors Influencing the Maintenance of Drug Reinforcement 19
   3.1. Behavioral and Environmental Effects 19
   3.2. Biochemical Factors 24
4. Dependence Potential 27
   4.1. Observational Measures of Withdrawal 28
   4.2. Altered Performance Measures during Withdrawal 31
   4.3. Relationship between Drug-Seeking Behavior and
        Withdrawal 32
   References 34

Chapter 2

The Dependence Syndrome Concept as Applied to Alcohol and
Other Substances of Abuse
    Therese A. Kosten and Thomas R. Kosten

1. A New Look at the Dependence Syndrome 47
   1.1. Comparing Alcohol to Other Substances of Abuse 47
   1.2. Comparing Dependence to Other Constructs 48
2. Diagnosis and the Dependence Syndrome 49
   2.1. Creating Diagnostic Guidelines for Dependence 49
   2.2. The Instrument for Data Collection Is Theory Bound 50

3. Observation and Theory in the Dependence Syndrome 51
   3.1. The Operational Definitions 51
   3.2. Borrowing Ideas from Hunger 51
4. Motivation Theory 52
   4.1. Relationship of Motivation to Other Theories 52
   4.2. Defining Motivation 53
   4.3. Acquired Motivation 54
   4.4. The Motivational Aspects of Dependence 56
5. Methodology 56
   5.1. Assessment of Drug Dependence and Withdrawal 56
   5.2. Relating Biological Variables to Behavioral Variables 58
6. Results 59
   6.1. Dependence Correlates with Opiate Withdrawal Severity 59
   6.2. Unidimensionality of the Dependence Syndrome 60
   6.3. Internal Consistency of Dependence Scales 60
   6.4. Relating Biological to Behavioral Aspects of Dependence 62
   6.5. Dependence Item Comparisons across Substances 62
7. Conclusions and Future Directions 64
   7.1. How Constructs Are Useful for Dependence 64
   7.2. How Motivation Theory Is Useful for Dependence 65
   7.3. Limitations of Current Work and Future Directions 66
   References 66

Chapter 3

Operationalization of Alcohol and Drug Dependence Criteria by Means of a Structured Interview
   Linda B. Cottler and Susan K. Keating

1. Introduction 69
2. Development Originates with the Nomenclature 70
3. Structured Interviews with the Robins Influence 71
4. The Essentials of a Good Interview 74
5. The Evolution of Operationalizing Criteria 77
6. Operationalization—What It Looks Like 78
7. Discussion 81
   References 82

Chapter 4

From Basic Concepts to Clinical Reality: Unresolved Issues in the Diagnosis of Dependence
   Thomas F. Babor, Barbara Orrok, Neil Liebowitz, Ronald Salomon, and Joseph Brown

1. Introduction 85
2. The Concept of Dependence 87
   Case 1: John B. 87

3. Polysubstance Use 89
   Case 2: Joe H. 89
4. The Primary–Secondary Distinction 91
   4.1. Case 3: Allen T. 91
   4.2. Case 4: George B. 92
5. Other Psychopathology 94
   5.1. Case 5: Gerald A. 94
   5.2. Case 6: Betty B. 94
6. Use of the Multiaxial System 97
   Case 7: Alex B. 97
7. Conclusion 101
   References 103

II. Social Deviancy and Alcohol Dependence 105

Alfonso Paredes, Section Editor

Chapter 5

A Review of Correlates of Alcohol Use and Alcohol Problems in Adolescence
Kathleen K. Bucholz

1. Introduction 111
2. Demographic Correlates 113
   2.1. Age 113
   2.2. Gender 113
   2.3. Ethnicity 113
   2.4. Religion 114
   2.5. Socioeconomic Status 114
3. Parental Attributes 115
4. Peer Influences 116
5. Personality and Personal Values 118
   Measures of Conventionality 118
6. Psychiatric Correlates 119
   6.1. General Deviant Behavior 119
   6.2. Depressive Symptoms 120
7. Conclusion 120
   References 121

Chapter 6

Drug Use and Its Social Covariates from the Period of Adolescence to Young Adulthood: Some Implications from Longitudinal Studies
Kazuo Yamaguchi

1. Introduction 125
2. Social Covariates of Drug Use 126
   2.1. Age 126

2.2. Age of Onset 127
2.3. Historical Period 129
2.4. Family and Work Roles 131
2.5. Causation and Selection Effects of Illicit Drug Use on Drug
       Users' Patterns of Role Transitions 136
2.6. Influence of Significant Others 138
2.7. Indirect Effects in the Dynamic Relationship between Drug
       Use and Life Events 139
3. Concluding Remarks 140
   References 142

Chapter 7

Longitudinal Patterns of Alcohol Use by Narcotics Addicts
Yih-Ing Hser, M. Douglas Anglin, and Keiko Powers

1. Introduction 145
2. Literature Review 146
   2.1. Considerations of Background Characteristics 146
   2.2. Patterns of Alcohol Use among Opiate Users 147
   2.3. Abuse of Alcohol by Opiate Addicts Maintained on
         Methadone 148
   2.4. Consequences of Alcohol and Opiate Use 149
3. Longitudinal Patterns of Alcohol Use and Related Behaviors
   among Narcotics Addicts 150
   3.1. Sample Characteristics 151
   3.2. Longitudinal Patterns of Use 158
   3.3. Alcohol-Related Deaths 164
4. Discussion 167
   References 169

Chapter 8

Problem Drinking and Alcohol Problems: Widening the Circle of Covariation
Stanley W. Sadava

1. Introduction 173
2. Consumption and Consequences 174
   2.1. Interrelationships and Causality 174
   2.2. Adolescent Consumption and Consequences in Adulthood .. 177
3. Alcohol-Specific and Non-Alcohol-Specific Causes 179
4. Behavioral Specificity 182
   4.1. Concurrent Use of Other Drugs 182
   4.2. Other Problem Behaviors 184
5. Psychosocial Variables and Vulnerability 186

6. Personality and Vulnerability 187
7. Gender and Vulnerability 189
8. Family and Vulnerability 190
9. Stress, Drinking, and Vulnerability 192
10. Conclusions 194
    References 196

III. Biological Issues: Ethanol–Drug Interactions 203
Richard A. Deitrich, Section Editor

Chapter 9

Behavioral Aspects of Alcohol–Tobacco Interactions
James P. Zacny

1. Introduction 205
2. Documenting the Relationship between Alcohol and Tobacco
   Consumption 206
   2.1. Descriptive Studies 206
   2.2. Experimental Studies 207
3. Possible Mechanisms Underlying the Relationship between
   Alcohol and Tobacco Consumption 210
4. Joint Effects of Alcohol and Tobacco on Behavior 211
5. Alcohol/Tobacco Association and Drug Relapse 214
6. Alcohol/Tobacco Association and Disease 216
7. Summary 216
   References 217

Chapter 10

Interactions of Ethanol and Nicotine at the Receptor Level
Allan C. Collins

1. Introduction 221
2. Behavioral Interactions between Alcohol and Nicotine 222
   2.1. Ethanol–Nicotine Self-Administration 222
   2.2. Physiological and Behavioral Interactions 222
   2.3. Cross-Tolerance between Ethanol and Nicotine 223
3. Mechanisms of Ethanol–Nicotine Interactions 224
   3.1. Structure of the Nicotinic Receptors 224
   3.2. Effect of Lipids on Nicotinic Receptor Function 225
   3.3. Ethanol's Effects on Nicotinic Receptor Binding 226
   3.4. Effects of Ethanol on Nicotinic Receptor Function 227

    4. Conclusions 228
       References 229

Chapter 11

Interactions between Alcohol and Benzodiazepines
   Leo E. Hollister

    1. Introduction 233
    2. Clinical Considerations of Interactions 234
       2.1. Concurrent Abuse 234
       2.2. Cross-Tolerance 234
       2.3. Driving Ability 235
       2.4. Overdoses 235
    3. Experimental Studies of Interactions 236
       3.1. Pharmacokinetics 236
       3.2. Pharmacodynamics 237
    4. Conclusions 238
       References 239

IV. Emerging Clinical Issues in the Treatment of Alcohol and/or Other Drugs of Abuse 241

   Edward Gottheil, Section Editor

Chapter 12

Cultural Factors in the Choice of Drugs
   Dwight B. Heath

    1. Introduction 245
    2. Psychoactive Drugs and the Human Animal 246
    3. The "Drug-of-Choice" Phenomenon at a Cultural Level 247
       3.1. Changing Patterns of Drug Use 248
       3.2. Intracultural Variation 249
    4. Implications for Culture and Choice 250
       4.1. Culture as Metaphor 251
       4.2. Education as Prevention 252
       References 254

Chapter 13

Self-Regulation and Self-Medication Factors in Alcoholism and the Addictions: Similarities and Differences
   E. J. Khantzian

    1. Introduction 255
    2. The Challenge of Self-Regulation 256

3. Old and New Theories of Human Distress 258
   3.1. Drives and Conflict 258
   3.2. Affects and Structure 258
   3.3. Development and Adaptation 258
4. Common Factors in Alcoholism and the Addictions 259
   4.1. Affects 260
   4.2. Well-Being and Self-Esteem 261
   4.3. Relationships.. 261
   4.4. Self-Care 262
5. Drugs and Self-Medication 263
   5.1. Stimulants 263
   5.2. Opiate–Analgesics 264
6. Alcohol and Self-Medication 265
   6.1. Affects and Alcohol 266
   6.2. Well-Being, Self-Esteem, and Alcohol 267
   6.3. Relationships and Alcohol 268
7. Conclusion.. 268
   References 269

Chapter 14

Treating Combined Alcohol and Drug Abuse in Community-Based Programs
Robert L. Hubbard

1. Introduction 273
2. Estimations and Nature of Alcohol and Drugs and Extent of
   Combined Use 274
3. Combined Alcohol and Drug Problems in Two Samples of
   Community Programs 275
4. Issues in Treating Combined Alcohol and Drug Abuse 277
   4.1. Diagnosis 277
   4.2. Treatment 279
   4.3. The Recovery Process 280
5. Summary 281
   References 281

Chapter 15

Structured Outpatient Treatment of Alcohol vs. Drug Dependencies
Arnold M. Washton

1. Introduction 285
2. Outpatient vs. Inpatient Treatment 287
3. When Is Outpatient Treatment Appropriate? 288
4. Alcoholism vs. Drug Addiction Treatment 289
   4.1. Treatment Philosophy and Goals 289

    4.2. Treatment Techniques 291
  5. Ingredients of Effective Outpatient Treatment 294
  6. Stages of Outpatient Treatment 299
    6.1. Assessment and Crisis Intervention 299
    6.2. Early Abstinence 301
    6.3. Relapse Prevention 302
    6.4. Advanced Recovery 302
  7. Final Comment 303
    References 304

Chapter 16

**Behavioral Treatment of Alcohol and Drug Abuse: What Do We
Know and Where Shall We Go?**
Reid K. Hester, Ted D. Nirenberg, and Ann M. Begin

  1. Introduction 305
  2. Assessment of Alcohol and Drug Abuse 306
  3. Behavioral Treatments for Alcohol and Drug Abuse 307
    3.1. Aversion Therapies 308
    3.2. Behavioral Self-Control Training 310
    3.3. Behavioral Marital and Family Therapy 312
    3.4. The Community Reinforcement Approach/Contingency
        Management 313
    3.5. Social Skills Training 315
    3.6. Stress Management Training 316
    3.7. Cue Exposure 317
  4. Similarities in Behavioral Alcohol and Drug Abuse Treatment 318
  5. Future Directions in Treatment and Research 319
  6. Summary 320
    References 320

Contents of Previous Volumes 329

Index 339

The Nature of the Syndrome

Thomas F. Babor, Section Editor

The concept of dependence has had a long and tangled history, with different scientific disciplines, theoretical approaches, and methodological procedures all contributing to a diversity of explanations that are at once professionally embarrassing and intellectually stimulating. Is dependence a biological condition, a personality disorder, a form of psychopathology, a learned behavior, a social construction of reality, or a culturally conditioned form of social imitation? The diversity implicit in this question gives testimony to the lack of agreement about the nature of dependence. Despite the difficulty that psychiatrists, psychologists, pharmacologists, biologists, sociologists, and anthropologists have experienced in communicating with each other about the nature of alcohol and drug dependence, there has been substantial progress in the past decade in the development of concepts, methods, and theories that all disciplines can use to conduct research and to debate its findings.

The chapters in this section deal with two of the most intriguing and fundamental questions in the field of alcohol and drug studies: What is the nature of dependence, and how can it be measured? They speak directly to the complexities of developing scientific and clinical information about substance use disorders by carefully reviewing current knowledge about basic concepts, research methods, and diagnostic implications. When they are read, as they should be, as a complementary series of articles, they tell a fascinating story about the way in which basic and applied research is attempting to explore the nature of dependence. Ranging from behavioral pharmacology to psychiatric epidemiology, and from laboratory experimentation to clinical diagnosis, the articles in this section demonstrate the value of interdisciplinary collaboration, and the need for complementarity between research and practice, method and theory, laboratory studies and clinical observation.

The first chapter, by Marilyn Carroll, Maxine Stitzer, Eric Strain, and Richard Meisch, sets the stage for subsequent articles by painstakingly re-

Thomas F. Babor • Department of Psychiatry, University of Connecticut School of Medicine, Farmington, Connecticut 06032.

viewing the remarkable achievements of behavioral pharmacology research during the past 20 years. Although it is one of the youngest disciplines to contribute to an understanding of alcohol and drug dependence, its contributions have been enormously valuable for both researchers and clinicians. Applying research techniques developed for the investigation of human and animal learning mechanisms, behavioral pharmacologists have identified a number of variables that are responsible for the initiation, maintenance, and control of psychoactive substance use. These variables include the type of psychoactive substance, the dose taken, the response costs involved, the route of administration, the schedule of access, the organism's prior history and functioning, and the environmental context of substance use.

By integrating the principles of learning and conditioning derived from psychological learning theory, this research has shown that nearly all dependence-producing drugs have the ability to serve as positive reinforcers, a phenomenon that goes beyond their connection with the relief of withdrawal symptoms. It also shows that the mechanisms of acquisition involved in drug self-administration may be quite different from those that maintain the behavior. Most important, this body of research provides a clear cause for optimism regarding the potential of behavioral science to understand the underlying mechanisms of alcohol and drug dependence. Animal models developed to study genetic factors, alternative reinforcers, dosage effects, withdrawal signs, and a variety of other variables related to dependence permit the exploration of a broad range of hypotheses relevant to human drug self-administration and have already exercised an influence on diagnostic criteria and treatment modalities.

The second chapter, by Therese and Thomas Kosten, adds theoretical and clinical depth to the basic science issues raised by a behavioral pharmacology approach to drug dependence. While animal models provide valuable insights into the mechanisms of acquisition, maintenance, and extinction of drug-seeking behaviors, descriptive research using phenomenological methods has emerged as an important source of clinical data from human subjects. In their exploration of the generalizability of the alcohol dependence syndrome concept to other psychoactive substances, especially cocaine and heroin, the Kostens point out the difficulties involved in measuring hypothetical constructs and the merits of going beyond psychological learning theory to account for the complexity of substance use disorders. Because there is no consensus about the learning mechanisms involved in dependence or the biological substrate of drug-seeking behavior, advances in our understanding of dependence will probably have to await the integration of different theoretical approaches, such as learning principles, motivation theory, and neurobiological models.

Like the first chapter, Chapter 2 emphasizes the importance of theory in the design and interpretation of research on dependence. Not only does theory open up a much broader fund of knowledge to guide the formulation of hypotheses, it also suggests constructs that provide organizing principles for operational definitions and predictions.

Drawing on the results of an interview study of alcohol and polydrug users, the authors suggest that the provisional symptoms of the DSM-III-R dependence concept do indeed cluster in time, in the same individuals, and in a similar way across many psychoactive substances. The data also suggest that the syndrome concept may not apply equally well to all psychoactive substances, but that this may be less a fault of the concept than a basic pharmacological property of substances such as hallucinogens and cannabis.

Although the phenomenological method has its advantages, there is always the risk that the tools we create may eventually lead us astray or so influence the measurement of what we are studying that the data are little more than methodological artifacts. Fortunately, Chapter 2 makes a compelling case for the need to consider dependence as motivated behavior that can be studied by several different methods. Because research relying exclusively on phenomenological methods can be affected by a variety of biases and other sources of error, it is refreshing to see an ingenious attempt to provide external validation of the kind of verbal report methods that so much clinical research relies on. By incorporating a direct measure of biological dependence on opiates (i.e., withdrawal symptom severity following a challenge dose of the opiate antagonist naloxone), this chapter illustrates an important methodological tool for bridging the gap between different disciplinary orientations and methological approaches.

The third chapter in this section, by Linda Cottler and colleagues, seeks to bridge the gap between concepts and measurement, giving an inside view of how the methods of descriptive epidemiology are applied to the study of dependence in population studies and clinical research. Also communicated in this chapter is the fascinating notion that the tools of the trade eventually may shape the way we conceptualize dependence, if only because concepts that do not permit operationalization and objective measurement no longer have credibility. In what is clearly an attempt to wed phenomenology and positivism, psychiatric epidemiologists have advanced the art of interviewing to the point where much of the data we interpret in clinical research is obtained through the objective measurement of subjective experience.

The chapter begins with a discussion of problems associated with the design of an epidemiological instrument that will eventually be used for the definition, estimation, and investigation of alcohol and drug dependence. The problems in constructing such an instrument include the lack of a unifying concept of dependence, the need to develop clearly specified criteria, and the translation of criteria into questions and response categories that ultimately have some objectively verifiable external referent. Fortunately, advances in psychiatric interviewing techniques and questionnaire survey design have made the epidemiologist's task much easier. Standardized questions, memory aids, improved training techniques for interviewers, systematic procedures for evaluating the reliability (consistency) of interviewers and respondents, and the application of test validation procedures to determine accuracy all have contributed to the development of a new generation of psychiatric interviews. These instruments, epitomized by the Substance Abuse Module of the Composite International Diagnostic Interview, promise to provide valuable data about the clustering of dependence symptoms into an identifiable syndrome, the similarity of dependence symptoms across substances, and the generalizability of dependence concepts across cultures.

One concept that has recently become a focal point for discussions of psychoactive substance use is the syndrome concept of drug dependence first advanced as a provisional definition of alcohol dependence and later generalized to other substances.[1,2] The final chapter in this series, by Thomas Babor and his colleagues, attempts to bridge the gap between basic concepts and clinical reality by discussing the syndrome concept from the viewpoints of patients and therapists. This is not always the most scientific way to explore the nature of dependence, but it is an approach supported by the truism that the behavioral sciences begin with the careful observation of individual cases. To the extent that the study of dependence is often motivated by the wish to relieve human suffering, it is appropriate to highlight the case history as a way of placing dependence in the broader context of life span development, psychiatric disorder, environmental stressors, and social influence.

None of these chapters makes a compelling case for a definitive explanation of the nature of dependence, but each describes in its own way the significant progress that has been made in areas such as theory, methodology, and clinical description. It is only after such progress has been made that the nature of the syndrome will be understood.

References

1. Edwards G, Gross MM: Alcohol dependence: Provisional description of a clinical syndrome. *Br Med J* 1:1058–1061, 1976.
2. Edwards G, Arif A, Hodgson R: Nomenclature and classification of drug- and alcohol-related problems: A WHO memorandum. *Bull WHO* 59:225–242, 1981.

The Behavioral Pharmacology of Alcohol and Other Drugs

Emerging Issues

Marilyn E. Carroll, Maxine L. Stitzer, Eric Strain, and Richard A. Meisch

Abstract. Alcohol and other drugs are compared with respect to their abuse liability and dependence potential. Drug-reinforced behavior is defined, and factors related to the establishment of this behavior that have received increasing experimental attention in recent years are reviewed. Acquisition techniques, schedule of access, route of self-administration, and organism factors, such as species, gender, and genetic background, are discussed. Other areas of emerging interest are the effect of feeding regimens, alternative reinforcers, and social conditions on drug-reinforced behavior. Also, biochemical factors such as neurochemical alterations, hormonal changes, and alcohol and other drug combinations, are considered. Finally, dependence potential is considered in terms of observational changes and performance alterations that seem to be sensitive indicators of the protracted aspects of drug withdrawal. The relationship between drug-seeking behavior and withdrawal is examined.

1. Introduction

This chapter is focused on the abuse liability and dependence potential of alcohol and other drugs. Alcohol and drug intake are generally viewed as operant behavior with the drugs functioning as positive reinforcers. Reinforcers are defined as events or consequences that are presented contingent upon a response and subsequently increase the probability of responses leading to their delivery. This conceptual model of drug abuse has been successfully used in both animal and human laboratory studies of alcohol as well as other drugs. The terms *drug-reinforced behavior* and *drug self-administration* are often used interchangeably; however, in the case of oral drug intake, there

Marilyn E. Carroll • Department of Psychiatry, University of Minnesota Medical School, Minneapolis, Minnesota 55455. **Maxine L. Stitzer and Eric Strain** • Department of Psychiatry and Behavioral Sciences, Johns Hopkins University School of Medicine/Key Medical Center, Baltimore, Maryland 21224. **Richard A. Meisch** • University of Texas Health Science Center at Houston, Houston, Texas 77030.

can be important differences between the two forms of behavior. Drug self-administration occurs when an animal drinks a drug dissolved in water or a palatable vehicle. If the drug and vehicle intake does not exceed vehicle intake, the drug is not functioning as a reinforcer. This situation is less likely to occur with intravenous drug self-administration because animals do not typically self-inject saline or other vehicles unless they have self-administered a drug that increases all activity (e.g., lever pressing on active as well as inactive levers). Thus, in the case of the intravenous route, *drug self-administration* is more likely to be synonymous with *drug-reinforced behavior,* but if the terms are to be used correctly, several control conditions have to be applied to clearly demonstrate that a self-administered intravenously delivered drug is also functioning as a reinforcer.[1] For instance, when "active" and "inactive" levers are reversed, responding should "follow" the active lever. The rate of lever pressing should decline when infusions are delivered noncontingently upon responses but in the same pattern that they were previously self-administered. Finally, as is the case with oral self-administration, the drug solution should maintain higher rates of responding when the vehicle is substituted or presented concurrently. Often it is necessary to use intermittent reinforcement schedules to observe these drug–vehicle differences if the animals have a history of high rates of responding.

In this chapter alcohol and other drugs are compared with respect to factors related to the establishment of drug-reinforced behavior. With respect to the maintenance of drug-taking behavior, a number of emerging issues are considered. For example, recent work has been concerned with altering the availability of other reinforcing events in the environment, and dramatic increases and decreases in drug-reinforced behavior have ensued. The biochemical basis of drug abuse is of great interest not only for a better understanding of underlying mechanisms, but for the development of pharmacotherapy. The effects of an ethanol antagonist and opiate receptor antagonists on ethanol and other drug use are examined. Polydrug abuse has become more prevalent in recent years, and experimental studies of alcohol and other drug interactions are considered. Finally, there are new developments in the study of dependence and related withdrawal syndromes as defined in terms of both physiological changes and alterations in performance.

There are a number of excellent reviews concerning the behavioral pharmacology of alcohol[2–12] as well as reviews comparing alcohol and other drugs.[13–17] These reviews have identified and documented the importance of many variables that control drug-taking behavior, including type of drug, dose, response costs, route of self-administration, and environmental and history conditions. It is beyond the scope of the present chapter to identify and discuss all of these factors. However, this review will focus on a few of these variables that have received increasing amounts of experimental attention, as well as those that have been shown to have impact on the development of treatment strategies.

2. Factors Related to the Establishment of Alcohol and Other Drugs as Reinforcers

Ethanol-reinforced behavior can be divided, like operant behavior in general, into three phases: establishment, maintenance, and termination. Establishment of ethanol-reinforced behavior incorporates two distinct phases: (1) acquisition or learning of a new behavior that produces ethanol, and (2) exposure to ethanol in sufficient amounts and durations to establish reinforcing effects. This section discusses factors that influence the establishment of ethanol as a reinforcer, including (1) acquisition techniques, (2) schedule of access, (3) route of self-administration, and (4) antecedent conditions (e.g., organism factors).

2.1. Acquisition Techniques

Unlike certain reinforcers such as food or a saccharin solution (which experimental subjects will consume under a variety of circumstances), rats and rhesus monkeys will not spontaneously drink ethanol solutions, especially at concentrations above 8%.[8] Therefore, specific training procedures are necessary before ethanol will serve as a reinforcer. Such training procedures are also important in establishing other orally delivered drugs as reinforcers.[16]

There are two impediments to establishing orally delivered ethanol and other drugs as reinforcers. One is that the taste of many drug solutions is aversive, especially in concentrations that have behavioral effects. Given a choice between a drug solution and water, the animals will drink the water. The second problem is that there is a delay between ingestion of the drug solution and the onset of effects that follow absorption. This delay is on the order of minutes, and it is far longer than the delays between emissions of a response and delivery of a reinforcer that have been found to be optimal for learning to occur. A series of procedures has evolved that circumvents these difficulties and leads to the establishment of many orally delivered drugs, including ethanol, as reinforcers. Common elements include the use of food-deprived animals, the induction of drinking, and the gradual increase of drug concentrations.[18,19] In some cases; however, these three factors are not always necessary.[20]

2.1.1. Schedule-Induced Polydipsia. One of the first procedures used to establish ethanol as a reinforcer was schedule-induced polydipsia. *Schedule-induced polydipsia* is the term used to describe the excessive drinking that occurs when food-deprived rats intermittently receive small pellets of food and have access to water.[21] Under conditions of schedule-induced polydipsia rats will drink up to one-half of their body weight in water in a period of a little over 3 hr. A number of investigators have generated excessive drinking of ethanol and other drugs by substituting these drugs for water under conditions that generate polydipsic drinking.[22] Importantly, when the polydipsic drinking is terminated by no longer presenting food pellets, animals often persist in drinking substantial volumes of ethanol solutions, but no longer drink much water when it is substituted for or presented concurrently with the drug.[23-26] Subsequent tests, such as making ethanol available under intermittent reinforcement schedules, confirm that ethanol has come to function as a reinforcer.[18-27] Successful results have been obtained with other drugs[28] and with rhesus monkeys as well as rats.[29-31] The positive findings with other drugs demonstrate that the schedule induction procedure is effective with drugs that lack caloric value. These results, in turn, suggest that the establishment of ethanol as a reinforcer in this paradigm is not due to ethanol's caloric value, but rather to its reinforcing properties.

2.1.2. Postprandial Drinking.   A procedure related to schedule-induced polydipsia is postprandial drinking. This type of drinking can be reliably induced by giving food-deprived animals a limited ration of food. Once a stable pattern of water drinking is obtained, drug solutions, including ethanol solutions, can be substituted for water, and if necessary, the drug concentration can be gradually increased over time. Subsequently, the food access can be terminated, and the food is then given after the experimental session. As with schedule-induced polydipsia, water drinking drops to very low levels following removal of food from sessions, but drug drinking persists if the procedure has established the drug as a reinforcer.[18,32]

2.1.3. Reduced Food Rations.   A third procedure is related to the two previous procedures in that animals are food deprived and are trained to emit responses that activate liquid delivery devices. However, the procedure differs in that animals are not given food during the experimental session; thus, drinking is not induced by eating. The animals are simply provided with access to a drug solution; very low concentrations are often used initially if the drug has an aversive taste. Response rates gradually increase across sessions, and the concentration of the drug solution is then increased in steps. Confirmation that the drug is functioning as a reinforcer occurs when water is substituted for the drug solution and water consumption falls to levels below drug values. This procedure seems to work best with animals that have high operant levels of water drinking, possibly because these animals are the ones most likely to ingest the drug solution in significant quantities when it replaces water. Note that, as with the other procedures, the animals are not water deprived, and they have free access to water between sessions.[18,20,33]

2.1.4. Oral Substitution.   A fourth acquisition procedure is to add the drug to another solution that is already serving as a reinforcer.[34,35] For example, pentobarbital was added to an ethanol solution that was already functioning as a reinforcer for monkeys. The amount of pentobarbital was gradually increased across sessions. Once an intermediate pentobarbital concentration was reached, the amount of ethanol in the solution was gradually reduced across sessions until only the pentobarbital solution was present. Subsequent tests confirmed that pentobarbital had been established as a reinforcer.[34] Ethanol drinking has been initiated by a similar strategy; ethanol was added to a sucrose solution and then the sucrose concentration was gradually decreased to zero.[35]

2.1.5. Concurrent Access: Established Reinforcer and Ethanol. A fifth procedure is to introduce ethanol concurrently with another orally delivered drug that is functioning as a reinforcer. In a recent experiment five monkeys were trained to self-administer orally-delivered phencyclidine (0.25 mg/ml) and water under concurrent fixed-ratio 16 schedules. When increasing concentrations of ethanol (1, 2, 4, and 8% wt/vol) were substituted for water they were readily accepted from the first day of substitution, and they maintained rates of responding that were substantially higher than water. Figure 1 summarizes these results and shows that the high rates of ethanol self-administration were related to decreased phencyclidine intake in one (M-B2) of the five monkeys. These data suggest that this method may produce rapid acquisition of drug self-administration behavior; however, further work is needed to extend the generality of this method. It is possible that phencyclidine and ethanol share discriminative stimulus effects and/or similar reinforcing effects.

2.1.6. Intravenous Substitution. A final procedure has been to substitute an ethanol solution for another drug that is already functioning as an intravenously-delivered reinforcer. This approach is most feasible in studies that employ the intravenous route and thereby minimize taste factors. Ethanol functioned as a reinforcer for rhesus monkeys when it was substituted either for intravenously delivered cocaine or for methohexital.[37] The pattern of ethanol-reinforced behavior that developed did not differ from that of monkeys for whom ethanol was the initial reinforcing drug. Likewise, different procedures were used to generate self-administration of intravenously delivered phencyclidine in monkeys; despite the different procedures, the final performances were similar.[38,39]

Different acquisition procedures may lead to more rapid or consistent acquisition of drug-reinforced behavior, depending on a number of factors, such as, the drug history of the animal,[40,41] the taste of the drug, and operant levels of the animals. However, the different acquisition procedures lead to stable patterns of drug-reinforced responding and levels of drug intake that do not differ from one another. This finding has been best documented in the case of ethanol.[18] Thus, the specific manner in which ethanol is established as a reinforcer is not important in terms of subsequent behavior.[19,37] There is a parallel with the development of opioid dependence in humans. Jaffe[42] has noted that there may be very different circumstances that lead to initial opioid

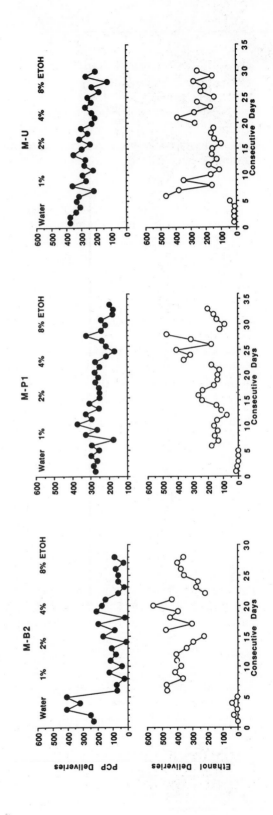

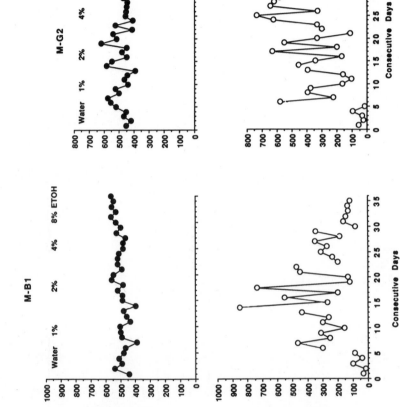

Figure 1. Ethanol and phencyclidine (PCP) deliveries are presented over a series of consecutive days when concurrent water was replaced with 1, 2, 4 and then 8% (wt/vol) ethanol. Both solutions were available under concurrent fixed-ratio 16 schedules during daily 3-hr sessions. Breaks between connected points indicate a change in ethanol concentration. The first five points represent the last five days of stable responding when PCP and water were concurrently available. The next point (open circle) represents the first day the five monkeys (M-B2, M-P1, M-U, M-B1, and M-G2) were exposed to ethanol.

use; however, over time similar patterns of drug taking emerge regardless of the original motivation for opioid use.

2.2. Schedule of Access: Limited vs. Unlimited

A major determinant of drug-reinforced behavior is the schedule of access, which differs from the schedule of reinforcement. The schedule of access refers to periods of drug availability, and it is defined by two parameters: the duration of the drug availability periods and the length of time between such periods.[8] When the interval between periods of drug access is zero, there is continuous or unlimited drug access. The effects of unlimited and limited drug access have been compared, and rhesus monkeys have generally been used in these studies. The principal finding has been that when access to ethanol is unlimited, ethanol intake is highly variable and often occurs in bouts that extend over several days, that are followed by periods of abstinence lasting a day or longer.[37,43–45] In contrast, when access is limited to a few hours each day, ethanol intake is very stable and regular.[37,43–45] Studies of ethanol drinking conducted with alcoholic humans have produced similar results.[46] Thus, if a stable baseline is needed for evaluating the effects of an independent variable, the use of limited access periods provides the necessary stability.[46]

Under unlimited-access conditions rhesus monkeys will self-inject large quantities of ethanol that produce physiological dependence.[37,43,45] After self-injecting ethanol for a number of days, rhesus monkeys will electively stop taking ethanol and consequently exhibit withdrawal signs.[37,43,45] This is an important finding, for it indicates that avoidance of withdrawal effects is not always a powerful determinant of self-administration. Similar findings occur when psychomotor stimulant drugs such as cocaine and amphetamine are studied.[47] Binges of drug taking last for several days followed by periods of self-imposed abstinence. However, other drugs such as opioids and barbiturates are self-administered in stable, regular patterns regardless of whether access is limited or unlimited.[47]

If ethanol access is limited to discrete periods throughout a 24-hr interval, higher rates of responding occur during the discrete periods than occur during unlimited access, but the total amount of ethanol consumed (g/kg) is greater during unlimited access.[47,48] For example, in one study the following conditions of ethanol availability were studied: 1 hr out of 24, 1 hr out of 8, 1 hr out of 4, and 1 hr out of 2.[49] The mean number of ethanol responses per 1-hr period increased as the time between access periods increased.[50] Comparable studies have not been conducted with drugs other than ethanol. Both rates of intake and total intake are important measures, but rate has often been neglected. The importance rate is that the magnitude and duration of drug effects depend on both the amount consumed and the rate of intake.

2.3. Route of Self-Administration

For rhesus monkeys ethanol can serve as a reinforcer when delivered via the oral,[30,31,51] intragastric,[52,53] and intravenous routes.[37,43,54–57] Similar findings have been demonstrated with other reinforcing drugs, such as pentobarbital,[58,59] phencyclidine,[29,40,60] ketamine,[61,62] and amphetamine.[61,63] Each route has both advantages and disadvantages. When the intravenous route is used, taste effects are avoided, and the delay between drug-reinforced behavior, such as lever pressing, and the onset of drug effects is minimized. A major disadvantage is the relatively short time that a catheter is patent; this is usually a period of months, thus precluding a long series of within-subject comparisons. The use of catheters is often complicated by the development of infections.

Doses of ethanol that maintain behavior via the intravenous route in monkeys range from 50 to 560 mg/kg. When the intragastric route is employed, problems associated with the taste of ethanol are circumvented, and the delay between responding and onset of drug effects is less than with the oral route. Moreover, there appear to be fewer problems with catheter patency. However, large doses of ethanol, 100–1000 mg/kg, are required to reinforce behavior, and only low rates of responding have been reported. Use of the oral route avoids the problems associated with catheters but poses two other problems: the aversive taste of intermediate and high ethanol concentrations and the delay that elapses between drinking and the onset of effects that follow absorption. These problems can be overcome by the use of certain training procedures (see Section 2.1 on acquisition techniques). The doses used can be calculated by multiplying the concentration used by the volume delivered upon completion of each reinforced response sequence. The product of the volume and concentration is then divided by the monkey's weight. The doses range from approximately 7 to 28 mg/kg,[51] and these are substantially less than the doses used with other routes of administration.

Why are smaller doses effective with the oral route? The answer may lie in the importance of taste stimuli as both conditioned reinforcers and discriminative stimuli for drug taking. Results described in the conditioned taste aversion literature demonstrate that learning can occur even when there are long temporal delays between the ingestion of sapid liquids and the onset of aversive or punishing effects. The establishment of orally delivered drugs as reinforcers demonstrates that similar learning may occur when the ingested liquid contains drugs and the delayed effects are reinforcing.[64] The taste of drug solutions probably serves as both a conditioned reinforcer and a discriminative stimulus by virtue of repeated pairing of taste stimuli with reinforcing effects. Data to support this interpretation are lacking for ethanol. However, with phencyclidine and its analogs the taste of the drug has been shown to serve as a conditioned reinforcer,[65] and it is plausible that the taste of other drug solutions functions in the same manner. Given that reinforcing effects also occur in the presence of a drug's taste, it follows that such taste effects also serve as discriminative stimuli.[66] An analogous case has been demonstrated with rats. In rats for whom ethanol has been established as a reinforcer, the odor of ethanol serves as a discriminative stimulus.[27]

An anomalous finding is that ethanol does not function as a reinforcer for rats when delivered intravenously,[67–69] but it does function as an excellent reinforcer when delivered orally. At present there is no explanation as to why this is the case. However, at least one factor can be ruled out. In three studies that attempted to establish intravenous ethanol self-administration in the rat, it was possible to obtain intravenous self-administration of other drugs such as pentobarbital and cocaine.[67–69] Thus, the failure to obtain intravenous ethanol self-administration cannot be attributed to faulty catherization technique. One study was particularly impressive in that rats self-administered the pharmacologically related drug, pentobarbital, and they also self-administered combinations of pentobarbital and ethanol.[68] However, responding was not maintained when ethanol alone was used. Since a range of ethanol doses was studied, it is unlikely that the failure was due to selection of an inappropriate dose. There are several reports of intravenous ethanol self-administration in the rat.[70–74] However, the doses used were so small and the rates of responding so low that it is not possible to attribute the behavior to the reinforcing effects of ethanol. Intragastric ethanol self-administration has also been reported in rats.[75–81] Complicated experimental designs and lack of control procedures make these studies difficult to interpret.

In other studies intravenously delivered ethanol functioned as a *negative* reinforcer[82,83] and as a punisher.[83] This result is important for several reasons. First, it indicates that one possible reason for failures to obtain reliable intravenous self-administration is that intravenously delivered ethanol can have aversive effects in the rat. Second, it extends the list of drugs that have been shown to function as both negative and positive reinforcers. For example, cocaine,[84] nicotine,[85] and pentazocine[86] can serve as positive reinforcers under some conditions and as negative reinforcers or punishers under other conditions. Third, a more extensive analysis of the conditions under which ethanol functions as a negative reinforcer (or as an aversive stimulus in punishment paradigms) may form the basis for developing treatment and prevention strategies.

2.4. Organism Factors

Previous sections have reviewed environmental conditions related to the establishment of alcohol and other drugs as reinforcers. There is convincing evidence to suggest that variables such as route of administration, reinforcement schedules, and the drug itself are fundamental determinants of drug-maintained behavior and their effects show generality across a number of species, including humans.[13,14] However, there has also been increasing evidence within the last decade that organism factors (e.g., species, gender, and genetic factors) are also important in the establishment of drugs as reinforcers.

2.4.1. Species.
Ethanol is one of the few drugs where species differences exist in intravenous self-administration. As discussed in Section 2.3, intravenously delivered ethanol is not reliably established as a reinforcer for

rats, but it is for monkeys. Weeks and Collins[87] have surveyed data on i.v. self-administration of 27 drugs, and results from studies of rats and monkeys concurred that the drugs were functioning as reinforcers for both species for 24 of the 27 drugs. Other than ethanol, the exceptions were nalorphine and ethylketazocine, which were active for rats but not monkeys.

Orally delivered ethanol can serve as a reinforcer for mice,[88,89] rats,[26,27] rhesus monkeys,[30,31] and baboons.[90] Three species, specifically mice, rats, and rhesus monkeys, have been widely studied in multiple experiments, and certain findings are common to all three species. For example, when ethanol concentration is varied, response rates and liquid deliveries are an inverted U-shaped function of concentration, whereas ethanol intake (g of ethanol per kg of body weight per session) rises with increases in concentration.[26,51,88] The high end of the concentration range that subjects will self-administer in operant behavior experiments includes values that are well beyond those found in two-bottle preference tests. In ethanol reinforcement studies, concentrations such as 32% (w/v) for rats and rhesus monkeys and 16% (w/v) for mice, are consumed in significantly greater volumes than water.[8,10] Thus, it does not appear that they are consumed solely on the basis of taste.

When fixed-ratio (FR) size is increased, the rate of ethanol-reinforced responding first increases and then decreases, while numbers of ethanol deliveries initially remain constant and then decrease.[27,91,92] The pattern of ethanol-reinforced responding under FR schedules is similar to that maintained by other reinforcers. The highest rate of responding and drinking is at the beginning of the session, and this initial burst is usually followed by a pause and then by subsequent bouts of drinking later in the session. This pattern is of interest, since it is the pattern that most rapidly results in maximal pharmacological effects. In summary, the striking similarity of results across species demonstrates the common determinants and generality of behavior reinforced by orally delivered ethanol. It is noteworthy that such cross-species generality has also been found with other reinforcing drugs.[15,41]

2.4.2. Gender.   Epidemiological studies based on a population of high-school students indicate that there are striking sex differences in the use of alcohol and other drugs, such as marijuana, cocaine, inhalants, and opiates other than heroin, while there are smaller sex differences in the use of stimulants, heroin, cigarettes, and tranquilizers. Generally, males represent a higher percentage of those using drugs, with the exception of tranquilizers and cigarettes.[93] The reasons for these differences are not known. Until recently, gender was a variable that received little attention in laboratory studies concerned with the reinforcing effects of alcohol and other drugs. In fact, in many nonhuman primate studies of alcohol self-administration, only male monkeys were used,[51,90,92] although intravenously delivered ethanol has been demonstrated to function as a reinforcer in female monkeys.[94]

In a recent study of ethanol drinking, free-fed male rhesus monkeys more readily acquired and maintained ethanol self-administration than female monkeys.[95] Of nine monkeys, all five males drank ethanol when access to a sweet, orange-flavored solution was contingent on ethanol drinking; however, only two of the four females responded to this contingency. An additional variable was drug history; one female was drug naïve and the other had a drug history. The three monkeys that sustained high rates of intake were male and they had a drug history. Of the two males that sustained moderate intakes, one had a drug history and one was naïve. None of the females continued to self-administer ethanol when behavioral contingencies were removed. These data indicate that both gender and drug history are important determinants of the acquisition and maintenance of ethanol self-administration.

Earlier studies of ethanol drinking as a function of gender in rats have been reviewed by others[8,96] and generally concur that female rats and mice drink more ethanol (per unit of body weight) than male rats. This has been attributed to higher rates of metabolism in female rats.[97] Gender differences have not yet been reported for self-administration of related sedative/hypnotic drugs, but other effects have been reported. For example, studies of physiological dependence on drugs such as pentobarbital,[98] barbital,[99] and methaqualone[100] revealed more severe withdrawal signs in female rats. Female rats consumed more caffeine (as a percentage of total liquid intake) than male rats, but when the rats were food deprived, males showed a more dramatic increase in percent of caffeine ingested.[101] Other studies have indicated that female rats drink more of a morphine solution than male rats[102,103] and more of a morphine–sucrose solution[104] than male rats. Taken together these studies show that gender is an important variable that may affect the generalizability of results from studies of the behavioral pharmacology of drugs of abuse. However, the direction of gender difference appears to vary with the species, the drug, and the experimental design.

2.4.3. Genetic Factors. Portions of this section are based on an earlier review.[105] Studies using the two-bottle-choice technique have repeatedly demonstrated genetic differences in ethanol drinking. In the first study, conducted by Mardones and colleagues,[106] rats were selectively bred for high and low ethanol drinking, and reliable differences emerged between lines. Large differences in ethanol intake were also found among inbred mouse strains.[107,108] Differences in ethanol drinking among selected lines and inbred strains of rats and mice are well documented, and a large body of literature exists.[109] Strain differences have also been found in oral morphine[110,111] and etonitazene intake.[112,113] Over the last 5 years operant conditioning methods and concepts have been used to analyze genetic differences in the reinforcing effects of ethanol.

2.4.3a. Selectively Bred Rats. At Indiana University, rats have been selectively bred for ethanol preference (P line) and for ethanol nonpreference (NP line). The intragastric self-administration of ethanol was studied in one experiment.[114] Rats from the P line intragastrically delivered self-infused ethanol up to 9.4 g/kg of body weight per day. When water was substituted for the ethanol solution, responding diminished, but when ethanol once again replaced water, responding returned to previous levels. Thus, for the rats in the P line, ethanol appeared to serve as a reinforcer. In contrast, rats in the NP line self-administered only 0.7 g/kg per day. As the investigators noted, as the intragastric route was used, these findings indicate that the reinforcing effects of ethanol are postabsorptive and not due to ethanol's taste or smell.

In recent years the techniques used to establish ethanol and other drugs as orally effective reinforcers[16] have been applied to the study of genetic differences. Several series of experiments have been conducted. One series concerned the establishment of ethanol as a reinforcer for alcohol-accepting (AA) and alcohol-nonaccepting (ANA) rats. These rats were selectively bred from an original foundation stock based on high and low ethanol drinking in a two-bottle-choice paradigm.[115] In one operant conditioning study, a variant of previous procedures was used.[116] The AA and ANA rats were maintained at 75% of their free-feeding weight and were induced to drink water in the operant chamber by giving them food in their home cage 60 min prior to the start of the session. Once a stable pattern of water-reinforced responding was present, they were given a sequence of increasing ethanol concentrations: 0.5, 1, 2, 4, and 5.7%. After behavior was stable at 5.7%, the time of feeding was shifted from before to after the session.

During the induced drinking phase both the AA and ANA lines consumed progressively larger amounts of ethanol (g/kg) as the concentration was increased. At 5.7% the AA rats ingested 1.5 g/kg and had a mean blood ethanol level of 176 mg/dl. The ANA rats consumed 0.9 g/kg and had a mean blood ethanol level of 116 mg/dl. Thus, both strains consumed enough ethanol to produce pharmacological effects. However, when access to food was shifted to after the sessions, responding of the AA rats was maintained by 5.7% ethanol, while responding of the ANA rats dropped to low levels. Thus, ethanol came to function as a reinforcer for the AA but not for the ANA rats. The differential maintenance of behavior was confirmed by subsequent manipulations that compared water- and ethanol-maintained responding. In the AA rats, but not in the ANA rats, ethanol consistently maintained high rates of lever pressing that substantially exceeded water control levels.[116] In a related experiment, ethanol concentration was varied between 8 and 32% (w/v), and responding by AA rats was well maintained at all concentrations.[117]

2.4.3b. Inbred Rats. The establishment and maintenance of ethanol-reinforced behavior have been studied in two inbred rat strains, the Lewis and Fischer 344 rats.[118] These lines were studied because they have had no common ancestors for at least 75 years, thereby maximizing their possible genetic divergence. Ethanol was established as a reinforcer using procedures similar to that used in the previously described study.[116] For both the Lewis and the Fischer 344 strains, ethanol maintained higher response rates and was consumed in larger volumes than the water vehicle. In addition, in both strains

blood ethanol levels increased with increases in ethanol concentration. However, Lewis rats drank substantially more ethanol than Fischer rats. The typical inverted U-shaped function between ethanol concentration and number
of ethanol deliveries was observed for the Lewis rats, whereas for the Fischer
rats much smaller differences were seen between ethanol- and water-main-
tained responding. In another experiment, ethanol deliveries were made contingent on completion of an FR response requirement. For the Lewis strain, as
the FR size was increased, the number of responses generally increased in
direct proportion to the FR value, so that the number of deliveries remained
constant, especially at the lower FR values. However, at higher FR, a decrease
in ethanol deliveries and blood ethanol levels occurred. Similar results were
obtained with the Fischer 344 rats, but the rate of responding was lower and
less consistent. Behavioral activation, as measured in an open field test, was
seen in Lewis rats but not in Fischer 344 rats. Taken together these findings
show that ethanol serves as a strong positive reinforcer for the Lewis rats and
as a weak positive reinforcer for the Fischer 344 rats, and that genotype is a
determinant of the degree to which ethanol functions as a reinforcer.

2.4.3c. *Inbred Mice.* In another series of studies, two inbred mouse
strains, the C57BL/6J and the BALB/cJ mice, were studied.[119] As in related
experiments, ethanol drinking was initially induced by maintaining the mice
at a reduced body weight, and when a stable pattern of water drinking was
established, a series of increasing ethanol concentrations (1, 2, 4, and 8% w/v)
replaced water. Mice from both strains drank substantial amounts of ethanol.
At 8%, C57BL/6J mice had blood levels of 269 mg/dl, and the BALB/cJ mice
had blood levels of 183 mg/dl. However, when access to food was switched to
after the session, large differences between strains emerged. The C57BL/6J
persisted in drinking substantial amounts of ethanol (2.45 g/kg per 30-min
session), whereas the BALB/cJ mice drank very little (0.57 g/kg per 30-min
session). Subsequent tests confirmed that ethanol had come to serve as a
reinforcer for the C57BL/6J mice but probably not for the BALB/cJ mice.[119]

These findings were systematically replicated in a second experiment in
which ethanol concentration was varied from 1 to 32%. At 8 and 16%, responding by the C57BL/6J mice reliably exceeded water control values,
whereas responding by the BALB/cJ mice never rose above the water (vehicle)
values. The C57BL/6J's pattern of responding was similar to that seen when
ethanol serves as a reinforcer for other species: the highest rate of responding
occurred at the beginning of the session, responding over the session was
negatively accelerated.[120] In a third experiment with C57BL/6J and BALB/cJ
mice, ethanol deliveries occurred under an intermittent schedule of reinforcement, specifically an FR schedule.[91] For the C57BL/6J mice, as FR value was
increased in the sequence 1, 2, 4, and 8, there were almost directly proportional increases in response rate at 8 and 16% but not at 0% (water). For the
BALB/cJ mice, at no condition did ethanol maintain responding at levels that
significantly exceeded vehicle responding. Thus, ethanol functioned as an
effective reinforcer for the C57BL/6J mice and as a marginal or ineffective

reinforcer for the BALB/cJ mice. In these experiments and those with the rats, the differences between strains in the reinforcing effects of ethanol paralleled differences found in earlier preference studies of ethanol drinking. This suggests that there may be common aspects to ethanol-reinforced behavior as measured in operant chambers with liquid delivery systems and ethanol drinking as measured in home cages with drinking bottles.

2.4.3d. *Interaction between Genotype and Other Factors.* Drug-reinforced behavior, including ethanol-reinforced behavior, is complex in that it is a learned operant behavior that is determined by many variables, including the animal's experimental history, the dose of the drug, deprivation states, and schedule of reinforcement. This means that there are many possible points at which strains may differ. For example, two strains may show identical behavior at a low drug dose but differences at high doses. Also, strains may have equivalent drug intakes under an FR 1 schedule but different intakes at higher ratio values. A third example is that strains may show equivalent performance under an intermittent schedule of reinforcement but differ in the amount of responding emitted when the drug is replaced by its vehicle. Such differences may be correlated with other variables, such as the probability of resuming drug self-administration when the drug is again made available.

In summary, genetic factors are important determinants of the reinforcing effects of ethanol and probably all abused drugs. The effects of genotype can be large in magnitude. However, in relation to the entire range of variables that affect the acquisition of drug-reinforced behavior, it is not known precisely how important genetic factors are. Furthermore, the mechanisms responsible for these genetic effects are not known. It is unlikely, however, that strain and selected line differences are due solely to acceptance or rejection of novel-tasting substances, since genetic factors are also important determinants of drug action when drugs are simply administered parenterally to an organism by the experimenter.[121]

The complexity of drug reinforced behavior has several implications for the analysis of genetic determinants. First, comparisons among strains should be made using several independent variables and a range of values of each independent variable (e.g., a range of drug doses). Second, the complexity of the behavior increases the number of possible mechanisms that may account for strain differences. Third, the complexity of the behavior means that the use of involved genetic methods such as selective breeding studies will be more difficult. However, the importance of genotype is such that genetic studies should be pursued despite these difficulties.

3. Factors Influencing the Maintenance of Drug Reinforcement

The maintenance of ethanol-reinforced behavior and behavior reinforced by other drugs is influenced by a number of current conditions as well as those that are antecedent to acquisition of drug-reinforced behavior. These current circumstances are divided into two groups, although there is considerable overlap. The first set of factors that are discussed are changes in the external environment, such as feeding conditions, presence or absence of alternative reinforcers, and social factors. The second group consists of changes that occur within the animal, such as neurochemical alterations through other drugs or diet, hormonal cycles in female rats, and the combination of alcohol with other drugs (agonists and antagonists).

3.1. Behavioral and Environmental Effects

Previous reviews of drug-reinforced behavior have discussed factors that play a major role in the maintenance of drug-taking behavior, such as stimulus control, reinforcement schedule, punishment, type of drug, dose or magnitude of reinforcement, and conditioned reinforcement.[13,14] The present chapter includes three variables, feeding conditions, alternative reinforcers, and social conditions. Data have been accumulating in recent years to suggest that these also may be major determinants of drug-reinforced behavior.

3.1.1. Altered Feeding Conditions.

In animals, reducing the daily allotment of food results in marked increases in self-administration of drugs that are abused by humans, such as alcohol,[27] d-amphetamine,[61,122] opioids, cocaine,[123,124] phencyclidine,[20,31] and barbiturates.[40,59] The magnitude of this effect is nearly the same across all of these drugs; there is at least a twofold increase in intake at low to moderate doses and concentrations. The generality of these findings has been extended to several different species, routes of self-administration, and schedules of reinforcement. There are only a few corroborating observations from human studies. Clinical findings suggest that reduced food intake is implicated in relapse to cigarette smoking,[125] to quantities of alcohol used,[126] to the high prevalence of drug abuse in patients with eating disorders,[127] and to a variety of other forms of substance abuse,[128] including coca leaf chewing.[129]

A number of control procedures have indicated that the increased drug intake due to reduced food availability is not explained by general increases in activity or liquid intake, pharmacokinetic changes, effects of specific drugs on feeding behavior, palatability of the drugs, differences in tolerance development, or caloric replacement. Many of these specific hypothesis concerning the effects of reduced feeding have been ruled out as the generality of the findings has increased. Furthermore, food deprivation effects may extend beyond the drug self-administration period. For example, during extinction, when saline has replaced cocaine in the i.v. infusion pumps, reduced food availability dramatically increased responding that was previously rewarded by cocaine in rats.[130] Also, reduced food access increased responding in monkeys when the amount of phencyclidine presented at the end of the session was fixed and not dependent on the rate of responding.[131,132]

The limitations of the food deprivation phenomenon have revealed important information. For instance, food deprivation facilitates intake of drugs such as nicotine[133,134] or caffeine[101] that are not easily established as reinforcers in animals or low doses of drugs, such as cocaine[135,136] and d-amphetamine,[133] that function as reinforcers for humans and laboratory animals. However, reduced food access had no effect on self-administration of drugs with equivocal[86] reinforcing effects in animals but that are abused by humans, such as delta-9-THC[137] and diazepam,[133] or on drugs that do not function as reinforcers for animals or humans (e.g., perphenazine).[133] In addition, intake of drugs such as orally delivered cocaine and phencyclidine was comparable to water levels in rats, but the drugs did not function as reinforcers via this route and food deprivation decreased rather than increased the rats' intake. Thus, reduced food intake enhances the reinforcing effects of drugs, but it does not induce increased self-administration of drugs that have not been demonstrated to function as reinforcers under a particular route of administration. Studies of complete dose–response functions for drugs that function as reinforcers show that the difference in self-administration between free and restricted feeding is greatest at low doses and gradually diminished as the dose increases. At the higher doses, where reinforcing effects would be expected to be greater,[33,140] reducing food intake has little or no facilitory effect on drug intake.[60,135,137]

Most of these results also support the statement that reduced feeding specifically increases the reinforcing effects of drugs. Alcohol and other drugs that function as reinforcers are not unique in their relationship to reduced food intake. There are previous reports of increased behavior maintained by other nonfood events, such as light onset,[139] wheel running,[140] electrical stimulation of the brain,[141] and saccharin presentation.[142] These results suggest that the food and drug interaction may be more generally conceived as a form of reinforcer interaction.

Interpretations of the food deprivation effect on drug-reinforced behavior have been complicated by the recent finding that the effects of reduced feeding may change over time or as a function of feeding and drug history.[138] For example, rats drinking ethanol eventually increase their consumption if the drug is available for an extended period of time while the animals remain food satiated.[143] Recent studies with monkeys responding for orally delivered ethanol (R. A. Meisch and S. Schrader, personal communication) and phencyclidine[138] show that over extended periods of food satiation and drug access, the drugs are consumed in greater quantities during food satiation than they are during food deprivation.

In conclusion, the feeding condition has emerged as a powerful determinant of drug-reinforced behavior. There is a specific interaction between the availability of food and drugs that function as reinforcers. Animal studies have shown that reduced food availability produces similar changes in the overall rate and pattern of drug-reinforced behavior in most drugs (including alcohol) that are abused by humans. There is anecdotal evidence from human studies that concurs with laboratory findings; however, the next step is clearly to systematically replicate and extend this animal work to human subjects.

3.1.2. Availability of Concurrent/Competing Reinforcing Events.   The reduction of drug-reinforced behavior by concurrent availability of other reinforcers is considered to be a form of reinforcer interaction. The effect of competing reinforcers on alcohol intake has been recently reviewed.[144] There are a number of investigations concerning the effects of introducing dietary reinforcers on drug-rewarded behavior.[145] The results are in a direction that would be predicted from a reinforcer interaction hypothesis, specifically that drug intake is generally reduced by the addition of palatable and/or caloric substances to the drug-taking situation. For instance, oral alcohol intake is reduced by providing rats with palatable sucrose solutions.[146–150] More specific analyses of macronutrients and alcohol intake reveal an inverse relationship between alcohol and carbohydrate intake and a positive correlation between protein and alcohol intake.[151] The results of a dietary recall study conducted with patients in an alcoholism treatment program concur with these laboratory findings. Patients were grouped according to the number of days they stayed sober after their last drink. Those who stayed sober longer selected diets twice as high in sugar (e.g., added to beverages) and other carbohydrates than the low-sobriety group.[126]

Substances other than food, such as money[152] or video-game playing have been reported to reduce alcohol intake in normal human subjects.[144] Food, palatable noncaloric liquids, and ethanol all function similarly as alternative reinforcers to reduce drug (e.g., phencyclidine) intake in monkeys. Figure 2 shows the effect of providing free food[153] (top frame), saccharin[154] (center frame), and ethanol[37] (lower frame) to monkeys that had access to 0.25 mg/ml phencyclidine (PCP) and water under concurrent FR 16 schedules. In the initial experiment the monkeys were maintained on reduced food rations at 85% of their free-feeding weight. This function served as the baseline condition for the top two frames as the experiments were conducted at nearly the same time. The concentration-response function was redetermined several years later for the third comparison (lower frame). Food, saccharin and ethanol all substantially reduced PCP-maintained behavior at lower PCP concentrations, but they had relatively little effect at the higher PCP concentrations. Although a caloric replacement interpretation is not ruled out in the case of food and ethanol, the similar results with a noncaloric substance, saccharin, argue against this hypothesis.

A recent experiment with rats showed that i.v. cocaine self-administration was also reduced by presentation of a glucose and saccharin solution.[155] In contrast, when this solution was removed in other groups of rats that had also been self-administering intravenously delivered cocaine[155] or etonitazene,[135] drug-maintained responding increased. These studies have also demonstrated that an alternative reinforcer, such as a glucose and saccharin drinking solution, can delay the acquisition of i.v. cocaine self-administration,

Figure 2. A comparison of data from three experiments in which alternative substances were available during PCP self-administration sessions is presented. In the top frame PCP deliveries are plotted across a range of PCP concentrations (0.03, 0.06, 0.12, 0.25, 0.5 and 1.0 mg/ml), when food was freely available (FS) and when the monkeys were maintained at 85% of their free-feeding body weight (FD). In the center frame the same (FD) PCP function (PCP and water) is contrasted with the number of PCP deliveries earned when a saccharin solution (0.03% wt/vol) was concurrently available (PCP and Sacc). This experiment was conducted immediately after the one that is depicted in the top frame. The lower frame shows a retest of the concurrent PCP and water (FD) condition that was conducted several years later in the same three monkeys, and these data are compared to a condition in which PCP and ethanol (8% wt/vol) were available under concurrent FR 16 schedules (PCP and ETOH). The abbreviations in parentheses indicate whether the monkeys were food satiated (FS) by allowing them free access to food or food deprived (FD) by maintaining them at 85% of their free feeding weight. Open circles indicate the condition in which food and water were concurrently available and the monkeys were food deprived. Filled circles represent conditions under which alternative reinforcers were available, e.g., food (upper frame), saccharin (center frame) and ethanol

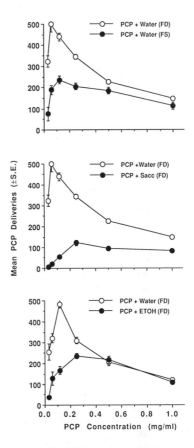

(lower frame). Each point refers to a mean of the last five days of stable behavior for three monkeys (M-B2, M-G2, and M-P1). The vertical bars represent the mean standard errors across the three monkeys.

and similarly, the availability of i.v. cocaine can prevent the development of high rates of glucose and saccharin drinking.[155]

Another method of suppressing drug-reinforced behavior has been to make an alternative reinforcer contingent on the absence of drug taking. For instance, alcohol-reinforced behavior has been reduced in rats by delaying food availability as a consequence of drug-maintained responding.[156,157] Clinical experiments have shown that removal of reinforcers as a consequence of drug self-administration[46,158] or presentation of nondrug reinforcers contingent on the absence of drug taking[159–162] effectively reduced alcohol and other drug use. Skinner[163] acknowledged the desirability of reducing or terminating behavior by reinforcing an alternative behavior rather than by punishment or extinction. Recent work suggests that positive consequences or incentives have equivalent efficacy to aversive consequences in reducing other drug use in methadone patients.[164] In summary, modification of drug-reinforced behavior by manipulating access to alternative events in the environment appears to be an effective means of reducing drug-taking behavior.

3.1.3. Social Factors. Alcohol use in human social settings has been widely studied.[165-168] There are a number of variables that control the amount of alcohol consumed, such as the group size,[169,170] modeled consumption rates,[171] sociable or unsociable model status,[172] cost of alcohol,[173,174] and naturalistic[175,176] or seminaturalistic[177] bar settings. The complex interactions among these and other variables in a given social setting determine whether alcohol drinking will be enabled or inhibited.

Animal work has the potential for systematic manipulation of social variables over extended periods of time; however, there are few animal models of social effects on ethanol drinking and other drug use. Generally, the studies show that social isolation increases intake of ethanol but not of the vehicle. One series of studies showed that rats housed in an isolated environment self-administer more morphine than colony-housed animals.[178,179] Similarly, a study of socially reared juvenile rhesus monkeys showed that animals that were intermittently separated from three other monkeys in their social group drank more alcohol when they were separated than when they were together.[180] A control group that was continuously separated drank less than the intermittently separated group (during isolation). Crowley and Andrews[181] compared different acquisition procedures for establishing alcoholic-like drinking in primate (*Macaca nemestrina*) social groups. They found that dominant animals consumed large amounts, while the low-ranked animals did not develop these high rates of drinking owing to their limited access to the area containing the drinking spouts.[181]

3.2. Biochemical Factors

This section provides examples of changes that occur within the animal due to administration of a different drug or diet or due to naturally occurring changes such as hormone cycles, and how these biochemical alterations affect alcohol- and drug-reinforced behavior. A thorough review of this topic is provided by Asghar.[182]

3.2.1. Neurochemical Alterations. There are increasing reports that more specific dietary alterations are accompanied by neurochemical changes that are also implicated in drug effects. These neurochemical changes may be related to the interactive effects of drugs and dietary factors that have been described on the behavioral level. For example, the same glucose and saccharin solution that was reported above to reduce i.v. cocaine self-administration in rats produced tolerance to the analgesic effects of low doses of morphine in rats.[183] This and other sweet-tasting substances may release endogenous opioid peptides that compete with the reinforcing effects of cocaine.

Others have found a relationship between ingestion of a palatable food or liquid and opiate receptor binding in the whole brain[184] and in the hypothalamus[185] of rats.

Another example of food constituents affecting a pharmacological response is found in the study of amino acid neurotransmitter precursors. For example, d-amphetamine self-administration is reduced in rats pretreated with tyrosine and l-tryptophan, a serotonin precursor.[186,187] Increased availability of serotonin via administration of reuptake inhibitors (e.g., fluoxetine and zimelidine, respectively) has also been shown to reduce alcohol[188] and morphine[189] intake in rats. Serotonin enhancing agents have also shown some efficacy for the treatment of alcoholism in humans.[190,191] In a double-blind, placebo-controlled crossover experiment with 13 heavy drinkers, zimelidine (200 mg) was found to increase the number of days of abstinence and decrease the daily number of drinks consumed[192] and fluoxetine reduced alcohol intake in male inpatient alcoholics.[193] In another study fluvoxamine improved episodic memory in patients with alcoholic amnesia.[194]

Serotonin reuptake inhibitors, such as citalopram,[195] fluoxetine,[196] and others,[197] also reduce behavior rewarded by intracranial self-stimulation in animals. Recent data from this laboratory indicate that l-tryptophan and fluoxetine treatments reduce i.v. cocaine self-administration in rats in a dose-dependent manner, and cocaine self-injection rapidly returns to baseline rates when these treatments are terminated.[198] Only the highest doses of l-tryptophan or fluoxetine produced small decrements in food intake and behavior maintained by a glucose and saccharine solution.[198]

The implications for the effects of drug- and dietary-induced neurochemical changes on drug abuse are very important not only for a better understanding of the etiology of the disease, but for the development of pharmacotherapy to reduce drug intake and prevent relapse to drug use. For instance, serotonin reuptake blockers have been reported to be a useful adjunct to behavioral strategies and psychotherapy for reducing relapse to cocaine use.[199,200] An important issue to be considered is that the interaction between drugs of abuse and specific neurotransmitter pools may differ substantially during the different phases of drug dependence: acquisition, maintenance, and termination (abstinence).

3.2.2. Hormonal Changes. Studies with female rats have shown that ethanol drinking decreases during the estrous cycle.[201] Rats given high levels of synthetic estrogens also reduce voluntary alcohol intake.[96] However, comparable studies with other drugs are limited. Recent work showed an increase in cocaine self-administration during estrous.[202] This finding was dependent upon the reinforcement schedule; no differences were found with a fixed-ratio schedule of drug delivery, while significant differences were noted with a progressive-ratio schedule. In addition to a potential interaction between sex hormones and drug self-administration, there is the possibility that hormones may influence the effects of an antagonist while not altering the baselines rates of self-administration maintained by the agonist.[202]

There has been an interest in fluctuations in gonadal hormones and alcohol intake in women; however, the data do not strongly indicate a relationship between cycle phase and pattern of alcohol use.[203,204] Clinical reports indicate that alcoholic women who increase their consumption during the premenstrual phase also report premenstrual dysphoria.[205,206] Two prospective investigations reported no relationship between alcohol intake and the premenstrual phase,[207,208] while another reported increased consumption during the luteal phase.[209] Ethanol metabolism was examined in female social drinkers, and it was found that those taking oral contraceptives showed a decreased ethanol disappearance rate compared to another group of women who were not taking oral contraceptives.[210] Both groups were tested at three phases during the menstrual cycle; however, the relatively small changes in estrogen levels in normally menstruating women did not alter the rates of ethanol metabolism.[210] Existing data suggest that the effects of hormonal changes on drug-reinforced behavior may be specific to the species or drug tested and dependent on the schedule of access and amount of drug consumed. Further research is needed to clearly define a relationship between female drinking patterns and hormonal cycles.

3.2.3. Alcohol and Other Drug Combinations.   Two major areas of emerging research concerning drug combinations may have considerable importance for our understanding and treatment of drug dependence. The first is the issue of polydrug abuse, alcohol and other psychoactive drugs (agonists). Second is the effect of antagonists such as the alcohol antagonist (RO 15-4513) as well as opioid antagonists and neurotransmitter blockers.

3.2.3a. Polydrug Abuse.   Polydrug abuse has become common among recreational drug users, and alcohol is the drug that is most often used with other drugs. With several exceptions, there have been few prospective human studies or animal laboratory investigations describing interactions of the reinforcing effects of alcohol with a variety of other drugs. Clinical laboratory studies have demonstrated a strong association between cigarette smoking and alcohol consumption in alcoholic men[211–213] and male[214] and female social drinkers.[215] Others have shown that a history of alcohol abuse was associated with an intensified pattern of cigarette smoking, but current ethanol use was not related to an increased smoking pattern.[216] Alcohol consumption has not been shown to be closely related to marijuana use, but marijuana did suppress alcohol drinking.[217]

The examination of polydrug use with animal models is limited by procedural difficulties. The time required to conduct a careful parametric analysis of two or more concurrently self-administered drugs would exceed the catheter life reported for i.v. self-administration projects. The oral or intragastric route would be more desirable, but the number of orally delivered drugs that have been established as reinforcers is limited,[16] probably because of the rat's rejection of bitter tastes. Primates more readily accept oral delivery of a variety of drugs abused by humans than rats,[16] but reports of drug interactions have been limited. A recent investigation of oral ethanol and phencyclidine self-administration indicated that a behaviorally active, self-administered dose of phencyclidine had no effect (compared with water vehicle) on ethanol intake across a range of concentrations.[36] The phencyclidine intake was nearly the same regardless of the concurrent ethanol concentration.[36] On the other hand, intake of low phencyclidine concentrations was reduced by an 8% ethanol solution, and intake of this fixed ethanol concentration was slightly suppressed by the higher phencyclidine concentrations. Generally, the intake of these two drugs was additive; each drug was consumed at high rates as if water had been concurrently available. These results emphasize the possibility of increased toxicity in human polydrug abusers.

Another example of attempts to study drug interaction has been the parenteral administration of a second drug during ethanol self-administration. For instance, injections of chlordiazepoxide (a drug known for its dipsogenic effect)[218] reduced ethanol-reinforced responding and intake, but it did not significantly alter responding maintained by a 1% sucrose solution or water.[219] Thus, these results appear to be due to specific drug interaction rather than a conditioned taste aversion or a nonspecific suppression in liquid intake. Other investigators have found that injections of low doses of morphine increased ethanol consumption in rats.[220] Further work such as this is needed to identify other drug combinations that may lead to excessive intake of alcoholic beverages in humans.

3.2.3b. Antagonist Effects.   There has been great interest in the potential of the imidazobenzodiazepine R0 15-4513 as an ethanol antagonist.[221] An animal study reported in 1986[222] shows that injection of this drug rapidly reverses alcohol intoxication. A recent review discusses the behavioral and biochemical actions of ethanol and R0 15-4513 as a potential antagonist.[221]

There has also been considerable interest in examining the possible involvement of the opiate system in alcohol drinking. Opiate antagonists have been shown to decrease ethanol intake in rats and monkeys using oral,[223–225] intragastric,[226] and intravenous[227] self-administration methods. There have been few studies of the effects of opiate antagonists on self-administration of other nonopiate drugs; however, one study demonstrated increased intravenous cocaine self-administration after naltrexone pretreatment in rats.[228] Others have shown that opiate antagonists reduce consumption of a saccharin solution in rats. That alcohol, cocaine, and other drugs as well as palatable substances may act on common neural substrates mediating reward is supported by a report that chronic intake of glucose and saccharin intake in rats produces tolerance to the analgesic effects of low doses of morphine.[183]

There is a considerable amount of literature revealing effects of opiate antagonists on other behavioral effects of alcohol. For instance, opiate antagonists reversed the psychomotor effects of ethanol,[229–231] chlordiazepoxide,[232,233] and diazepam,[234] as well as ethanol intoxication and coma in humans.[235–338] Others have reported no effect[239] or that naltrexone potentiated an ethanol-induced performance deficit.[240,241] There are also an increasing number of reports that opiate antagonists potentiate effects of other nonopiate drugs, such as cocaine,[242] methylxanthines,[243] LSD,[244–247] DMT,[245] DOM,[246] and mescaline.[248]

4. Dependence Potential

In the following sections both physiological changes and performance alterations are considered as parts of the same withdrawal process. Changes in performance that occur during drug withdrawal were originally described by Schuster and Thompson.[249,250] These performance alterations are compared to physiological changes or a consistent stereotyped syndrome of physiological effects that may also be behavioral (e.g., jumping, shaking). There is currently a trend toward more quantitative, objective measures of withdrawal. Performance measures have been useful for isolating and studying withdrawal effects of drugs that do not produce a physiological syndrome or for examining protracted withdrawal effects of low doses of drugs that do not produce physiological changes during withdrawal.

4.1. Observational Measures of Withdrawal

This section describes the classical observable alcohol withdrawal syndrome in humans and laboratory animals. Observational rating scales that are used to quantify these signs and symptoms are also reviewed. Finally, factors influencing withdrawal severity (e.g., dietary changes) are discussed.

4.1.1. Signs and Symptoms of Withdrawal.   In humans, alcohol withdrawal has been characterized as a sequence of stages of varying severity, involving signs, symptoms, and verbal reports.[251] Tremors begin a few hours after abstinence initiation and are typically seen as morning shakes after a night of sleeping. The next stage consists of convulsions, or "rum fits," which occur 13–24 hr following cessation. These are grand mal seizures which can occur in flumes and are susceptible to photic stimulation. Alcoholic hallucinosis may occur with tremors and/or seizures, and they peak at 24 hr. Finally, delirium tremens occurs at 72–96 hr. This phase is characterized by disrupted consciousness, autonomic hyperactivity, agitation, and visual and tactile hallucinations. It is relatively rare, and can be fatal.

Much of the parametric research on alcohol withdrawal has been conducted with animal models, rats and mice being the most extensively studied. Withdrawal in rats appears to follow a characteristic sequence, as described in detail by Hunter and co-workers.[252] In a series of preconvulsive stages (2–5 hr postwithdrawal), rats initially show evidence of piloerection and stiffening of the tail. In subsequent hours, tail arching and an ataxic gait may be observed, as well as a disrupted sleep pattern. There is then a period of motoric disturbance, with hypoactivity, rigidity of extensor muscles, and fasiculations. At this time (5–8 hr postwithdrawal) there is also hyperactivity in response to stimuli. Episodes of sudden sprawling, spontaneous vocalizations, whole-body rigidity, and severe tremors may be seen. Spontaneous convulsions, in some cases leading to death, occur in a small percentage of animals.

4.1.2. Observational Rating Systems. The signs and symptoms of withdrawal discussed in the preceding section have been used in observational rating systems to quantify dependence levels by assessing withdrawal intensity after drug exposure. Unfortunately, there is considerable variation across studies with regard to experimental methodologies. For example, mice, rats, dogs, cats, monkeys, chimpanzees, and humans have all been employed to investigate alcohol withdrawal; each species may have a different sensitivity and/or spectrum of specific withdrawal signs.[253] Another source of variation in withdrawal testing is the route of exposure. Animals have been exposed to alcohol via inhalation, intragastric, intraperitoneal, and oral routes prior to withdrawal testing, with potential differences in the intensity and time course of ensuing withdrawal symptoms. Finally, different studies have used a variety of specific observational rating systems to characterize withdrawal states. A previous paper[253] has reviewed the observational methods typically used for quantifying alcohol withdrawal states in animals. The measurement domains include (1) motoric symptoms (e.g., tremor, rigidity, abnormal tail signs), (2) behavioral signs (e.g., changes in activity levels, reactivity, startle, irritability, spontaneous vocalizations, and real or apparent hallucinatory behavior), (3) gastrointestinal signs (vomiting, retching, diarrhea), (4) autonomic symptoms (e.g., heart rate, respiration, or temperature changes, sweating, salivation, piloerection), and (5) seizures or convulsions. One consensus emerging from this methodological variation is that the most useful observational signs of withdrawal from ethanol appear to be those that reflect underlying central nervous system (CNS) hyperexcitability. Thus, in humans, observations of tremor and convulsions play a key role in defining alcohol withdrawal. Tremor is also a reliable withdrawal sign in primates.[254,255] Commonly employed methods for testing hyperexcitability in animals involve rating behavioral reactions to acoustic, electrical, or handling stimuli.[253] Finally, in rodent models, convulsions and seizures can be reliably elicited by standardized handling techniques, such as picking mice up by the tail,[256] or by use of acoustic stimuli.[257,258] Seizures can be graded in intensity, latency of onset, number, duration or threshold for production and therefore provide a sensitive semi-quantitative index of withdrawal severity.

Alcohol withdrawal symptoms across species can thus be seen to have similar characteristics. Both humans and rats exhibit restlessness, tremor, sleep disturbance, tachycardia, hyperthermia, and CNS hyperexcitability. Qualities such as these can also be found in the withdrawal states for other drugs, such as sedative/hypnotics. Furthermore, it has been shown that barbiturates and benzodiazepines will suppress withdrawal symptoms in animals made physically dependent on alcohol.[259] However, animal models for human aspects of alcohol withdrawal such as alcoholic hallucinosis and delirium tremens have not been found, suggesting a certain limitation to these analogies.

The commonality of withdrawal signs and symptoms suggests that drug withdrawal, in general, might be mediated by some common final pathway, with different drug types influencing the path to different degrees. However, withdrawal from opiates is characterized by a different set of signs and symptoms (including nausea and vomiting, muscle aches, lacrimation, rhinorrhea, yawning, diarrhea, pupillary dilation, gooseflesh, and sweating). While opiate antagonists may influence factors associated with alcohol intoxication (see Section 3.2.3b), the withdrawal states of alcohol and opiates appear to be distinct. Alcohol does not relieve opiate withdrawal symptoms, nor do opiates alleviate alcohol withdrawal symptoms. Hence, it appears that alcohol and opiate withdrawal effects operate through different mechanisms.[260]

4.1.3. Factors Influencing Withdrawal Severity.   Dietary changes, such as an absence of protein in meals or temporary fasting, can slow alcohol metabolism in the rat[261] and hence may prolong blood alcohol levels after the last administration of alcohol. Even well-nourished rats will lose weight when given alcohol, although the loss is not as much as in rats deprived of nutrients.[262] Thus, diet and weight loss must be controlled in order to avoid confounding effects on measures of withdrawal. In studies where weight loss was not a factor, alcohol exposure dose has been shown to influence withdrawal intensity. For example, Goldstein[256] administered alcohol to mice by inhalation and found increasing severity of convulsions during handling up to a blood alcohol concentration of 1.86 mg/ml, but not higher. Exposure duration has also been identified as an important determinant of withdrawal intensity, with graded increases in withdrawal intensity generally related to increasing exposure durations.[263–265] In studies where exposure dose and duration have been combined into a total exposure index, there has been a clear orderly relationship between total exposure and withdrawal intensity.[256,264]

A more severe withdrawal reaction can be observed if the rate of decrease in blood alcohol concentration is accelerated.[264] Route of administration may also play a role in determining the severity of withdrawal.[266] However, variations across routes of administration may simply reflect differences in consistency or magnitude of blood alcohol levels achieved. Pattern of administration over time is another factor that may influence withdrawal severity. In rats given alcohol by inhalation, Goldstein found that breaks of sobriety lasting at least 24 hr resulted in a complete remission of dependence in mice.[263] However, other investigators have observed greater withdrawal severity during second exposure to alcohol even when a substantial period of sobriety has intervened,[267,268] suggesting a more permanent change in sensitivity to physical dependence as a result of exposure history. In humans, clinical evidence suggests that withdrawal severity varies with the intensity of the preceding drinking episode,[269] and that an intermittent pattern of drinking is related to more severe withdrawal symptoms.[270]

With regard to the development of physical dependence, one interesting observation emerging from the animal studies is that withdrawal signs can be reliably elicited following single-dose exposure to ethanol.[256,271] This observation contradicts the commonly held belief that withdrawal phenomena can be observed only after prolonged exposure to dependence-producing drugs. It suggests instead that physical dependence is graded rather than a discrete phenomenon that begins with the first drug exposure and progresses in intensity or severity with repeated or prolonged exposures.

4.2. Altered Performance Measures during Withdrawal

An advantage of studying drug withdrawal with performance measures is that objective, quantitative results can be compared across conditions of drug exposure, species, different drugs, and a number of other variables. Sensitive behavioral measures have also revealed that abstinence syndromes may last considerably longer that the 2–3 days which are typically the duration of physiological symptoms. The definition of an abstinence syndrome in terms of disruptions in performance is important because human drug users report avoidance of withdrawal symptoms as a major cause of relapse to drug use.

One of the first studies of withdrawal-induced performance alteration was conducted by Thompson and Schuster.[250] They had trained monkeys to respond on levers for food, to receive intravenous injections of morphine, and to avoid electric shock. After 30 days morphine access was terminated, and responding maintained by food and avoidance of electric shock was reduced. When morphine access was restored after 2 days of abstinence, rates of responding returned to preabstinence levels. Similar experiments were subsequently conducted with rhesus monkeys[272] and rats,[273] but the abstinence period was longer. Holtzman and Villarreal[272] reported a suppression in food-reinforced responses in rhesus monkeys that gradually recovered over 7 days. Ford and Balster[273] found a biphasic effect; initially response rates maintained by food on a Differential Reinforcement of Low Rates (DRL) schedule decreased, and after 3 or 4 days they were greater than control levels. In these studies overt signs of physiological dependence were noted during the first 2 or 3 days, but disruptions of operant behavior lasted for 6 or 7 days. Thus, the performance measures revealed a more protracted time course of the withdrawal effect.

At about this same time Ahlenius and Engel[274] reported a similar study with ethanol withdrawal in rats using a DRL schedule similar to that used by Ford and Balster.[273] After several months of chronic ethanol exposure, ethanol was replaced with water for 3 days, and during that time response rates increased, thereby reducing the number of food reinforcers. Behavior returned to baseline levels when ethanol was reinstated. The results of a more recent study concurred with this finding.[275] Rats that were trained to lever-press for food, water, and ethanol in a three-lever operant chamber increased their responding on the food lever when ethanol was withdrawn. Studying a related drug, chlordiazepoxide, McMillan and Leander[276] also found increases in behavior maintained by food under a fixed interval (FI) schedule when the drug was removed from rats' drinking water. The increases began on the second day of withdrawal and continued until the 14th day. In contrast, Brady and others[277] reported suppressed food intake in baboons that began 8 days after discontinuation of diazepam and continued for 15 days. Reaction time to visual and auditory stimuli was increased during this time and peaked on the 10th day of withdrawal.

Subsequently, there have been other reports of performance alterations upon removal of drugs that are not known to produce classical withdrawal physiological syndromes like those that follow termination of chronic alcohol or opiate use. For instance, in one study, Leith and Barrett[278] trained rats to press a lever for electrical stimulation of the medial forebrain bundle. Amphetamine increased self-stimulation, and tolerance developed. After an increasing dose regimen, amphetamine treatment was terminated for 4 days. On the second day marked suppression in responding was reported, but it returned to pretreatment levels by the fourth day. When amphetamine was reinstated, the facilitory effect on brain self-stimulation immediately returned. A similar study has been reported by Simpson and Annau[279] in which electrical stimulation of the brain was reduced by terminating amphetamine self-administration for 4 days. These authors have also generalized their results to iproniazid, a monoamine oxidase inhibitor. When this group terminated chronic administration of chlorpromazine, a neuroleptic that reduced brain self-stimulation rates, there was a rebound increase in self-stimulation rates above pretreatment baselines. Houser[280] showed decreases in avoidance behavior in squirrel monkeys after chronic administration and subsequent withdrawal of amphetamine and α-methyl-p-tyrosine.

There have been similar demonstrations of performance alterations following drug withdrawal with other operant behavioral baselines and other drugs that are not associated with marked physiological withdrawal syndromes, such as caffeine,[281,282] THC,[283,284] phencyclidine,[285–288] ketamine,[287] and cocaine.[289,290] The significance of these studies is that withdrawal-induced performance can occur after discontinuation of chronic drug exposure or intermittent drug exposure[286] in the absence of overt signs of physiological distress. The performance disruptions can last 8–10 days or longer, and they are often quite severe.[285] Recent evidence suggests that performance deficits produced by withdrawal of one drug may be enhanced by adding withdrawal of a second drug.[282]

4.3. Relationship between Drug-Seeking Behavior and Withdrawal

It is clear from the voluminous literature on the physiological dependence and withdrawal that the vast majority of studies have involved passive administration and termination of the drug in question, the drugs have not been shown to be functioning as reinforcers. Testing for physiological and behavioral withdrawal symptoms is typically conducted in the absence of available drug for self-administration. Thus, an important omission from this analysis of drug withdrawal are the effects on drug-seeking behavior or drug self-administration. This is an unfortunate omission since, at least in humans, it is thought that drug-seeking behavior, motivated by the urge to relieve unpleasant withdrawal symptomatology, is a critical aspect of dependence and relapse. Thus, there is a gap in our understanding of dependence and withdrawal with regard to the effects of withdrawal states on drug reinforcement and drug self-administration behavior.

Evidence accumulated to date suggests that ethanol may differ from other drugs, particularly opiates, with regard to effects of withdrawal on drug seeking and drug reinforcement. For example, evidence from both experimental and anecdotal reports indicates that ethanol drinking by human abusers may not consistently occur in the presence of ethanol withdrawal. Thus, humans tend to engage in "binge" or "spree" patterns of drinking followed by periods of voluntary abstinence that are maintained in spite of emerging withdrawal signs.[265] In contrast, drug use tends to be more regular and consistent with opiates, which suggests that the emergence of withdrawal signs may more reliably set the occasion for additional drug-seeking and drug self-administration behavior in opiate abusers. These observations suggest that drug seeking and drug reinforcement may be more reliably enhanced by physiological dependence on opiates than by physiological dependence on alcohol.

Wasaka and co-workers[291] reported a study in which progressive ratio performance was used to assess the reinforcing properties of a variety of drugs during periods of chronic drug treatment vs. periods of saline pretreatment (induced abstinence). When testing was conducted with the opiate drugs morphine or dihydrocodeine, the animals worked much harder to obtain infusions during the induced withdrawal condition than during the drug pretreatment condition (e.g., progressive ratios attained were four to six times higher during induced abstinence). In contrast, only small increments in progressive ratios (1.5–1.7 times higher) were obtained during induced abstinence when the test was conducted with either pentazocine or pentobarbital. Yanagita[292] similarly observed no increase in progressive ratio performance during withdrawal from cocaine. These data, although limited to observations under a single set of behavioral parameters and single chronic dosing levels, suggest that drug reinforcement was enhanced during withdrawal from opiate agonists to a greater extent than during withdrawal from other drugs.

Other animal studies have provided evidence that opiates are self-administered during withdrawal,[293] but attempts to demonstrate the reinforcing effect of ethanol during ethanol withdrawal have been unsuccessful[294] (Winger, personal communication). For example, Winger (personal communication) trained rhesus monkeys to self-administer ethanol intravenously during 3-hr daily sessions. When ethanol-reinforced responding was stable, physiological dependence was induced by passive infusions of additional ethanol, and withdrawal signs, particularly tremor, could be observed prior to daily self-administration sessions. Ethanol self-administration was suppressed in the presence of these withdrawal signs, particularly during the first 24 hr of withdrawal when tremors were at their peak intensity, and returned to normal only after withdrawal signs had subsided.

One difficulty encountered in interpreting studies of drug self-administration during withdrawal is that withdrawal may produce performance impairment that could interfere with responding maintained by a variety of reinforcers, including drug reinforcers. Thus, it is possible that drugs simply differ in the amount of behavioral impairment they produce during withdrawal independently of their effects on drug-seeking or drug reinforcement. Additional research using sensitive techniques to assess drug reinforcement that do not rely heavily on motoric responding (e.g., choice studies) are needed to further clarify the effects of withdrawal on drug reinforcement and drug seeking. Nevertheless, it is intriguing that animals have failed in experimental settings to take advantage of the opportunity to relieve withdrawal symptoms by self-administering ethanol. Further experimental work is needed to understand the relationship between drug reinforcement (self-administration) and withdrawal states.

ACKNOWLEDGMENTS. Current research reported in this chapter was supported by National Institute on Drug Abuse grants DA 00944, DA 02486, and DA 03240. The authors are grateful to Sylvie T. Lac for library research and to Marcia Smith and Becky Dethmers for assistance with preparation of the manuscript.

References

1. Meisch RA: Factors controlling drug reinforced behavior. *Pharmacol Biochem Behav* 27:367–371, 1987.
2. Amit Z, Smith BR, Sutherland EA: Oral self-administration of alcohol: A valid approach to the study of self-administration and human alcoholism, in Bozarth MA (ed): *Methods of Assessing the Reinforcing Properties of Abused Drugs.* New York, Springer-Verlag, pp 143–160.
3. Cicero TJ: A critique of animal analogs of alcoholism, in Majchrowicze, Noble EP (eds): *Biochemistry and Pharmacology of Ethanol,* Vol 2. New York, Plenum Press, pp 553–560.
4. Cicero TJ: Animal models of alcoholism? in Eriksson K, Sinclair JD, Kiianmaa K (eds): *Animal Models in Alcohol Research.* New York, Academic Press, pp 99–117.
5. Eriksson K, Sinclair JD Kiianmaa K (eds): *Animal Models in Alcohol Research.* New York, Academic Press, 1980.
6. McClearn GE: Animal models of genetic factors in alcoholism, in Mell NK (ed): *Advances in Substance Abuse: Behavioral and Biological Research.* Greenwich CT, JAI Press, pp 185–217.
7. Mello NK: Animal models for the study of alcohol addiction. *Psychoneuroendocrinology* 1:347, 1976.
8. Meisch RA: Ethanol self-administration: Infrahuman studies, in Thompson T, Dews PB (eds): *Advances in Behavioral Pharmacology,* Vol 1. New York, Academic Press, 1977, p 35.
9. Meisch RA: Animal studies of alcohol intake. *Br J Psychiatry* 141:113, 1981.

10. Meisch RA: Alcohol self-administration by experimental animals, in Smart RG, Cappell HD, Glaser FB, Israel Y, Kalant H, Popham RE, Schmidt W, Sellers EM (eds): *Research Advances in Alcohol and Drug Problems*, Vol 8. New York, Plenum Press, 1984, p 23.

11. Myers RD: Psychopharmacology of alcohol. *Annu Rev Pharmacol* 18:125, 1978.

12. Pohorecky LA: Animal analog of alcohol dependence. *Fed Proc* 40:2056, 1981.

13. Griffiths RR, Bigelow GE, Henningfield JE: Similarities in animal and human drug taking behavior, in Mello NK (ed): *Advances in Substance Abuse*, Vol 1. Greenwich CT, JAI Press, 1980, pp 1–90.

14. Johanson CE: Drugs as reinforcers, in Blackman DE, Sanger DJ (eds): *Contemporary Research in Behavioral Pharmacology*. New York, Plenum Press, 1978, pp 325–390.

15. Johanson CE, Schuster CR: Animal models of drug self-administration, in Mello NK (ed): *Advances in Substance Abuse: Behavioral and Biological Research*, Vol 2. Greenwich, CT, JAI Press, 1981, pp 219–298.

16. Meisch RA, Carroll ME: Oral drug self-administration: Drugs as reinforcers, in Bozarth MA (ed): *Methods of Assessing the Reinforcing Properties of Abused Drugs*. New York, Springer-Verlag, 1987, pp 143–160.

17. Winger G, Young AM, Woods JH: Ethanol as a reinforcer. Comparison with other drugs, in Kissin B, Begleiter (eds): *The Biology of Alcoholism: The Pathogenesis of Alcoholism*, Vol 7. New York, Plenum Press, 1983, pp 107–131.

18. Meisch RA: The function of schedule-induced polydipsia in establishing ethanol as a reinforcer. *Pharmacol Rev* 27:465–473, 1975.

19. Samson HH: Initiation of ethanol-maintained behavior: A comparison of animal models and their implication to human drinking, in Thompson T, Dews PB, Barrett JE (eds): *Neurobehavioral Pharmacology*, Vol 6. Hillsdale, NJ, Lawrence Erlbaum Associates, 1987, p 221.

20. Carroll ME: Rapid acquisition of oral phencyclidine self-administration in food-deprived and food-satiated rhesus monkeys: Concurrent phencyclidine and water choice. *Pharmacol Biochem Behav* 17:341–346, 1982.

21. Falk JL: Production of polydipsia in normal rats by an intermittent food schedule. *Science* 133:195–196, 1961.

22. Sanger DJ: Drug taking as adjunctive behavior, in Goldberg SR, Stolerman IP (eds): *Behavioral Analysis of Drug Dependence*. Orlando, FL, Academic Press, 1986, p 123.

23. Freed EX, Carpenter JA, Hymowitz N: Acquisition and extinction of schedule-induced polydipsia consumption of alcohol and water. *Psychol Rep* 26:915–922, 1970.

24. Freed EX, Lester D: Schedule-induced consumption of ethanol: Calories or chemotherapy? *Physiol Behav* 5:555–560, 1970.

25. Meisch RA: Increased rate of ethanol self-administration as a function of experience in Harris LS (ed): *Proceedings of the Committee on Problems of Drug Dependence*. Washington, DC, National Academy of Sciences–National Research Council, 1969, p 6266.

26. Meisch RA, Thompson T: Ethanol intake in the absence of concurrent food reinforcement. *Psychopharmacologia (Berlin)* 22:72–79, 1971.

27. Meisch RA, Thompson T: Ethanol as a reinforcer: Effects of fixed-ratio size and food deprivation. *Psychopharmacologia (Berlin)* 28:171–183, 1973.

28. Meisch RA, Stark LJ: Establishment of etonitazene as a reinforcer for rats by the use of schedule-induced drinking. *Pharmacol Biochem Behav* 7:195–203, 1977.

29. Carroll ME, Meisch RA: Oral Phencyclidine (PCP) self-administration in rhesus monkeys: Effects of feeding conditions. *J Pharmacol Exp Ther* 214:339–346, 1980.

30. Henningfield JE, Meisch RA: Ethanol as a positive reinforcer via the oral route for rhesus monkeys: Maintenance of fixed-ratio responding. *Pharmacol Biochem Behav* 4:473–475, 1976.

31. Meisch RA, Henningfield JE, Thompson T: Establishment of ethanol as a reinforcer for rhesus monkeys via the oral route: Initial results. *Adv Exp Med Biol* 59:323–342, 1975.

32. Roehrs TA, Samson HH: Ethanol reinforced behavior assessed with a concurrent schedule. *Pharmacol Biochem Behav* 15:539–544, 1981.

33. Lemaire GA, Meisch RA: Pentobarbital self-administration in rhesus monkeys: Drug concentration and fixed-ratio size interactions. *J Exp Anal Behav* 42:37–49, 1984.

34. Lemaire G, Meisch RA: Oral drug self-administration in rhesus monkeys: Interactions between drug amount and fixed-ratio size. *J Exp Anal Behav* 44:377–389, 1985.
35. Samson HH: Initiation of ethanol reinforcement using a sucrose-substitution procedure in food- and water-sated rats. *Alcoholism (NY)* 10:436–442, 1986.
36. Carroll ME: Self-administration of orally-delivered phencyclidine and ethanol under concurrent fixed-ratio schedules in rhesus monkeys. *Psychopharmacology* 93:1–7, 1987.
37. Winger GD, Woods JH: The reinforcing property of ethanol in the rhesus monkey: I. Initiation, maintenance and termination of intravenous ethanol-reinforced responding. *Ann NY Acad Sci* 215:162–175, 1973.
38. Balster RL, Johanson CE, Harris RT, Schuster CR: Phencyclidine self-administration in the rhesus monkey. *Pharmacol Biochem Behav* 1:167–172, 1973.
39. Pickens R, Thompson T, Muchow DC: Cannabis and phencyclidine self-administration by animals, in Goldberg L, Hoffmeister (eds): *Psychic Dependence*, Bayer Symposium IV. Berlin, Springer-Verlag, 1973, p 78.
40. Carroll ME, Stotz DC, Kliner DJ, et al: Self-administration of orally-delivered methohexital in rhesus monkeys with phencyclidine or pentobarbital histories: Effects of food deprivation and satiation. *Pharmacol Biochem Behav* 20:145–151, 1984.
41. Young AM, Herling S: Drugs as reinforcers: Studies in laboratories animals, in Goldberg SR, Stolerman IP (eds): *Behavioral Analysis of Drug Dependence*. Orlando, FL, Academic Press, 1986, p 9.
42. Jaffe, JH: Drug addiction and drug abuse, in Gilman AG, Goodman LS, Gilman A (eds): *Goodman and Gilman's The Pharmacological Basis of Therapeutics*, ed 6. New York, Macmillan, 1980, p 535.
43. Deneau G, Yanagita T, Seever MH: Self-administration of psychoactive substances by the monkey. *Psychopharmacologia (Berlin)* 16:30–48, 1969.
44. Henningfield JE, Meisch RA: Ethanol drinking by rhesus monkeys with concurrent access to water. *Pharmacol Biochem Behav* 10:777–782, 1979.
45. Woods JH, Ikomi F, Winger G. The reinforcing property of ethanol, in Roach MK, McIsaac W, Creaven PJ (eds): *Biological Aspects of Alcohol*. Austin, University of Texas Press, 1971, p 371.
46. Bigelow GR, Griffiths R, Liebson I. Experimental models for the modification of human drug self-administration: Methodological developments in the study of ethanol self-administration by alcoholics. *Fed Proc* 34:1785–1792, 1975.
47. Pickens R, Meisch RA, Thompson T: Drug self-administration: An analysis of the reinforcing effects of drugs, in Iversen LL, Ivesen SD, Snyder SH (eds): *Handbook of Psychopharmacology*, Vol 12. New York, Plenum Press, 1978, p 1.
48. Marcucella H, Munro I, MacDonall JS: Patterns of ethanol consumption as a function of the schedule of ethanol access. *J Pharmacol Exp Ther* 230:658–664, 1984.
49. Marcucella H, Munro I: Patterns of ethanol and water consumption as a function of restricted ethanol access and feeding condition. *Psychopharmacology (Berlin)* 89:145–149, 1986.
50. Marcucella M, Munro I: Ethanol consumption of free feeding animals during restricted ethanol access. *Alcohol Drug Res* 7:405–414, 1987.
51. Henningfield JE, Meisch RA: Ethanol drinking by rhesus monkeys as a function of concentration. *Psychopharmacology (Berlin)* 57:133–136, 1978.
52. Altshuler HL, Talley L: Intragastric self-administration of ethanol by the rhesus monkey: An animal model of alcoholism, in Seixas FA (ed): *Currents in Alcoholism*, Vol 1. New York, Grune & Stratton, 1977, p 243.
53. Altshuler HL, Weaver S, Phillips P: Intragastric self-administration of psychoactive drugs by the rhesus monkey. *Life Sci* 17:883–890, 1975.
54. Yanagita T, Takahashi S: Dependence liability of several sedative-hypnotic agents evaluated in monkeys. *J Pharmacol Exp Ther* 185:307–316, 1973.
55. Carney JM, Llewellyn ME, Woods JH: Variable interval responding maintained by intravenous codeine and ethanol injections in the rhesus monkey. *Pharmacol Biochem Behav* 5:577–582, 1976.

56. DeNoble VJ, Begleiter H: Alcohol self-administration in monkeys (*Macaca radiata*): The effects of prior alcohol exposure. *Pharmacol Biochem Behav* 8:391–397, 1978.

57. Karoly AJ, Winger GD, Ikomi F, Woods JH: The reinforcing property of ethanol in the rhesus monkey. *Psychopharmacology (Berlin)* 58:19–25, 1978.

58. Goldberg SR, Hoffmeister F, Schlichting UU, Wuttke W: A comparison of pentobarbital and cocaine self-administration in rhesus monkeys: Effects of dose and fixed-ratio parameter. *J Pharmacol Exp Ther* 179:277–283, 1971.

59. Meisch RA, Kliner DJ, Henningfield JE: Pentobarbital drinking by rhesus monkeys: Establishment and maintenance of pentobarbital-reinforced behavior. *J Pharmacol Exp Ther* 217:114–120, 1981.

60. Balster RL, Johanson CE, Harris RT, et al: Phencyclidine self-administration in the rhesus monkey. *Pharmacol Biochem Behav* 1:167–172, 1973.

61. Carroll ME, Stotz DC: Oral *d*-amphetamine and ketamine self-administration by rhesus monkeys: Effects of food deprivation. *J Pharmacol Exp Ther* 227:28–34, 1983.

62. Moreton JE, Meisch RA, Stark L, Thompson T: Ketamine self-administration by the rhesus monkey. *J Pharmacol Exp Ther* 203:303–309, 1977.

63. Balster RL, Schuster CR: A comparison of *d*-amphetamine, *l*-amphetamine, and methamphetamine self-administration in rhesus monkeys. *Pharmacol Biochem Behav* 1:67–71, 1973.

64. Meisch RA, Carroll ME: Establishment of orally delivered drugs as reinforcers for rhesus monkeys: Some relations to human drug dependence, in Thompson T, Johanson CE (eds): *Behavioral Pharmacology of Human Drug Dependence*. NIDA Research Monograph No. 37, DHHS Publication No. (ADM) 81–1137. Washington, DC, U.S. Government Printing Office, 1981, p 197.

65. Carroll ME, Oral self-administration of phencyclidine analogs by rhesus monkeys: Conditioned taste and visual reinforcers. *Psychopharmacology (Berlin)* 78:116–120, 1982.

66. Carroll ME, Meisch RA: Concurrent etonitazene and water intake in rats: Role of taste, olfaction and auditory stimuli. *Psychopharmacology* 64:1–7, 1979.

67. Collins RJ, Weeks JR, Cooper MM, et al: Prediction of abuse liability of drugs using IV self-administration by rats. *Psychopharmacology (Berlin)* 82:60–13, 1984.

68. DeNoble VJ, Mele PC, Porter JH: Intravenous self-administration of pentobarbital and ethanol in rats. *Pharmacol Biochem Behav* 23:759–763, 1985.

69. Grupp LA: An investigation of intravenous ethanol self-administration in rats using a fixed ratio schedule of reinforcement. *Physiol Psychol* 9:359–363, 1981.

70. Numan R. Multiple exposures to ethanol facilitates intravenous self-administration of ethanol by rats. *Pharmacol Biochem Behav* 15:101–108, 1981.

71. Smith SC, Davis WM: Intravenous alcohol self-administration in the rat. *Pharmacol Res Commun* 6:397–402, 1974.

72. Smith SG, Werner TE, Davis WM: Comparison between intravenous and intragastric alcohol self-administration. *Physiol Psychol* 4:91–93, 1976.

73. Smith SG, Werner TE, Davis WM: Intravenous drug self-administration in rats: Substitution of ethyl alcohol for morphine. *Psychol Rec* 25:17–20, 1975.

74. Sinden JD, LeMagnen J: Parameters of low-dose ethanol intravenous self-administration in the rat. *Pharmacol Biochem Behav* 16:181–183, 1982.

75. Amit Z, Stern HH: Alcohol ingestion without oropharyngeal sensations. *Psychonomic Sci* 15:162–163, 1969.

76. Deutsch JA, Cannis JT: Rapid induction of voluntary alcohol choice in rats. *Behav Neural Biol* 30:292–298, 1980.

77. Hardy WT, Deutsch JA: Preference for ethanol in dependent rats. *Behav Biol* 20:482–492, 1977.

78. Smith SG, Werner TE, Davis WM: Alcohol-associated conditioned reinforcement. *Psychopharmacologia (Berlin)* 53:223–226, 1977.

79. Smith SG, Werner TE, Davis WM: Intragastric drug self-administration by rats exposed successively to morphine and ethanol. *Drug Alcohol Depend* 7:305–310, 1981.

80. Smith SG, Werner TE, Davis WM: Technique for intragastric delivery of solutions: Application for self-administration of morphine and alcohol by rats. *Physiol Psychol* 3:220–224, 1975.

81. Waller MB, McBride WJ, Gatto GJ, Lumeng L, Li T-K: Intragastric self-infusion of ethanol by ethanol-preferring and -nonpreferring lines of rats. *Science* 225:78–80, 1984.

82. Grupp LA: Ethanol as the negative reinforcer in an active avoidance paradigm. *Prog. Neuropsychopharmacol.* 5:241–244, 1981.

83. Grupp LA, Stewart RB: Active and passive avoidance behaviour in rats produced by intravenous infusions of ethanol. *Psychopharmacology* 79:318–321, 1983.

84. Spealman, RD: Behavior maintained by termination of a schedule of self-administered cocaine. *Science* 204:1231–1232, 1979.

85. Henningfield JE, Goldberg SR: Nicotine as a reinforcer in human subjects and laboratory animals. *Pharmacol Biochem Behav* 19:989–992, 1983.

86. Hoffmeister F, Wuttke W: Self-administration: Positive and negative reinforcing properties of morphine antagonists in rhesus monkeys, in Braude MC, Harris LS, May EL, Smith JP, Villarreal JE (eds): *Advances in Biochemical Psychopharmacology*, Vol 8. New York, Raven Press, 1974.

87. Weeks JR, Collins J: Screening for drug reinforcement using intravenous self-administration in the rat, in MA Bozarth (ed): *Methods of Assessing the Reinforcing Properties of Abused Drugs.* New York, Springer-Verlag, 1987, pp 35–44.

88. Elmer GI, Meisch RA, George FR: Oral ethanol reinforced behavior in inbred mice. *Pharmacol Biochem Behav* 24:1417–1421, 1986.

89. Meisch RA, Thompson, T: Ethanol intake in the absence of concurrent food reinforcement. *Psychopharmacologia (Berlin)* 22:72–79, 1971.

90. Henningfield JE, Ator NA, Griffiths RR: Establishment and maintenance of oral ethanol self-administration in the baboon. *Drug Alcohol Dependence* 7:113–124, 1981.

91. Elmer GI, Meisch RA, Goldberg SR, George FR: Fixed-ratio schedules of oral ethanol self-administration in inbred mouse strains. *Psychopharmacology (Berlin)* 96:431–436, 1988.

92. Meisch RA, Henningfield JE: Drinking of ethanol by rhesus monkeys: Experimental strategies for establishing ethanol as a reinforcer. *Adv Exp Med Biol* 85B:443–463, 1977.

93. Johnston LD, O'Malley PM, Bachman JG: *Use of Licit and Illicit Drugs by America's High School Students 1975–1984*, DHHS Publication No. (ADM) 85-1394, Washington DC, U.S. Government Printing Office, 1985.

94. Mello NK, Bree MP, Mendelson JH, et al: Alcohol self-administration disrupts reproductive function in female macaque monkeys. *Science* 221:677–679, 1983.

95. Grant KA, Johanson CE: Oral ethanol self-administration in free-feeding rhesus monkeys. *Alcoholism: Clin Exp Res*, 12:780–784, 1988.

96. Eriksson K: Factors affecting voluntary alcohol consumption in the albino rat. *Ann Zool Fennici* 6:227, 1969.

97. Eriksson K: Inheritance of behavior towards alcohol in normal and motivated choice situations in mice. *Ann Zool Fennici*, 8:400–405, 1971.

98. Suzuki T, Koike Y, Yoshii T et al: Sex differences in the induction of physical dependence on pentobarbital in the rat. *Jpn J Pharmacol* 39:453–459, 1985.

99. Suzuki T, Koike Y, Yoshii T, et al: Sex differences in physical dependence on barbital in rats. *Jpn J Psychopharmacol* 6:373–380, 1986.

100. Suzuki T, Koike Y, Misawa M: Sex differences in physical dependence on methaqualone in the rat. *Pharmacol Biochem Behav* 30:483–488, 1988.

101. Heppner CC, Kemble ED, Cox WM: Effects of food deprivation on caffeine consumption in male and female rats. *Pharmacol Biochem Behav* 24:1555–1559, 1986.

102. Alexander BK, Coambs RB, Hadaway PF: The effect of housing and gender on morphine self-administration in rats. *Psychopharmacology* 58:175–179, 1978.

103. Hill SY: Addiction liability of tryon rats: Independent transmission of morphine and alcohol consumption. *Pharmacol Biochem Behav* 9:107–110, 1978.

104. Hadaway PF, Alexander BK, Coombs RB, Beyerstein B: The effect of housing and gender on preference for morphine–sucrose solutions in rats. *Psychopharmacology* 66:87–91, 1979.

105. Meisch RA, George FR: Influence of genetic factors on drug-reinforced behavior in animals, in Pickens R, Svikis D (eds): *Biological Vulnerability to Drug Abuse*. National Institute on Drug Abuse, Research Monograph Series, No. 88, DHHS Publication No. (ADM) 88-90, Washington DC, U.S. Government Printing Office, 1988, pp 9–14.

106. Mardones RJ, Segovia MN, Hederra DA: Heredity of experimental alcohol preference in rats. II. Coeffecient of heredity. *Q J Stud Alcohol* 14:1–2, 1953.

107. McClearn GE, Rodgers DA: Differences in alcohol preference among inbred strains of mice. *Q J Stud Alcohol* 20:691–695, 1959.

108. McClearn GE, Rodgers DA: Genetic factors in alcohol preference of laboratory mice. *J Comp Physiol Psychol* 54:116–119, 1961.

109. Deitrich RA, Spuhler K: Genetics of alcoholism and alcohol actions, in Smart RG, Cappell HD, Glaser FB, Israel Y, Kalant H, Popham RE, Schmidt W, Sellers EM (eds): *Research Advances in Alcohol and Drug Problems*, Vol 8. New York, Plenum Press, 1984, p 47.

110. Eriksson K, Kiianmaa, K: Genetic analysis of susceptibility to morphine addiction in inbred mice. *Ann Med Exp Biol Fenn* 49:73–78, 1971.

111. Horowitz GP, Whitney G, Smith JC, Stephan FK: Morphine ingestion: Genetic control in mice. *Psychopharmacology (Berlin)* 52:119–122, 1977.

112. Carroll ME, Pederson MC, Harrison RG: Food deprivation reveals strain differences in opiate intake of Sprague–Dawley and Wistar rats. *Pharmacol Biochem Behav* 24:1095–1099, 1986.

113. George FR, Meisch RA: Oral narcotic intake as a reinforcer: Genotype x environmental interactions. *Behav Genet* 14:603, 1984.

114. Waller MB, McBride WJ, Gatto GJ, Lumeng L, Li T-K: Intragastric self-infusion of ethanol by ethanol-preferring and -nonpreferring lines of rats. *Science* 225:78–80, 1984.

115. Eriksson K: Genetic selection for voluntary alcohol consumption in the albino rat. *Science* 159:739–741, 1968.

116. Ritz MC, George FR, deFiebre CM, Meisch RA: Genetic differences in the establishment of ethanol as a reinforcer. *Pharmacol Biochem Behav* 24:1089–1094, 1986.

117. Ritz MC, George FR, Meisch RA: Ethanol self-administration in ALKO rats: I. Effects of selection and concentration. *Alcohol* 6:227–233, 1989.

118. Suzuki T, George FR, Meisch RA: Differential establishment and maintenance of oral ethanol reinforced behavior in Lewis and Fischer 344 inbred rat strains. *J Pharmacol Exp Ther* 245:164–170, 1988.

119. Elmer GI, Meisch RA, George FR: Mouse strain differences in operant self-administration of ethanol. *Behav Genet* 17:439–451, 1987.

120. Elmer GI, Meisch RA, George FR: Differential concentration-response curves for oral ethanol self-administration in C57BL/6J and BALB/cJ mice. *Alcohol* 4:63–68, 1987.

121. Broadhurst PL: *Drugs and the Inheritance of Behavior*. New York, Plenum Press, 1978.

122. Takahashi RN, Singer G, Oei TPS: Schedule-induced self-injection of d-amphetamine by naive animals. *Pharmacol Biochem Behav* 9:857–861, 1968.

123. Carroll ME, France CP, Meisch RA: Intravenous self-administration of etonitazene, cocaine and phencyclidine in rats during food deprivation and satiation. *J Pharmacol Exp Ther* 217:241–247, 1981.

124. Carroll ME, France CP, Meisch RA: Food deprivation increases oral and intravenous drug intake in rats. *Science* 205:319–321, 1979.

125. Hall SM, Ginsberg D, Jones RT: Smoking cessation and weight gain. *J Coun Clin Psychol* 54:342–346, 1986.

126. Yung L, Gordis E, Holt J: Dietary choices and likelihood of abstinence among alcoholic patients in an outpatient clinic. *Drug Alcohol Dependence* 12:355–362, 1983.

127. Hatsukami D, Gust S, Keenan R: Physiological and subjective changes from smokeless tobacco withdrawal. *Clin Pharmacol Ther* 41:103–107, 1987.

128. Franklin JC, Schiele BC, Brozek J, et al: Observations on human behavior in experimental semistarvation and rehabilitation. *J Clin Psychol* 4:28–45, 1948.

129. Hanna JM, Hornick CA: Use of coca leaf in southern Peru: Adaptation or addiction. *Bull Narc* 29:63–74, 1977.
130. Carroll ME: The role of food deprivation in the maintenance and reinstatement of cocaine-seeking behavior in rats. *Drug Alcohol Dependence* 16:95–109, 1985.
131. Carroll ME: Performance maintained by orally-delivered phencyclidine under second order, tandem and fixed-interval schedules in food-satiated and food-deprived rhesus monkeys. *J Pharmacol Exp Ther* 232:351–359, 1985.
132. de la Garza R, Bergman J, Hartel CR: Food deprivation and cocaine self-administration. *Pharmacol Biochem Behav* 15:141–144, 1981.
133. de la Garza R, Johanson CE: The effects of food deprivation on the self-administration of psychoactive drugs. *Drug Alcohol Dependence* 19:17–27, 1987.
134. Lang WJ, Latiff AA, McQueen A, et al: Self-administration of nicotine with and without a food delivery schedule. *Pharmacol Biochem Behav* 1:65–70, 1977.
135. Carroll ME, Boe IN: Effect of dose on increased etonitazene self-administration by rats due to food deprivation. *Psychopharmacology* 82:151–152, 1984.
136. Papasava M, Singer G: Self-administration of low-dose cocaine by rats at reduced and recovered body weight. *Psychopharmacology* 85:419–425, 1985.
137. Takahashi RN, Singer G: Effects of body weight levels on cannabis self-injection. *Pharmacol Biochem Behav* 13:877–881, 1980.
138. Carroll ME: Concurrent access to two concentrations of orally-delivered phencyclidine: Effects of feeding conditions. *J Exp Anal Behav* 47:347–362, 1987.
139. Segal EF: Confirmation of a positive relation between deprivation and number of responses emitted for light reinforcement. *J Exp Anal Behav* 2:165–169, 1959.
140. Symons JP: Wheel-running activity during ad-lib and food-deprivation conditions in four inbred mouse strains. *Bull Psychon Soc* 1:78–80, 1978.
141. Katz JH, Baldrighi G, Roth K: Appetitive determinants of self-stimulation. *Behav Biol* 23:500–508, 1978.
142. Hursch SR, Beck RC: Bitter and sweet saccharin preferences as a function of food deprivation. *Psychol Rec* 29:419–422, 1971.
143. Meisch RA, Thompson T: Ethanol intake as a function of concentration during food deprivation and satiation. *Pharmacol Biochem Behav* 2:589–596, 1974.
144. Vuchinich RE, Tucker JA: Contributions from behavioral theories of choice to an analysis of alcohol abuse. *J Abnor Psy* 97:181–195, 1988.
145. Carroll ME, Meisch RA: Increased drug-reinforced behavior due to food deprivation, in Thompson T, Dews PB, Barrett JE (eds.): *Advances in Behavioral Pharmacology*, Vol. 4, Academic Press, New York, 1984, pp 47–88.
146. Gentry RT, Dole VP: Why does a sucrose choice reduce the consumption of alcohol in C57BL/6J mice? *Life Sci* 40:2191–2194, 1987.
147. Lester D, Greenberg LA: Nutrition and the etiology of alcoholism: The effect of sucrose, saccharin and fat on the self-selection of ethyl alcohol by rats. *Q J Stud Alcohol* 13:553–560, 1952.
148. Samson HH, Falk JL: Alteration of fluid preference in ethanol-dependent animals. *J Pharmacol Exp Ther* 190:365–376, 1974.
149. Samson HH, Lindberg K: Comparison of sucrose-sucrose to sucrose-ethanol concurrent responding in the rat: Reinforcement schedule and fluid concentration effects. *Pharmacol Biochem Behav* 20:973–977, 1984.
150. Samson HH, Roehrs TA, Tolliver GA: Ethanol reinforced responding in the rat: A concurrent analysis using sucrose as the alternative choice. *Pharmacol Biochem Behav* 17:333–339, 1982.
151. Forsander DA, Sinclair JD: Protein, carbohydrate, and ethanol consumption: Interactions in AA and ANA rats. *Alcohol* 5:233–238, 1988.
152. Vuchinich RE, Tucker JA, Rudd EJ: Preference for alcohol consumption as a function of amount and delay of alternative reward. *J Abnor Psy* 96:259–263, 1987.
153. Carroll ME, Stotz DC: Increased phencyclidine self-administration due to food deprivation: Interaction with concentration and training conditions. *Psychopharmacology* 84:299–303, 1984.

154. Carroll ME: Concurrent phencyclidine and saccharin access: Presentation of an alternative reinforcer reduces drug intake. *Exp Anal Behav* 43:131–144, 1985.

155. Carroll ME, Lac ST, Nygaard SL: A concurrently available nondrug reinforcer prevents the acquisition or decreases the maintenance of cocaine-reinforced behavior. *Psychopharmacology,* 97:23–29, 1989.

156. Poling A, Thompson T: Effects of delaying food availability contingent on ethanol-maintained lever pressing. *Psychopharmacology* 51:289–291, 1977.

157. Poling A, Thompson T: Suppression of ethanol-reinforced lever pressing by delaying food availability. *J Exp Behav* 28:271–283, 1977.

158. Griffiths R, Bigelow G, Liebson I: Suppression of ethanol self-administration of alcoholics by contingent time-out from social interactions. *Behav Research Ther* 12:327–334, 1974.

159. Boudin HM: Contingency contracting as a therapeutic tool in the deceleration of amphetamine use. *Behav Ther* 3:604–608, 1972.

160. Cohen M, Liebson A, Faillace LA: The modification of drinking of chronic alcoholics, in Mello NK, Mendelson JH (eds): *Recent Advances in Studies of Alcoholism.* NIMH publication No. HSM 71-9045. Washington, DC: U.S. Government Printing Office, 1971, pp 745–766.

161. Stitzer ML, Bigelow GE, Lawrence C, et al: Medication take-home as a reinforcer in a methadone maintenance program. *Addict Behav* 2:8–14, 1977.

162. Stitzer ML, Bigelow GE, Liebson IA, et al: Contingency management of supplemental drug use during methadone maintenance treatment, in Grabowski J, Stitzer ML, Henningfield JE (eds): *Behavioral Intervention Techniques in Drug Abuse Treatment.* NIDA Research Monograph No. 46. Washington, DC, U.S. Government Printing Office, 1984, pp 84–103.

163. Skinner BF: *Science and Human Behavior.* New York, Macmillan, 1953.

164. Iguchi M, Stitzer, ML, Bigelow GE, et al: Contingency management and methadone maintenance: Effects of reinforcing and aversive consequences on illicit polydrug use. *Drug Alcohol Dependence* 22:1–7, 1988.

165. Calahan D, Cisin I, Crossley H: *American Drinking Practices.* New Brunswick, NJ, Rutgers Center of Alcohol Studies, 1969.

166. Harford TC, Ganes LS (eds): Social Drinking Contexts, NIAAA Monograph No. 7, DHHS publication no (ADM) 81-1097. Washington DC, U.S. Government Printing Office, 1981, pp 1–244.

167. Stitzer ML, Griffiths RR, Bigelow GE, et al: Social stimulus factors in drug effects in human subjects in Thompson T, Johanson CE (eds): *Behavioral Pharmacology of Human Drug Dependence,* NIDA Research Monograph No. 37. Washington DC, U.S. Government Printing Office, 1981, pp 130–154.

168. Watson DW, Sobell MB: Social influences on alcohol consumption by black and white males. *Addict Behav* 7:87–91, 1982.

169. Rosenbluth J, Nathan PE, Lawson DM: Environmental influences on drinking by college students in a college pub: Behavioral observation in the natural environment, *Addict Behav* 3:117 1978.

170. Storm T, Cutler RE: Observations of drinking in natural settings. *J Stud Alcohol* 42:972–997, 1981.

171. Caudill BD, Marlatt GA: Modeling influences in social drinking: An experimental analogue. *J Consult Clin Psychol* 43:405–415, 1975.

172. Collins RL, Parks GA, Marlatt GA: Social determinants of alcohol consumption: The effects of social interaction and model status on the self-administration of alcohol. *J Consult Clin Psychol* 53:189–200, 1985.

173. Babor TF, Mendelson JH, Greenberg I, et al: Experimental analysis of the "happy hour": Effects of purchase price on alcohol consumption. *Psychopharmacology* 58:35–42, 1978.

174. Babor TF, Brglas S, Mendelson JH, et al: Alcohol, affect, and the disinhibition of verbal behavior. *Psychopharmacology* 80:53–60, 1980.

175. Reid JB: Study of drinking in natural settings, in Marlatt GA, Nathan PE (eds): *Behavioral Approaches to Alcoholism.* New Brunswick, NJ, Rutgers Center of Alcohol Studies, 1978, pp 58–74.

176. Samson HH, Fromme K: Social drinking in a simulated tavern: An experimental analysis. *Drug Alcohol Dependence* 14:141–163, 1984.
177. Caudill BD, Lipscomb TR: Modeling influences on alcoholics' rates of alcohol consumption. *J Appl Behav Anal* 13:355–365, 1980.
178. Alexander BK, Coambs RB, Hadaway PF: The effect of housing and gender on morphine self-administration in rats. *Psychopharmacology* 58:175–179, 1978.
179. Hadaway PF, Alexander BK, Coambs RB, Beyerstein B: The effect of housing and gender on preference for morphine-sucrose solutions in rats. *Psychopharmacology* 66:87–91, 1979.
180. Kraemer GW, McKinney WT: Social separation increases alcohol consumption in rhesus monkeys. *Psychopharmacology* 86:182–189, 1985.
181. Crowley TJ, Andrews AE: Alcoholic-like drinking in simian social groups. *Psychopharmacology* 92:196–205, 1987.
182. Asghar K: Role of dietary and environmental factors in drug abuse. *Alcohol Drug Res* 7:61–83, 1986.
183. Bergmann F, Lieblich I, Cohen E, et al: Influence of intake of sweet solutions on the analgesic effect of a low dose of morphine in randomly bred rats. *Behav Neural Biol* 44:347–353, 1985.
184. Marks-Kaufman R, Harmon M, Barbate GF: The effects of dietary sucrose on opiate receptor binding in lean and obese mice. *Fed Proc* 44:424 1985.
185. Dum J, Gramsch CH, Herz A. Activation of hypothalamic beta-endorphin pools by reward-induced by highly palatable food. *Pharmacol Biochem Behav* 18 443–447, 1983.
186. Geis LS, Smith DG, Smith FL, et al: Tyrosine influence on amphetamine self-administration and brain catecholamines in the rat. *Pharmacol Biochem Behav* 25:1027–1033, 1986.
187. Smith FL, Yu DS, Smith DG, Leccese AP, et al: Dietary tryptophan supplements attenuate amphetamine self-administration in the rat. *Pharmacol Biochem Behav* 25:849–855, 1986.
188. Zabik JE, Binkerd K, Roache JD: Serotonin and ethanol aversion in the rat, in Naranjo CA, Sellers EM (eds): *Research Advances in New Psychopharmacology Treatments for Alcoholism.* New York, Elsevier, 1985, pp 87–105.
189. Rockman GE, Amit Z, Bourque C, et al: Reduction of voluntary morphine consumption following treatment with zimelidine. *Arch Int Pharmacodyn* 244:123–129, 1980.
190. Sinclair JD: The feasibility of effective psychopharmacological treatments for alcoholism. *Br J Addic* 82:1213–1223, 1987.
191. Tollefson GD: Serotonin and alcohol: interrelationships. *Psychopathology* 22(Suppl.):1–78, 1989.
192. Naranjo CA, Sellers EM, Roach CA, Woodley DV, Sanchez-Craig M, Sykora K: Zimelidine-induced variations in alcohol intake by nondepressed heavy drinkers. *Clin Pharmacol Ther* 35:375–381, 1984.
193. Gorelick DA: Effect of fluoxetine on alcohol consumption. *Alcoholism* 10:113, 1986.
194. Martin PR, Adinoff B, Bone GAH, et al.: Fluvoxamine (F) treatment of alcoholic chronic organic brain syndromes (COBS). *Clin Pharmacol Ther* 41:211, 1987.
195. Heel RC, Morley PA, Brogden RN, et al: Zimelidine: A review of its pharmacologic properties and therapeutic efficacy in depressive illness. *Drugs* 24:169–206, 1982.
196. Cazala P: Effects of Lilly 110140 (fluoxetine) on self-stimulation behavior in the dorsal and ventral regions of the lateral hypothalamus in the mouse. *Psychopharmacology* 71:143–146, 1980.
197. Atrens DM, Ungerstedt U, Ljungberg T: Specific inhibition of hypothalamic self-stimulation by selective reuptake blockade of either 5-hydroxytryptamine or noradrenaline. *Psychopharmacology* 52:177–180, 1977.
198. Carroll ME, Lac ST, Acensio M, et al: Fluoxetine or dietary L-tryptophan reduce intravenous cocaine self-administration in rats. *The FASEB Journal* 3:A419, 1989.
199. Gawin FH, Ellinwood EH: Cocaine and other stimulans: actions, abuse, and treatment. *N Engl J Med* 18:1173, 1988.
200. O'Brien CP: Pharmacological and behavioral treatments of cocaine dependence: Controlled studies. *Clin Psychol* 49:17, 1988.

201. Aschkenasy-Lelu P: Action de la sous-alimentation et de l'inanition sur la consommation d'alcool du rat et leur action genitale. *Arch Sci Physiol* 14:165–174, 1960.
202. Roberts DCS, Loh EA, Vickers GJ: Self-administration of cocaine on a progressive ratio schedule in rats: Dose response relationship and effect of haloperidol pretreatment. *Psychopharmacology,* 97:535–538, 1989.
203. Mello NK: Some behavioral and biological aspects of alcohol problems in women, in Kalant OJ (ed): *Alcohol and Drug Problems in Women,* Research Advances in Alcohol and Drug Problems, Vol V. New York, Plenum Press, 1980, pp 263–298.
204. Mello NK: Drug use patterns and premenstrual dysphoria, in Ray B, Braude M (eds): *Women and Drugs: A New Era for Research,* NIDA Research Monograph No 65 DHHS Publication NO (ADM) 86-1447. Washington DC, U.S. Government Printing Office, 1986, pp 31–48.
205. Belfer ML, Shader RI. Premenstrual factors as determinants of alcoholism in women, in Greenblatt M, Schuckit MA (eds): *Alcohol Problems in Women and Children.* New York, Grune & Stratton, 1976, pp 97–102.
206. Podolsky E: The woman alcoholic and premenstrual tension. *J Am Med Wom Assoc* 18:816–818, 1963.
207. Griffin ML, Mello NK, Mendelson JH, et al: Alcohol use across the menstrual cycle among marijuana users. *Alcohol* 4:457–462, 1987.
208. Sutker PB, Goist KC, King AR: Acute alcoholic intoxication in women: Relationship to dose and menstrual cycle phase. *Alcoholism: Clin Exp Res* 11:74–79, 1987.
209. Harvey SM, Beckman LJ: Cyclic fluctuation in alcohol consumption among female social drinkers. *Alcoholism: Clin Exp Res* 9:465–476, 1985.
210. Jones MK, Jones BM: Ethanol metabolism in women taking oral contraceptives. *Alcoholism: Clin Exp Res* 8:24–28, 1984.
211. Griffiths RR, Bigelow GE, Liebson I: Facilitation of human tobacco self-administration by ethanol: A behavioral analysis. *J Exp Anal Behav* 25:279–292, 1976.
212. Henningfield JE, Chait LD, Griffiths RR, Cigarette smoking and subjective response in alcoholics. Effects of pentobarbital. *Clin Pharmacol Ther* 33:806–812, 1983.
213. Henningfield JE, Chait LD, Griffiths RR: Effects of ethanol on cigarette smoking by volunteers without histories of alcoholism. *Psychopharmacology* 82:1–5, 1984.
214. Mello NK, Mendelson JH, Sellers ML, et al: Effect of alcohol and marijuana on tobacco smoking. *Clin Pharmacol Ther* 27:202–209, 1980.
215. Mello NK, Mendelson JH, Palmieri SL: Cigarette smoking by women: Interactions with alcohol use. *Psychopharmacology* 93:8–15, 1987.
216. Keenan RM, Hatsukami DK, Pickens RW et al.: The relationship between chronic ethanol exposure and cigarette smoking in the laboratory and the natural environment. *Psychopharmacology,* in press, 1989.
217. Mello NK, Mendelson JH, Kuehnle JC, et al: Human polydrug use: marijuana and alcohol. *Pharmacol Exp Ther* 207:922–935, 1978.
218. Cooper SJ: Effects of opiate agonists and antagonists on fluid intake and saccharine choice in the rat. *Neuropharmacology* 22:323–328, 1983.
219. Samson HH, Grant KA: Chlordiazepoxide effects on ethanol self-administration: Dependence on concurrent conditions. *J Exp Anal Behav* 43:353–364, 1985.
220. Reid L, Hubbell C: Opioids' modulation of alcohol intake, in Harris LS (ed): *Problems of Drug Dependence, 1987,* NIDA Research Monograph No 81. Washington, DC, U.S. Government Printing Office, 1988, p 304.
221. Ticku MK, Kulkarni SK: Molecular interactions of ethanol with GABAergic system and potential of R015-4513 as an ethanol antagonist. *Pharmacol Biochem Behav* 30:501–510, 1988.
222. Suzdak PD, Glowa JR, Crawley JN, et al: A selective imidazobenzodiazepine antagonist of ethanol in the rat. *Science* 234:1243–1247, 1986.
223. De Witte P: Naloxone reduces alcohol intake in a free-choice procedure even when both drinking bottles contain saccharin, sodium or quinine substances. *Neuropsychobiology* 12:73–77, 1984.

224. Myers RD, Borg S, Mossberg R: Antagonism by naltrexone of voluntary alcohol selection in the chronically drinking macaque monkey. *Alcohol* 3:383–388, 1986.
225. Samson HH, Doyle TF: Oral ethanol self-administration in the rat: Effect of naloxone. *Pharmacol Biochem Behav* 22:91–99, 1985.
226. Sinden JD, Marfaing-Jallat P, LeMagnen J: The effect of naloxone on intragastric ethanol self-administration. *Pharmacol Biochem Behav* 19:1045–1048, 1983.
227. Altshuler HL, Phillips PE, Feinhandler DA: Alteration of ethanol self-administration by naltrexone. *Life Sci* 26:679–688, 1980.
228. Carroll ME, Lac ST, Walker MJ, et al: Effects of naltrexone on intravenous cocaine self-administration in rats during food satiation and deprivation. *J Pharmacol Exp Ther* 238:1–7, 1986.
229. Harris RA, Erikson CK: Alteration of ethanol effects by opiate antagonists. *Curr Alcohol* 5:17–28, 1979.
230. Ho AKS, Ho CC: Toxic interactions of ethanol with other central depressants: Antagonism by naloxone to narcosis and lethality. *Pharmacol Biochem Behav* 11:111–114, 1979.
231. Kiianmaa K, Hoffman PL, Tabakoff B: Antagonism of the behavioral effects of ethanol by naltrexone in BALB/c, C57BL/6, and DBA/2 mice. *Psychopharmacology* 79:291–294, 1983.
232. Duka T, Cumin R, Haefely W, et al: Naloxone blocks the effects of diazepam and meprobamate on conflict behavior in rats. *Pharmacol Biochem Behav* 15:115–117, 1981.
233. Koob GF, Strecker RE, Bloom FE: Effects of naloxone on the anti-conflict properties of alcohol and chlordiazepoxide. *Subst Alcohol Actions-Misuse* 1:447, 1980.
234. Herling S: Naltrexone blocks the response-latency increasing effects but not the discriminative effects of diazepam in rats. *Eur J Pharmacol* 88:121–124, 1983.
235. Jeffcoate WJ, Herbert M, Cullen MH, et al: Prevention of effects of alcohol intoxication by naloxone. *Lancet* 2:1157–1159, 1979.
236. Jeffreys B, Flanagan RJ, Volans GN: Reversal of ethanol-induced coma with naloxone. *Lancet* 1:308–309, 1980.
237. Mackenzie AI: Naloxone in alcohol intoxication. *Lancet* 1:733–734, 1979.
238. Sorenson SC, Mattisson KI: Naloxone antagonist in severe alcohol intoxication. *Lancet* 2:668–669, 1978.
239. Jorgenson HA, Hole K: Does ethanol stimulate brain opiate receptors? Studies on receptor binding and naloxone inhibition of ethanol-induced effects. *Eur J Pharmacol* 75:223–229, 1981.
240. Galizio M, Smaltz SC, Spencer BA: Effects of ethanol and naltrexone on free-operant avoidance behavior in rats. *Pharmacol Biochem Behav* 21:423–429, 1984.
241. Harris RA, Snell D: Interactions between naltrexone and non-opiate drugs evaluated by schedule-controlled behavior. *Neuropharmacology* 19:1087–1093, 1980.
242. Carroll ME, Lac ST, Walker MJ et al: Effects of naltrexone on intravenous cocaine self administration in rats during food satiation and deprivation. *J Pharmacol Exp Ther* 238:1–7, 1986.
243. Collier HoJ, Cuthbert NJ, Francis DL: Character and meaning of quasi-morphine withdrawal phenomena elicited by methylxanthines. *Fed Proc* 40:1512–1518, 1981.
244. Fertziger AP, Fischer R: Interaction between narcotic antagonist (naloxone) and lysergic acid diethylamide (LSD) in the rat. *Psychopharmacology,* 54:313–314, 1977.
245. Ruffing DM, Domino EF: Effects of selected opioid agonists and antagonists on DMT- and LSD-25-induced disruption of food-rewarded bar pressing behavior in the rat. *Psychopharmacology* 75:226–230, 1981.
246. Rech RH, Mokler DJ, Commissaris RL, et al: Behavioral Interactions of opioid agonists and antagonists with serotonergic systems, in Harris LS (ed): *Problems of Drug Dependence, 1983,* NIDA Research Monograph 49. Washington DC, U.S. Government Printing Office, 1984, pp 179–184.
247. Conner JD: Naloxonic potentiates behavioral disruption by hallucinogens in monkeys. *Pharmacologist* 27:167, 1985.

248. Commissaris RL, Moore KE, Rech RH: Naloxone potentiates the disruptive effects of mescaline on operant responding in the rat. *Pharmacol Biochem Behav* 13:601–603, 1980.
249. Schuster CR: Variables affecting the self-administration of drugs by rhesus monkeys, in Vaglborg H (ed): *Use of Nonhuman Primates in Drug Evaluation*, Austin, University of Texas Press, 1968, pp 283–299.
250. Thompson T, Schuster CR: Morphine self-administration, food-reinforced and avoidance behaviors in rhesus monkeys. *Psychopharmacologia (Berlin)* 5:87–94, 1964.
251. Victor M, Adams RD: The effect of alcohol on the nervous system. *Res Publ Assoc Res Nerv Ment Dis* 32:526–573, 1953.
252. Hunter BE, Riley JN, Walker DW: Ethanol dependence in the rat: a parametric analysis. *Pharmacol Biochem Behav* 3:619–629, 1975.
253. Friedman HJ: Assessment of physical dependence on and withdrawal from ethanol in animals, in Rigter H, Crabbe JC (eds): *Alcohol Tolerance and Dependence*. Amsterdam, Elsevier/North-Holland Biomedical Press, 1980.
254. Pieper WA, Skeen MJ: Alcohol withdrawal reactions in rhesus monkeys, in Gross MM (ed): *Alcohol Intoxication and Withdrawal*, Vol IIIb. New York, Plenum Press, 1977.
255. Tarika JS, Winger G: The Effects of ethanol, phenobarbital, and baclofen on ethanol withdrawal in the rhesus monkey. *Psychopharmacology* 70:201–208, 1980.
256. Goldstein DB: Relationship of alcohol dose to intensity of withdrawal signs in mice. *J Pharm Exp Ther* 180:203–215, 1972.
257. Noble EP, Gillies R, Vigran R, et al: The modification of the ethanol withdrawal syndrome in rats by di-*n*-propylacetate. *Psychopharmacolgia (Berlin)* 46:127–131, 1976.
258. Lieber CS, De Carli LM: Ethanol dependence and tolerance: A nutritionally controlled experimental model in the rat. *Res Com Chem Path Pharm* 6:983–991, 1973.
259. Goldstein DB: An animal model for testing effects of drugs on alcohol withdrawal reactions. *J Pharmacol Exp Ther* 183:14–22, 1972.
260. Wise RA: The role of reward pathways in the development of drug dependence. *Pharmacol Ther* 35:227–263, 1987.
261. Owens AH, Marshall EK: The metabolism of ethyl alcohol in the rat. *J Pharmacol Exp Ther* 115:360–370, 1955.
262. Baker TB, Cannon DS, Berman RF, Atkinson CA. The effect of diet on ethanol withdrawal symptomatology. *Addict Behav* 2:35–46, 1977.
263. Goldstein DB: Rates of onset and decay of alcohol physical dependence in mice. *J Pharmacol Exp Ther* 190:377–383, 1974.
264. LeBourhis B, Aufrere G: Pattern of alcohol administration and physical dependence. *Alcoholism: Clin Exp Res* 7(4):378–381, 1983.
265. Mucha RF, Pinel PJ, Van Oot PH: Simple method for producing an alcohol withdrawal syndrome in rats. *Pharmacol Biochem Behav* 3:765–769, 1975.
266. Mello NK, Mendelson JH: Clinical aspects of alcohol dependence, in Martin WR (ed): *Drug Addiction I*. Berlin, Springer-Verlag, 1977.
267. Branchey M, Rauscher G, Kissin G: Modifications in the response to alcohol following the establishment of physical dependence. *Psychopharmacologia (Berlin)* 22:314–322, 1971.
268. Poldrugo F, Snead OC: Electroencephalographic and behavioral correlates in rats during repeated ethanol withdrawal syndromes. *Psychopharmacology* 83:140–146, 1984.
269. Victor M: The Alcohol withdrawal syndrome. *Postgrad Med* 47:68–72, 1970.
270. Mello NK, Mendelson JH: Experimentally induced intoxication in alcoholics: A comparison between programmed and spontaneous drinking. *J Pharmacol Exp Ther* 173:101–116, 1970.
271. Sanders B: Withdrawal-like signs induced by a single administration of ethanol in mice that differ in ethanol sensitivity. *Psychopharmacology* 68:109–113, 1980.
272. Holtzman SG, Villarreal J: Operant behavior in the morphine-dependent rhesus monkey. *J Pharmacol Exp Ther* 184:528–541, 1973.
273. Ford RD, Balster RL: Schedule-controlled behavior in the morphine dependent rat. *Pharmacol Biochem Behav* 4:569–573, 1976.

274. Ahlenius S, Engel J: Behavioral stimulation induced by ethanol withdrawal. *Pharmacol Biochem Behav* 2:847–850, 1974.

275. Beardsley PM, Kalant H, Stiglick A, et al: Effects of ethanol self-administration and withdrawal in rats responding for food and water, in Harris LS (ed): *Problems of Drug Dependence, 1987*, NIDA Research Monograph No. 81. Washington DC, U.S. Government Printing Office, 1988, p 306.

276. McMillan DE, Leander JD: Chronic chlordiazepoxide and pentobarbital interactions on punished and unpunished behavior. *J Pharmacol Exp Ther* 207:515–520, 1978.

277. Brady JV, Griffiths RR, Heinz RD, et al: Assessing drugs for abuse liability and dependence potential in laboratory primates, in Bozarth MA (ed): *Methods of Assessing the Reinforcing Properties of Abused Drugs*. New York, Springer-Verlag, 1987, pp 45–86.

278. Leith NJ, Barrett RJ: Amphetamine and the reward system: Evidence for tolerance and post-drug depression. *Psychopharmacologia (Berlin)* 46:19–25, 1976.

279. Simpson DM, Annau, Z. Behavioral withdrawal following several psychoactive drugs. *Pharmacol Biochem Behav* 7:59–64, 1977.

280. Houser VP: Modulation of avoidance behavior in squirrel monkeys after chronic administration and withdrawal of *d*-amphetamine or *a*-methyl-*p*-tyrosine. *Psychopharmacologia (Berlin)* 28:213–234, 1973.

281. Carney JM: Effects of caffeine, theophylline and theobromine on schedule controlled responding in rats. *Br J Pharmacol* 75:451–454, 1982.

282. Carroll ME, Hagen EW, Acensio M, et al: Behavioral dependence on caffeine and phencyclidine in rhesus monkeys: Interactive effects. *Pharmacol Biochem Behav* 31:927–932, 1989.

283. Beardsley PM, Balster RL, Harris LS: Behavioral dependence in rhesus monkeys following chronic THC administration, in Harris LS (ed): *Problems of Drug Dependence, 1984*. Washington DC, U.S. Public Health Service, 1985, pp 111–117.

284. Branch MN, Dearing ME, Lee DM: Acute and chronic effects of delta-9-tetrahydrocannibinol on complex behavior of squirrel monkeys. *Psychopharmacology* 7:247–256, 1980.

285. Slifer BL, Balster RL, Woolverton WL: Behavioral dependence produced by continuous phencyclidine infusion in rhesus monkeys. *J Pharmacol Exp Ther* 230:339–406, 1984.

286. Carrol ME: A quantitative assessment of phencyclidine dependence produced by oral self-administration in rhesus monkeys. *J Pharmacol Exp Ther* 242:405–412, 1987.

287. Beardsley PM, Balster RL: Behavioral dependence upon phencyclidine and ketamine in the rat. *J Pharmacol Exp Ther* 242:203–211, 1987.

288. Wessinger WD: Behavioral dependence on phencyclidine in rats. *Life Sci* 41:355–360, 1987.

289. Carroll ME, Lac ST: Cocaine withdrawal produces behavioral disruptions in rats. *Life Sci* 40:2183–2190, 1987.

290. Woolverton WL, Kleven MS. Evidence for cocaine dependence in monkeys following a prolonged period of exposure. *Psychopharmacology* 94:288, 1988.

291. Wakasa Y, Takada K, Yanagita T: Influence of physical dependence on reinforcing effect of drugs. Committee on Problems of Drug Dependence meeting, Falmouth, MA, June 1988.

292. Yanagita T: An Experimental framework for evaluation of dependence liability of various types of drugs in monkeys. *Pharm Fut Man* 1:7–17, 1973.

293. Woods JH, Down DA, Villarreal JE: Changes in operant behavior during deprivation- and antagonist-induced withdrawal states, in Goldberg L, Hoffmeister F (eds): *Psychic Dependence*. Berlin, Springer-Verlag, 1973.

294. Myers RD, Staltman WP, Martin GE: Effects of ethanol dependence induced artificially in the rhesus monkey on the subsequent preference for ethyl alcohol. *Physiol Behav* 9:43–48, 1972.

The Dependence Syndrome Concept as Applied to Alcohol and Other Substances of Abuse

Therese A. Kosten and Thomas R. Kosten

Abstract. The dependence syndrome concept has been defined by both behavioral and biological changes that occur with excessive substance use. Originally developed for alcohol, this concept was adopted for diagnosing dependence on other substances of abuse, although little research had been done to test its validity for other drugs. This chapter addresses the validity of the dependence concept across drug classes in the following ways. First, we compare the dependence items for three different drugs, alcohol, opiates, and cocaine, in measures of internal consistency. Second, biological items are correlated with behavioral items to assess the usefulness of defining dependence by both biological and behavioral criteria. Finally, we draw upon ideas developed in motivational theory and apply these to the dependence syndrome concept. These analyses, while supporting the validity of the concept, lead to suggestions for refining the concept of dependence.

1. A New Look at the Dependence Syndrome

1.1. Comparing Alcohol to Other Substances of Abuse

The dependence syndrome concept, proposed by Edwards and Gross,[1] is a hypothetical construct defined by various behavioral and physiological alterations that can occur when a person abuses alcohol. Although originally hypothesized for alcohol abuse, the dependence syndrome construct was broadened and is now the basis for the *Diagnostic and Statistical Manual*, Third Edition, Revised (DSM-III-R) criteria for all psychoactive substance use disorders, including opioids and cocaine.[2] The dependence syndrome may be particularly informative when abuse of opioids is contrasted to abuse of cocaine. Both drugs are associated with substantial psychosocial or behavioral effects, yet physiological alterations have been associated with opioids but usually not with cocaine.[3,4] Recent debate has arisen about the physiological manifestations of cocaine withdrawal and tolerance, but the clear, stereotyped

Therese A. Kosten and Thomas R. Kosten • Substance Abuse Treatment Unit, Department of Psychiatry, Yale University School of Medicine, New Haven, Connecticut 06519.

withdrawal syndrome associated with both alcohol and opioids forms an interesting contrast to the predominantly "psychological" symptoms of cocaine withdrawal.[4]

The psychological and behavioral aspects of the dependence syndrome are different than the earlier criteria used to define substance dependence. Unlike earlier definitions of substance dependence, social consequences of drug using are not criteria for dependence in DSM-III-R.[5] Instead, physiological manifestations of chronic drug use are emphasized along with a psychological construct of dependence that is not easily translated into operational definitions. This construct includes salience, compulsion, and sterotypy in the narrowing of behaviors associated with the drug use.[6] The Structured Clinical Interview for DSM-III-R (SCID) has attempted to translate these concepts into specific questions with some success, but many issues remain to be addressed in methodology for testing the dependence construct.[7] This chapter examines some of these methodological and theoretical issues involved in the process of developing measures of hypothetical constructs.

One approach we take to address these issues is to compare alcohol, the substance for which the dependence syndrome was originally devised, to cocaine and opiates. We believe that a comparison of alcohol to these two drugs is useful for two reasons. First, because the degree to which these three drugs affect physiological processes differs, a comparison across all three drugs provides a good test of the validity of both the biological and the behavioral aspects of dependence. Second, we will be able to examine the generalizability of the construct from alcohol to two other severely debilitating, yet fairly common, substances of abuse.[8,9] This chapter also compares the relative usefulness of the operational definitions and postulates of the dependence syndrome for substance abuse in general.

1.2. Comparing Dependence to Other Constructs

The second way in which we propose to view dependence in a new way is by placing it in the framework of another theory, motivation. This is accomplished by borrowing ideas from classic studies and theories of motivational psychology[10,11] and by drawing inferences from related fields of study in motivation, such as hunger. We believe that comparing substance dependence to motivational constructs is instructive both for substance abuse research and for testing the general applicability of the dependence syndrome concept.

Much of the theoretical work on the dependence syndrome has drawn on learning and conditioning theories. For example, the work of Siegel[12] and Wikler[13] on classical conditioning of drug responses has influenced the conceptualization of the dependence syndrome.[14] According to this proposal, dependence is believed to develop in parallel with tolerance. Tolerance has more than a pharmacological definition in the dependence syndrome context and includes both the physical effects of the drug (biological responses) and the subject's learned responses to the environmental cues associated with taking the drug (behavioral responses). These environmental cues are believed to become conditioned stimuli through their association with some effect of the drug, the unconditioned stimulus.

The explanations vary about the conditioning effects on drug taking. Siegel has provided evidence that compensatory physiological responses become conditioned to environmental cues,[12] although others have not entirely supported his hypothesis.[15] Siegel suggests that when the addicted subject is exposed to the conditioned environmental cues (such as drug paraphernalia or drug-taking friends), s/he exhibits physiological responses that are opposite to those caused by the drug itself. Siegel hypothesized that these conditioned compensatory responses, which he believes prepare the addict for the pharmacological onslaught of the drug, can explain craving and tolerance.[12] Craving or withdrawal distress is often associated with symptoms that are also opposite to the drug effects, and these symptoms can lead to drug taking.[3] Wikler's explanation, which has been elaborated upon further by Eikelboom and Stewart,[16] differs from that of Siegel's. Wikler states that conditioned cues elicit visceral withdrawal responses similar to those responses that occur with pharmacological withdrawal.[13] Conditioned responses include physiological reflexes that are adapative responses to the initial drug effects and the compensatory feedback responses referred to by Siegel. Both Wikler and Eikelboom and Stewart emphasize that what is conditioned are central nervous system events mediated through afferent receptors. Events that occur outside of the central nervous system (e.g., changes in blood glucose levels) are not included. In addition, Wikler includes both external events and internal mood states as possible conditioned stimuli.

Whatever the ultimate conditioning explanations of drug use are, these studies have demonstrated two points. First, the behavioral aspects of drug abuse are clearly important and must be major considerations in an overall theory of substance abuse. Moreover, the relationship between behavioral and biological factors has been shown to be important. Second, understanding a new construct such as dependence can be enhanced by drawing on evidence and concepts from other, more established psychological theories. Learning theory, for example, has been fruitful for research, and motivation theory may also provide insights into drug dependence. Motivational factors are an integral part of many learning theories, such as Hull's,[17] yet they appear to have been somewhat neglected in considering drug-taking behavior.[18] This chapter examines dependence within the theoretical framework of motivation.

2. Diagnosis and the Dependence Syndrome

2.1. Creating Diagnostic Guidelines for Dependence

In psychiatry, we are frequently attempting to quantify phenomena that obviously exist, but are difficult to operationalize. The process of operationalization usually starts by identifying the most "classic" cases of the phenomena and describing them in detail. The difficulty always arises with the borderline cases that do not clearly fit into the classical description we develop. Identifying and trying to limit the cardinal features of the phenomena is the function of nosology in psychiatry. This process of creating a nosology can be completely empirical, and DSM-III-R has generally tried to remain atheoretical in developing diagnostic criteria.

The decision to not use theories of etiology when defining DSM-III-R disorders was made so that clinicians, who vary in theoretical orientations, would not be hindered in making diagnoses. For example, a psychoanalytically oriented clinician would view the etiology of certain disorders differently than a biologically oriented clinician. Yet, both would likely agree on the patient's diagnosis. Diagnosing substance dependence differs from many psychiatric disorders in that a clinician of any orientation would recognize that biological factors influence the etiology of this disorder. Substance dependence has two obvious biological factors associated with its diagnosis in many substances of abuse—presence of the substance in biological fluids (e.g., blood, urine, breath) and sterotyped withdrawal syndromes.[3] Because these biological factors are not uniformly present with all drugs of abuse, particularly hallucinogens, broader behavioral or psychological criteria for diagnosis are needed.

To develop broader criteria for dependence diagnoses, an informed descriptive approach can be used. Statistical procedures using large groups of subjects, who exhibit biological criteria of dependence (e.g., opiate addicts or alcoholics), can be used to delineate the behavioral criteria associated with the diagnosis. This approach would select the behavioral criteria that best predict course of illness, treatment outcome, and familial patterns for the more "biological" dependences. We can then apply the behavioral criteria to the less biological dependences. However, at this point there is little information available on many of these substances, and an overriding syndrome concept based on one substance (alcohol) was adopted. Further descriptive studies on dependence diagnoses are necessary to substantiate the validity of this syndrome across different substances. Validity can also be assessed by demonstrating a convergence of evidence for the general syndrome concept using other approaches. Our suggested approach is to use guidelines from theories such as learning or motivation. The utility of general theories is that we can draw on a much larger body of knowledge in order to design appropriate tests of the validity and reliability of our nosology. These theories can also provide hypothetical constructs that help develop more precise operational definitions with specific predictions about outcome.

2.2. The Instrument for Data Collection Is Theory Bound

Data are descriptions of the observed phenomena or disorder based on the interaction between the observer and the patient or subject. Data collected on substance abuse will be constrained by the language used to describe this disorder, i.e., the dependence criteria. Two methods recently developed for use in substance abuse diagnostic research are the Composite International Diagnostic Interview (CIDI), which is administered by lay interviewers,[19] and the SCID, which is designed for use by trained clinicians.[7] The quality of the data obtained from this method is dependent on the ability of the interviewer to adequately probe for relevant information and on the communication skills of both the interviewer and the subject. These problems are also encountered when other structured interviews or self-report questionnaires are used. Given the inherent constraints in this type of method, we must strive for the best communication possible between observer and subject.

Not only does the quality of data depend on the method used to collect it, but the method then affects the quality of the explanations generated by these data. Explanations are the functional relationships between observations (e.g., the answers to our interview questions) and the manipulations (e.g., use of drugs by our patients). Hypothetical constructs such as drug dependence and hunger are explanations that are based on initial observations, but affect the quality of later observations, in part, because they direct or guide the methodology used to collect the observations. Thus, our instruments and any data about the dependence syndrome are theory bound by a hypothetical construct that is not atheoretical, but has an incomplete theoretical base.

3. Observation and Theory in the Dependence Syndrome

3.1. The Operational Definitions

In keeping with the generally atheoretical position of DSM-III-R, the substance dependence syndrome has been defined operationally by physiological changes and by alterations in behavior that are not necessarily etiologically connected to a particular theoretical orientation. These operationalizations have been tested in a few studies and found to be fairly satisfactory both in identifying substance abusers using the earlier criteria and in having good reliability and internal consistency.[8,9,20,21] In general, these criteria have distinguished the heavy from the occasional drug user, but further work is needed on the concept of dependence for other drugs besides alcohol. We will address the question of dependence on opioids and cocaine by (1) expanding on the premise that dependence can be defined by both behavior and biology and (2) using the motivation theories developed for feeding behavior (hunger) to guide our operationalizing of the hypothetical construct of dependence.

3.2. Borrowing Ideas from Hunger

We choose to compare dependence to hunger because they have certain characteristics in common. For example, hunger does not easily lend itself to operational definitions. We know that people eat when they experience hunger, but people also often eat when they are not hungry and may not eat when hungry. Thus, hunger cannot be operationalized simply as the behavior of eating. Hunger must also have a motivational component. Why is the person eating? Eating or hunger disorders might be conceptualized as eating when not hungry (e.g., obesity) or not eating when hungry (e.g., anorexia nervosa). While this would be an incomplete description of these two disorders, hunger does provide a model hypothetical construct for developing diagnostic criteria. In terms of substance abuse, dependence cannot be operationalized as simply taking psychoactive substances, since some people use drugs for hedonic experiences or curiosity with no physiological manifestations of dependence. We propose that an interaction between theory-based hypothetical constructs and empirical validation will allow us to distinguish the substance abuser from the occasional drug user or the hungry person from the nibbler.

The relevance of hunger to substance dependence is twofold. First, both hypothetical constructs have biological and behavioral aspects that do not always correspond well to each other, as illustrated earlier. Second, both can be related to motivation theory. Using an umbrella theory such as motivation, which was developed partly through feeding research, should provide another framework in which to view the construct of dependence and suggest areas outside of learning theory for testing this relatively new construct.

4. Motivation Theory

4.1. Relationship of Motivation to Other Theories

In considering the dependence syndrome within motivation theory, the theories of learning, affect, and arousal must also be considered. In Figure 1, motivation is shown as a convergence point for these other theories. This convergence reflects a long-standing trend in psychology to integrate these

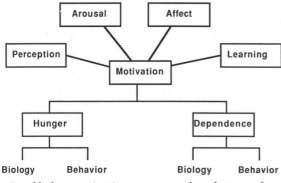

Figure 1. Schematic representation of the hypothetical construct of motivation to other constructs. Motivation is an integral part of many theories of learning, affect, arousal, and perception. The constructs of hunger and dependence, depicted below motivation, are examples of a type of motivation. Each type of motivation can be described by both biological and behavioral variables.

"prime movers" of behavior. Probably the most important early theory of learning, which was formulated by Hull,[17] viewed behavior as the result of complex interactions between learned mechanisms and motivation states.

Two other theories have been used as interacting parts of motivation theory: arousal and affect. Arousal, as used by Hebb,[22] was considered to function as a general drive. It was considered to have a specific neural substrate in the reticular formation, which had just been described in the brain stem.[23] Another brain stem structure noted for its far-reaching effects is the locus ceruleus. This neural structure has been considered an important contributor to opioid withdrawal and perhaps to other withdrawal syndromes, thus providing further neurobiological substrates for dependence.[24]

Affective arousal was a concept that Young introduced to supplement drive or motivation theories.[25] Affective disturbance, such as depression, is quite common among substance abusers and has frequently been described as a "motivating" factor not only for the abuse of drugs, but also for later seeking treatment.[26] Thus, a general, nonspecific arousal system and a more specific affective arousal system have been postulated as activating both animals and humans to behave, and these interactions with motivation seem particularly apt for substance abusers.

4.2. Defining Motivation

The middle area of Figure 1 shows motivation, our umbrella theory. Motivation is used to explain why the organism behaves in a particular way under particular circumstances. These circumstances include the internal state of the organism, the incentive or goal available, and the constraints on the behavior imposed by the present environmental situation. The first circumstance is represented by the biology box in the figure; the other two circumstances are subsumed under the behavior box. An example is an animal that has not had food for a day and is presented with a bad-tasting, quinine-adulterated chow that can only be reached by some painful means such as passing over a shock grid. How much food this animal will eat is different than the amount a similarly deprived animal would eat if the food were palatable and easily attainable.[10] It also differs from the amount a nondeprived animal would eat in any of these combinations of circumstances. To extrapolate to dependence, drug use is related to the presence of withdrawal symptoms (biology), previous experience in taking drugs to reduce these symptoms (behavior), and the difficulty involved in getting the drug (behavior). In these examples, changes in both biology and behavior are necessary to explain motivation.

The biological aspects of motivation are typically referred to as internal states or drives. Drives are reversible, temporary, and tend to energize behavior, which is directed, in part, to the specific goal (i.e., hunger leads to finding and eating food and dependence leads to finding and using drugs). Various theorists have developed explanations for the purpose of drives. Freud[27] believed that human behavior is directed at reducing stimulation arising from drives. (Drive is one translation of the German word *Trieb*.) Drive reduction is the basis of Hull's theory of learning,[17] which was elaborated upon by Miller.[10] And, as mentioned earlier, motivation or drive is also related to the constructs of learning, affect, and arousal.

Another distinction that should be made in terms of biology and behavior is between biological needs and psychological drives. A biological need is a deficiency or a deviation from homeostasis. This need may impel the organism to express certain behaviors that lead to correcting this deficiency. However, not all biological needs lead to psychological drives. Moreover, there are psychological drives for which there are no biological needs, such as curiosity or exploratory behavior. The psychological drive of curiosity may, in fact, be the original drive that leads to trying drugs. This is evidenced by the high scores on Zuckerman's sensation-seeking scale for opiate addicts (T. A. Kosten and B. J. Rounsaville, unpublished observations). This scale was developed by Zuckerman[28] as a measure of a person's innate desire for stimulation or arousal. Although we do not have longitudinal data, the higher scores for opiate addicts on this scale suggest that they have an innate need for a greater amount of stimulation, which is roughly equivalent to curiosity.

4.3. Acquired Motivation

Hunger differs from dependence in that the former is a primary motivation and the latter is an acquired motivation. Primary motivations arouse the organism to behave without the special training or experience that is needed for acquired motivation. Early theories concluded that motivation is acquired through classical conditioning. Based on empirical work, Miller[10] suggested that a previously neutral stimulus acquires motivating properties if it precedes in time the occurrence of an aversive event on a fairly regular basis. He found no evidence that motivation was acquired through association with a pleasurable event.

This explanation is challenged by the opponent-process theory of Solomon and Corbit[11] for two reasons. First, these authors argue that acquired motivation can occur by merely repeating the effective stimulus over time. For example, a person who is injected repeatedly with an opiate drug does not require conditioning processes to develop the biological characteristics of withdrawal and tolerance to the drug. Any change in the organism in this situation would not, strictly speaking, be due to learning; there is no neutral stimulus that was paired with the drug injection. However, this individual would be classified as having a substance neuroadaptation syndrome, not a substance dependence, according to the DSM-III-R criteria.[6] This distinction in classification reflects the decision to include both biological and behavioral alterations when diagnosing opiate dependence. Dependence is not defined by biological aspects only.

The second way that Solomon and Corbit differ from Miller is that they postulate that acquired motivation can be reinforced by either the offset of aversive states or the onset of pleasurable states.[11] Miller's theory speaks only of aversive states.[10] The acquisition of motivation reinforced by the onset of pleasurable states is consistent with the theory of Young.[25] Drug dependence may be acquired through either or both of these mechanisms. The onset of pleasurable states (euphoria, etc.) may reinforce drug-seeking behavior in the beginning stages, whereas the offset of aversive states (withdrawal symptoms) may reinforce the behavior at later stages of acquisition.

A two-stage process of acquired motivation is the model given by Solomon and Corbit.[11] The first process is associated with one type of affect (e.g., pleasure or fear) that is opposed by a second process of the opposite affect (e.g., pain or relief). The second, opposing process is the one most responsible for conditioning. For opiate addiction, the first process is associated with pleasurable affect; the second process is aversive. This explanation is supported by data describing the time course of symptoms in opiate addiction and by the work of Siegel[12] and Wikler.[13] However, motivation can also be acquired through a two-stage process in which the first stage is aversive and the second, opponent process is pleasurable. The data that support the latter explanation is derived, in part, from examining the time course of emotions described by sky divers. The first jump is associated with fear, which becomes offset by the opposing process of pleasure. With successive jumps, this second, pleasurable process becomes more salient and is responsible for conditioning the motivation to continue skydiving. This scenario described for skydiving may be more similar to what occurs with the acquisition of other drugs of abuse, such as hallucinogens or solvents, rather than the explanation given for opiate dependence. In either case, there is an acquired motivation, but treatment and prevention strategies for these other abused drugs may require very different approaches than those for alcohol or opiates.

The data needed to determine which of the two acquisition processes occur for the motivation to use drugs other than alcohol and opiates are difficult to obtain with current methodology. The postulates from these theories may not be clearly tested by the items in the DSM-III-R interview, because it is difficult to separate the pleasurable and aversive aspects that are due to drug taking from these aspects that are related to other activities. That is, one SCID item asks whether drug taking has led to abandoning other, presumably pleasurable activities, such as hobbies and visiting friends. An affirmative answer could reflect either of two occurrences. First, the former pleasures were abandoned owing to the competing euphoria of the drug use, which is commonly described in cocaine abusers. On the other hand, these former activities could be abandoned owing to the competing aversive state of withdrawal, as is commonly described by opioid addicts. The latter explanation is in accord with the postulate that stronger conditioning, and therefore acquisition of motivation, occurs, with the offset of aversive states. Since the dependence syndrome clearly specifies the existence of aversive states, such as withdrawal symptoms, this postulate can be at least partially supported by dependence syndrome data, but a clearer focus separating aversive from pleasurable states would be an important clarification in future work.

4.4. The Motivational Aspects of Dependence

The acquisition of the drug dependence drive may reflect different sources of motivation at different times during the course of drug use. The use of different types of drugs may also reflect different types of motivation. For these reasons, we should point out another distinction in types of motivation. Drive motivation is that motivation in which the organism is impelled to specific behaviors by the presence of a biological need. An incentive motivation is when the organism's behavior is directed not by the goal itself, but by the expectation of a reward for obtaining that goal. The drive to obtain drugs, dependence, is considered a drive motivation if we can demonstrate concurrent biological needs for the drug. This would include signs of withdrawal or tolerance, responses that may be elicited both by pharmacological effects and through conditioning. In the absence of biological needs, drugs may be used to obtain some other goal, such as approval from peers. Curiosity is another type of motivation that is considered an innate drive. Presumably it has a biological basis, yet it is considered to be devoid of biological needs.

Thus, three possible types of motivation lead to drug use: drive motivation, incentive motivation, and curiosity. The first has both behavioral and biological aspects, while the other two have only behavioral aspects. We need to determine which of these types of motivation should be used to classify drug dependence. Dependence criteria have not included those individuals who have just tried drugs out of curiosity and, thus, do not exhibit altered behavioral or biological responses. Nor have the criteria been designed to include those individuals who develop only biological aspects of drug use, as may occur when the drug is given for pain relief. Whether incentive motivation, where behavior, but not biology, is altered, is sufficient for dependence classification may differ depending on the class of psychoactive substance. Patients who use alcohol, opiates, and perhaps cocaine may require evidence for biological drive motivation in order to be considered dependent. In contrast, patients who use hallucinogens may not meet this requirement; their use may only be due to psychological drives. In this chapter, we are focusing on those drugs that have been identified as having a biological drive component. Understanding dependence on hallucinogens may require a different theoretical perspective.

5. Methodology

5.1. Assessment of Drug Dependence and Withdrawal

The 77 subjects reported in this chapter had sought treatment for substance abuse in the outpatient setting at the Yale Substance Abuse Treatment

Unit in New Haven, Connecticut. The sample was predominately male (65%) and white (64%) and the average age was 31 years. The rates of substance abuse or dependence for the three drugs relevant to this chapter were as follows: alcohol 44%, opiates 87%, and cocaine 74%. Many subjects abused more than one drug; the most common combinations of substances abused included all possible combinations of these three drugs.

The subjects were interviewed using the Structured Clinical Interview for the DSM-III-R Outpatient Version (SCID-OP) by graduate-level clinicians.[7] Subjects were asked to describe the presence and severity of behavioral and physiological symptoms of substance use. These items were rated, by the interviewer, on a three-point scale (1 = absent, 2 = possible, 3 = severe). For a subsample of the opioid addicts (N = 52) a Naloxone Challenge Test (NCT) was given to verify addiction. The subjects received an injection of naloxone hydrochloride (0.8 mg s.c.) in order to precipitate opiate withdrawal, and the resulting symptoms were rated using the scale developed by Wang et al.[29]

The data in this chapter are analyses of the SCID items. These items reflect the dependence construct and include both behavioral and biological questions. As shown in Table I, there are six behavioral items and three biological items. Of the six behavioral items, three reflect salience of drug use, two reflect compulsion to use drugs, and one is a readdiction liability question. Another item on readdiction liability was removed from the final version of the DSM-III-R criteria, but was retained for these analyses in order to have a more complete assessment of the dependence syndrome. Biological items were questions about whether the subject had experienced tolerance, withdrawal symptoms, or had used the drug for withdrawal relief.

Our analysis includes several measures of item-scale correlations as well as a measure of internal consistency, Cronbach's alpha.[30] We correlated each item with the total score based on the nine combined items. Correlations between items were used to compare biological variables with behavioral

Table I. Relationship between Dependence Syndrome Elements and SCID Items

SCID item	Dependence element	Type of element
1. Uses more than intended	Compulsion	Behavioral
2. Inability to decrease	Readdiction liability	Behavioral
3. Preoccupation with use	Compulsion	Behavioral
4. Impaired daily activity	Salience	Behavioral
5. Gave up nondrug activities	Salience	Behavioral
6. Continued use despite problems	Salience	Behavioral
7. Tolerance; need for increased amounts	Tolerance	Biological
8. Withdrawal symptoms	Withdrawal	Biological
9. Use for withdrawal relief	Withdrawal avoidance	Biological

variables. To make relative comparisons between these interitem correlations, we compared these correlations to how well the item correlated with the total score. Because individual items tend to correlate less well than combinations of items, we established a set of criteria to determine which of the single behavioral items correlated particularly well or poorly. The criterion for single items that had good correlations was that it account for an equivalent or greater amount of variance than the combined score (e.g., have an equal or greater correlation coefficient). The criterion for items that had poor correlations was that it account for 30% less variance than the combined scale correlations. The remaining items were considered to have similar levels of associations as the combined behavioral scale.

Previous research has demonstrated the usefulness of the dependence syndrome construct for drugs other than alcohol.[8,9,20,21] Our analysis shows that (1) quantity of drug use is not a good indicator of dependence, nor should we expect it to be one; (2) separation of the biological and the behavioral items is useful for understanding dependence; and (3) alcohol and cocaine are similar to each other and different from opiates in profile of biological and behavioral dependence.

5.2. Relating Biological Variables to Behavioral Variables

The biological components of drug dependence and their relationship to the amount of drug used differ across classes of drugs and within the same drug over the course of a drug-abusing career. As indicated previously, the strong pleasurable drives for continued drug use that occur early in a drug-abusing career may be markedly reduced as the addicted user tries to primarily avoid aversive states such as opioid withdrawal. In addition, these biological components have varying levels of correlation with the behavioral components of dependence. Moreover, we know from research in feeding behavior and its biological bases that there is often an inconsistency between behavior and biology. To address this inconsistency, Miller[31] has suggested that the amount of substance consumed (food or drug) is not meaningful unless effort involved in obtaining the goal is taken into account. A factor that reflects effort in obtaining the drug goal has been included in the dependence criteria: using the drug in spite of significant problems it causes. By including this motivational aspect of effort, the quantity and frequency of drug used may become more meaningful when related to the biological as well as to the behavioral components of dependence.

There have been attempts to find a correlation between the quantity of drug used and the degree of dependence.[9,20] In both studies, quantity of opiate use did not correspond to degree of dependence. In our study, we found that dependence did correlate with degree of naloxone-precipatated withdrawal. Although this relationship supports the validity of the dependence syndrome in opiate addiction, the degree of withdrawal did not correlate with quantity measures. While failure to establish a relationship between amount of drug (quantity and frequency) used and level or severity of dependence may be interpreted as not supporting the dependence concept, other considerations are important when using drug consumption data. First, consumption is difficult to measure. The data are based on the addicts' recall and can vary based on differences in purity across time and geographical locations. Second, as has been suggested by Miller,[31] use is not a good reflection of motivation (dependence) because other factors, such as how much effort was needed to obtain the drug, are not considered in these assessments. Effort to obtain illegal substances while hiding your habit could be considerable. Indeed, the alcohol and nicotine literature has been more successful in finding a correspondence between quantity and treatment success probably due to the relatively easy availability and acceptability of these licit drugs compared to the illicit drugs such as heroin and cocaine.[32,33]

Another important aspect of Miller's approach to the study of motivational constructs is to use intervening variables (roughly equivalent to hypothetical constructs) when there are two or more dependent variables and two or more independent variables.[31] To extrapolate his argument to opiate dependence, some examples of independent variables might be time since last drug use (deprivation level) or severity of precipitated withdrawal to a naloxone challenge (addiction level). Dependent variables or outcome variables related to this might include amount or frequency of drug used or effort put forth to obtain the drug. Examples of dependent variables that are in accord with the dependence construct would be salience of drug taking or compulsion to use drugs. Using an intervening variable or hypothetical construct such as dependence is one way to reduce the number of functional relationships. Moreover, it provides a test of the theoretical basis of the construct if different combinations of variables correlate well with each other. Since it is difficult to manipulate the independent variables in substance abuse research, we will use the biological items of the SCID instead. The behavioral items of the SCID will act as dependent or outcome measures. How well the biological items (independent variables) correlate with the behavioral items (dependent variables) will be a test of our intervening variable or hypothetical construct of dependence.

6. Results

6.1. Dependence Correlates with Opiate Withdrawal Severity

We performed a study in which we had a biological variable, other than SCID items, to correlate with the behavioral variables of the SCID. In this study, the biological variable was a measure of precipitated opiate withdrawal as determined by the Naloxone Challenge Test.[9] The amount of withdrawal symptoms evoked by the naloxone test correlated well with the opiate dependence score (0.30) which was based on the total score of the SCID items. The correlation improved when we removed the biological items from the scale (0.32), indicating that this biological variable of withdrawal severity was not simply an overlap with the biological items of the SCID. Furthermore, a biological indicator of addiction, such as severity of naloxone-precipitated withdrawal, relates well to the degree of dependence as measured by the SCID. Moreover, severity of withdrawal was particularly predictive of the behavioral aspect of the dependence syndrome. However, the results of one biological test are not sufficient for determining the presence of motivation or drug dependence.

6.2. Unidimensionality of the Dependence Syndrome

In a previous study, we showed support for the dependence syndrome concept across a number of different drugs.[8] We analyzed the SCID items for substance abuse diagnoses using scaling techniques and factor analysis. The dependence syndrome items loaded onto a single factor for the three drugs of alcohol, cocaine, and opiates, but not for other drugs, such as sedatives or stimulants. This indicates that for these three drugs the dependence concept is unidimensional. Moreover, the SCID items formed good approximations of Guttman scales for most of the drugs, giving further support for the uni-dimensionality of dependence. For alcohol, however, the approximation of unidimensionality was not as good as for opiates and cocaine. The reproducibility coefficient for alcohol was 0.85 and a score greater than 0.90 is considered excellent. Cocaine had a borderline excellent score of 0.90 and opiates showed excellent unidimensionality, with a coefficient of 0.94. These results support the usefulness of a dependence syndrome concept as a common concept across many drugs of abuse, especially opiates.

6.3. Internal Consistency of Dependence Scales

The item-scale correlations for the behavioral, biological, and combined scales were analyzed for internal consistency using Cronbach's alpha.[30] As shown in Table II, these values showed excellent internal consistency, with the exception of the biological items for alcohol. The value for this subscale showed moderate internal consistency (0.53). The item-scale correlations for the individual biological items for alcohol were modest, ranging from 0.56 for withdrawal relief to 0.74 for tolerance. In contrast, the biological-scale items for opiates had an impressive 0.96 value for internal consistency. Each biological item for opiates correlated with the total scale with values equal to or greater than 0.90. The withdrawal relief item correlated the best (0.96). For cocaine, the internal consistency for the biological subscale was quite high (0.87); individual scale items varied in the strength of their correlation from 0.64 for withdrawal relief to 0.90 for tolerance.

Next, we compared the internal consistencies of the behavioral subscales for the three substances. The behavioral scale for cocaine, which had an alpha value of 0.96, showed the best internal consistency across subscales and sub-

Table II. Item-Scale Correlations on Dependence Syndrome Items

Item	Alcohol	Cocaine	Opiate
Behavioral items			
Use more than intended	0.71	0.86	0.88
Inability to decrease use	0.72	0.84	0.92
Preoccupation with use	0.83	0.84	0.89
Impaired daily activity	0.76	0.91	0.86
Gave up nondrug activities	0.79	0.92	0.86
Continued use despite problems	0.85	0.91	0.79
Cronbach's alpha[a]	0.88	0.96	0.88
Biological items			
Tolerance	0.74	0.90	0.90
Withdrawal symptoms	0.61	0.75	0.91
Use for withdrawal relief	0.56	0.64	0.96
Cronbach's alpha	0.53	0.87	0.96
All items combined			
Cronbach's alpha	0.89	0.96	0.98

[a]Cronbach's alpha > 0.8 shows excellent consistency.

stances. All behavioral items for cocaine had item-scale correlations greater than 0.83. The behavioral items for opiates correlated at values greater than 0.79, with the item "continued use despite problems" exhibiting the worst item-scale correlation. Internal consistency of the behavioral subscale for opiates was excellent (0.88) and the value for the behavioral subscale for alcohol was identical. Yet, the item-scale correlations for alcohol were not as strong compared to the other two substances. The correlations ranged from 0.71 for "use more than intended" to 0.85 for "continued use despite problems." The complete, nine-item scale for each of these three substances showed excellent internal consistency; all alpha values were greater than 0.88.

Examining the biological and behavioral subscales of dependence separately provided useful insights into the characteristics of dependence for the three drugs. Alcohol was much less internally consistent than cocaine or opiates. When we separated the biological items from the behavioral items, cocaine had the most internal consistency for the behavioral items, while opiates had the most internal consistency for the biological items. Alcohol had the worst internal consistency for both cases. Interestingly, the internal consistencies for biological items compared to the behavioral items showed that the stronger relationship for biological items exists only in opiates. We had expected that alcohol would also show a stronger biological component for dependence. In fact, alcohol was similar to cocaine in that both substances showed more consistency in the behavioral component of dependence. However, alcohol's more consistent component is only as good as the poorer components of opiates and cocaine, which are the biological component and the behavioral component, respectively. Thus, alcohol is more similar to cocaine than it is to opiates, and opiates provide a very clear example of a dependence that has both biological and behavioral aspects.

6.4. Relating Biological to Behavioral Aspects of Dependence

To analyze the relationship between biological variables and behavioral variables we examined the correlation matrix for all items. Table III presents the correlations between the three biological items with the six behavioral items for each substance. The biological items are also compared to the combined behavioral subscale. With this analysis, we find another difference between opiates and both alcohol and cocaine. For the latter two substances, the biological item of tolerance has the best correspondence to behavior and it has the worst correspondence to behavior for opiates. Although this opiate correlation is comparatively low across biological variables, it is still higher than the tolerance correlation for either cocaine or alcohol. For cocaine and alcohol the worst correspondence between biology and behavior is with the withdrawal relief variable, which shows the best correspondence for opiates. All of these comparisons are relative to each other, since that is our only standard of comparison. And all of these correlations between specific biological items and the combination of the six behavioral items are quite good (all are greater than 0.45).

Next, we analyzed the individual behavioral item correlations with the three biological items. As stated earlier, we established a criterion by which we delineated items that correlated either well or poorly as compared to the correlations with the combined behavioral subscale. For alcohol, the behavioral item of "uses more" correlated very well with the biological item of tolerance (0.70). Intuitively, this finding makes sense and suggests that our measurements are fairly accurate. This is in contrast to the poor correlation between the same behavioral item and the other two biological variables of withdrawal and withdrawal relief (0.13 and 0.20). On the other hand, tolerance showed poor fit with the item "can't decrease." The biological variable, withdrawal relief, did correlate well with the "use despite problems" variable. We believe that this item reflects a measure of effort or motivation to obtain the substance. This finding suggests that the motivation to abuse alcohol is due, in part, to the presence of aversive states. This is in accord with the explanation for opiate dependence given by Solomon and Corbit.[11]

Overall, the behavioral items for cocaine correlated well with the biological items. In general, the tolerance item correlated best with the behavioral items. The motivational item of "use despite problems" was well correlated with all three biological items and was most strongly correlated for opiates. All three biological items correlated with this behavioral item at or above the same level as the combined behavioral subscale.

6.5. Dependence Item Comparisons across Substances

Further evidence for the similarities between alcohol and cocaine, in contrast to opiates, came when we compared the frequencies of report for each type of dependence item. In Table IV we grouped the six behavioral items into the three categories of compulsion, readdiction liability, and salience and also

Table III. Item Correlations between Behavioral and Biological Variables of the Dependence Syndrome: Type of Drug Effect

Substance	Biological variable	Uses more	Can't decrease	Preoccupation	Impairs activity	No other activity	Use despite problems	Combined behavioral variables
Alcohol	Tolerance	0.70	0.27	0.64	0.57	0.56	0.52	0.69
	Withdrawal	0.13	0.49	0.39	0.45	0.50	0.48	0.51
	Relief	0.20	0.46	0.34	0.32	0.39	0.55	0.48
Cocaine	Tolerance	0.82	0.70	0.82	0.79	0.80	0.72	0.86
	Withdrawal	0.63	0.62	0.48	0.50	0.51	0.67	0.64
	Relief	0.63	0.39	0.54	0.45	0.46	0.49	0.55
Opiate	Tolerance	0.05	0.87	0.77	0.76	0.83	0.90	0.90
	Withdrawal	0.07	0.85	0.73	0.85	0.93	0.94	0.94
	Relief	0.06	0.91	0.74	0.80	0.93	1.00	0.96

Table IV. Ranking the Frequencies of Reported Dependence Items by Substance

Dependence item	Substance of abuse		
	Alcohol	Cocaine	Opiate
Compulsion	3	4	1
Readdiction liability	4	2	3
Salience	1	1	4
Tolerance	2	3	6
Withdrawal	5	5	2
Withdrawal relief	6	6	5

listed the three biological items of tolerance, withdrawal, and withdrawal relief. The frequencies for which these categories of dependence were reported for each drug were rank-ordered. We can see that alcohol and cocaine are very similar in the ranking of items and both are different from opiates. Yet, for all three substances, the behavioral items tend to be reported more frequently. The exception for opiates was that the withdrawal item was ranked second in frequency of reports. For alcohol, the tolerance item was the exception and was also ranked second in reports. With cocaine, the behavioral items tended to be reported more frequently than the biological items as compared to the other two substances. This is consistent with the notion that cocaine has more behavioral than biological effects than alcohol or opiates.

With this analysis, we found no item, either biological or behavioral, that was not useful in defining dependence for any of the three substances. In general, tolerance was a good biological predictor of the behavioral aspects of dependence. The degree to which this is seen varies according to the substance. Tolerance certainly reflects "using more" of the substance. Yet this correlation was not particularly outstanding for cocaine compared to the combined score correlation. "Uses more" showed a relatively better correlation with withdrawal relief for cocaine. It is interesting that one of the two best behavioral item correlations and two of the three worst behavioral item correlations for alcohol was "uses more." Finally, the behavioral item of "use despite problems" fared well compared to the combined score across the substances. This item probably best reflects the degree of effort exerted to obtain the substance, one of the definitions of motivation (dependence).

7. Conclusions and Future Directions

7.1. How Constructs Are Useful for Dependence

Miller[31] states that for a hypothetical construct to be considered unidimensional, the construct would hold for examining the effects of different independent variables on different dependent variables or outcomes. In fact, there should be a perfect correlation such that one independent variable affects all outcomes similarly and these outcomes should be similarly affected by other independent variables. Discrepancies often occur, however, in the behavioral sciences. For example, the item of withdrawal symptoms may not predict whether the addict "uses more than intended" as well as the tolerance item does. Moreover, differences across substances may be seen in this pattern of correlations between dependence items. As Miller suggests, the use of multiple tests will enable us to see whether our initial conceptualization needs to be refined, because if only one or a few items were studied, this cross-checking would not have been clear. Thus, it would be useful to continue using the multiple items that are part of the SCID interview for diagnosing dependence. It is too soon to determine whether the concept of dependence should be modified. We need to test further the general usefulness of the concept across all drugs of abuse as well as to determine whether there are specific differences between drugs.

This chapter has examined the interrelationship of biological and behavioral aspects of the dependence syndrome for three of the most serious drugs of abuse—alcohol, opioids, and cocaine. All three of these drugs have fairly well-described biological as well as behavioral manifestations, and for opioids we used a direct measure of physiological dependence—withdrawal after challenge with the antagonist naloxone.[9] These two aspects of dependence were closely related, particularly for opioid abusers. This correspondence between these two aspects of dependence provides some additional support for its utility as a hypothetical construct around which to organize treatment and outcome evaluation, but a theoretical link might further guide future research.

7.2. How Motivation Theory Is Useful for Dependence

Motivation theory may provide a bridge between biology and psychological states, as this theory has for feeding behavior through the hypothetical construct of hunger. Motivation theory has been used as a bridge between biology and areas of learning theory, which has already been usefully applied to substance dependence. In general, motivation may link learning with the biological underpinnings of drug tolerance and withdrawal. While learning may establish connections between behavior patterns and drug administration, the acquired drive to seek out these drugs is not an inherent part of either learning theory or the pharmacology of these substances. This motivational link may be particularly important for drugs with less obvious biological concomitants of dependence, such as hallucinogens and solvents. Tolerance and withdrawal are not obvious elements of the abuse syndromes with these drugs, so examination of the dependence syndrome in these drugs requires a psychological focus with minimal biological standards to draw on.

By examining the dependence syndrome construct within the framework of motivation, we have identified a few relevant points that should help guide future work in refining this construct. First, we argued that it is more useful to determine a measure of effort involved in getting the substance rather than a quantity measure. Miller presented this case based on much empirical work with rats.[31] Studies comparing opiate dependence[9,20] or degree of opiate withdrawal[9] with a quantity measure of opiate use have failed to find a relationship. We suggest that measures of effort to get drugs be developed instead of trying to relate a pure quantity measure to dependence. Second, the work of Solomon and Corbit[11] suggests that we examine the time course of affect elicited by the drug. For opiates, the evidence suggests that when the subject first uses the drug, it elicits positive affect (euphoria); later use is associated with negative affect (withdrawal). The second affective process is responsible for acquisition of the motivation of dependence. Thus, an opiate user, to be considered dependent, should use drugs in order to counteract negative affect. Third, this theory of acquired motivation also suggests that more work is needed to define the dependence criteria so that we can separate the pleasurable and aversive aspects. The ambiguous item we discussed was "gave up nondrug activities." This item can reflect either that the drug use was more pleasurable than other activities or that the negative affect that leads to drug use is more salient than the pleasure derived from other activities. Determining which of the explanations is more accurate would allow us to assess whether the person has acquired the dependence motivation.

7.3. Limitations of Current Work and Future Directions

Defining a dependent person will be more difficult with other drugs such as hallucinogens and will also be more difficult in less selected populations than that used in this study. The analyses in this study were confined to treatment-seeking substance abusers, a small part of the total population of drug abusers. These SCID analyses need to be replicated using general psychiatric populations, as well as nonclinical samples where substance abuse is less prevalent, and where defining a "dependent" person will be more difficult. In defining dependence on any substance, the biological and behavioral components of the dependence syndrome need to be considered as interacting. Much of psychiatry is moving toward an increasing biological view of mental illness, and substance dependence has many quite obvious biological concomitants. It is hoped that future work will be able to capitalize on these biological concomitants as standards to assess the utility of continued psychological formulations of substance dependence.

ACKNOWLEDGMENTS. Support was provided by the National Institute on Drug Abuse grants P50-DA04050, R01-DA04505, and Research Career Award K02-DA00112 to TRK.

References

1. Edwards G, Gross MM: Alcohol dependence: Provisional description of the clinical syndrome. Br Med J 1:1058–1061, 1976.

2. American Psychiatric Association: *Diagnostic and Statistical Manual of Mental Disorders,* 3rd edition, revised (DSM-III-R). Washington DC, APA, 1987.

3. Kleber HD: Detoxification from narcotics, in Lowinson JH, Ruiz P (eds): *Subtance Abuse: Clinical Problems and Perspectives.* Baltimore, Williams & Wilkins, 1981.

4. Gawin FH, Kleber HD: Abstinence symptomatology and psychiatric diagnosis in cocaine abusers. *Arch Gen Psychiatry* 43:107–113, 1986.

5. American Psychiatric Association: *Diagnostic and Statistical Manual of Mental Disorders,* 3rd edition (DSM-III). Washington DC, APA, 1980.

6. Rounsaville BJ, Spitzer RL, Williams JBW: Proposed changes in DSM-III substance use disorders: Description and rationale. *Am J Psychiatry* 143:436–468, 1986.

7. Spitzer RL, Williams JBW, Gibbon M: The structured clinical interview for DSM-III-R-outpatient version (SCID-OP). Biometrics Research Department, New York State Psychiatric Institute, 722 West 168th Street, New York, NY 10032, 1987.

8. Kosten TR, Rounsaville BJ, Babor TR, et al: Substance use disorders in DSM-III-R. *Br J Psychiatry* 151:834–843, 1986.

9. Kosten TA, Jacobsen LK, Kosten TR: Severity of precipitated opiate withdrawal predicts drug dependence by DSM-III-R criteria. *Am J Drug Alcohol,* 15:237–250, 1989.

10. Miller NE: Studies of fear as an acquirable drive. I. Fear as motivation and fear-reduction as reinforcement in the learning of new responses. *J Exp Psychol* 38:89–101, 1948.

11. Solomon RL, Corbit JD: An opponent-process theory of motivation: I. Temporal dynamics of affect. *Psychol Rev* 81:119–145, 1974.

12. Siegel S: The role of conditioning in drug tolerance and addiction, in Keehn, JD (ed): *Psychopathology in Animals: Research and Treatment Implications.* New York, Academic Press, 1979.

13. Wikler A: Dynamics of drug dependence. *Arch Gen Psychiatry* 28:611–616, 1973.

14. Edwards G, Arif A, Hodgson R: Nomenclature and classification of drug- and alcohol-related problems: A WHO memorandum. *Bull WHO* 59:225–242, 1981.

15. Sherman JE: The effects of conditioning and novelty on the rat's analgesic and pyretic responses to morphine. *Learning Motivation* 10:383–418, 1979.

16. Eikelboom R, Stewart J: Conditioning of drug-induced physiological responses. *Psychol Rev* 89:507–528, 1982.

17. Hull CL: *Principles of Behavior.* New York, Appleton-Century, 1943.

18. Babor TF, Cooney NL, Lauerman RJ: The dependence syndrome concept as a psychological theory of relapse behavior: An empirical evaluation of alcoholic and opiate addicts. *Br J Addict* 82:393–405, 1987.

19. Robins LN, Wing J, Wittchen HU, Helzer JE, Babor TF, Burke J, Farmer A, Jablenski A, Pickens R, Regier DA, Sartorius N, Towle LH. The Composite International Diagnostic Instrument. *Arch Gen Psychiatry* 45:1069–1077, 1988.

20. Sutherland G, Edwards G, Taylor C, et al: The measurement of opiate dependence. *Br J Addict* 81:485–494, 1986.

21. Skinner HA, Goldberg AE: Evidence for a drug dependence syndrome among narcotic users. *Br J Addict* 81:479–484, 1986.

22. Hebb DO: Drives and the CNS (conceptual nervous system). *Psychol Rev* 62:243–254, 1955.

23. Magoun HW: *The Waking Brain.* Springfield, IL, Charles C Thomas, 1958.

24. Redmond DE Jr, Krystal JH. Multiple mechanisms of withdrawal from opioid drugs. *Annu Rev Neurosci* 7:443–478, 1984.

25. Young PT: The role of affective processes in learning and motivation. *Psychol Rev* 66:104–125, 1959.

26. Rounsaville BJ, Kosten TR, Weissman MW, et al: *Evaluating and Treating Depressive Disorders in Opiate Addicts.* NIDA Treatment Research Monograph Series, U.S. Dept. of Health and Human Services, Rockville, MD, 1985.

27. Freud S: Instincts and their vicissitudes, in Freud S: *Collected Papers, Vol IV.* London, Hogarth, 1950, pp 60–83.

28. Zuckerman M: *Sensation-Seeking: Beyond the Optimal Level of Arousal.* Hillsdale, NJ, Lawrence Erlbaum Associates, 1979.

29. Wang RIH, Wiesen RL, Lamid S, et al: Rating the presence and severity of opiate dependence. *Clin Pharmacol Ther* 16:653–658, 1974.
30. Cronbach LJ, Furby L: How should we measure "change"—Or should we? *Psychol Bull* 74:16–21, 1970.
31. Miller NE: Behavioral and physiological techniques: rational and experimental designs for combining their use, in Werner, Heidel (ed.) *The Handbook of Physiology, VI. The Alimentary Canal,* Washington, DC: American Physiological Society, 1967.
32. Hall SM, Benowitz NB, Jones RT: Blood cotinine levels as indicators of smoking treatment outcome. *Clin Pharmacol Ther* 35:810–814, 1984.
33. Babor TF, Mendelson JH: Empirical correlates of self-report drinking measures, in Galanter, M (ed): *Currents in Alcoholism, Vol VII.* New York, Grune & Stratton, 1980.

3

Operationalization of Alcohol and Drug Dependence Criteria by Means of a Structured Interview

Linda B. Cottler and Susan K. Keating

Abstract. There is growing concern worldwide about the extent of psychoactive substance abuse and dependence disorders. Epidemiological data are needed to assess the prevalence and severity of the problem. Collecting this type of data is possible with a highly structured and reliable diagnostic interview. The problems involved in developing such an interview are discussed in this chapter. They include the absence of a unified concept of psychoactive substance dependence and a lack of a standardized system of diagnostic criteria.

Recently a new instrument has been designed to assess psychoactive substance abuse and dependence disorders according to multiple diagnostic systems. The WHO/ADAMHA Composite International Diagnostic Interview Substance Abuse Module (CIDI-SAM) has been found to have excellent diagnostic reliability in a test–retest pilot study. This chapter describes the development and evolution of the interview and offers guidelines for operationalization of substance abuse and dependence criteria.

1. Introduction

There is worldwide concern about the prevalence and severity of psychoactive substance use. Epidemiological data are required in order to determine the extent of the problem, establish appropriate treatment programs, monitor trends in substance use, plan effective prevention programs, and discover correlates of substance abuse. With the advent of structured interviews, collecting epidemiological data is possible; however, the development of such an interview is difficult.

The problems associated with developing an interview to assess alcohol and drug dependence have been enumerated previously.[1–4] Among the problems are an absence of a unified concept of substance abuse and dependence—manifested by the number of existing diagnostic systems—and the

Linda B. Cottler and Susan K. Keating • Department of Psychiatry, Washington University School of Medicine, St. Louis, Missouri 63110.

considerable differences in the clarity of and detail in the criteria of these systems. Nevertheless, at present, a standardized interview, which serves a variety of diagnostic systems and is also reliable and acceptable across cultural lines, is unsurpassed in its ability to assess the severity of drug abuse and dependence.

An interview has been designed for the multicultural and multidiagnostic study of substance abuse and dependence—the WHO/ADAMHA Composite International Diagnostic Interview Substance Abuse Model (CIDI-SAM). This chapter describes this interview and the mechanics involved in developing questions that operationalize psychoactive substance use disorder criteria.

2. Development Originates with the Nomenclature

The development of any diagnostic interview should be based on the diagnostic criteria it hopes to assess; however, the criteria continue to evolve, resulting in, as Robins suggests, a symbiotic relationship between the developing diagnostic criteria and their assessment tools.[5] This relationship occurs because a lack of clarity in diagnostic concepts is sometimes only realized once the operationalization of these concepts is attempted, or because research data have generated empirical evidence for a change. In particular, the symbiotic relationship between the substance dependence criteria and the interviews that assess them has been strong. The recent change within the official nomenclature of American psychiatry—the *Diagnostic and Statistical Manual, Third Edition, Revised (DSM-III-R)*[6]—and the evolving *International Classification of Diseases,* Tenth Edition (ICD-10) have provided the atmosphere for further study.

Within several years of the DSM-III publication, the developers decided that there was sufficient evidence to warrant changes in the criteria, especially for substance abuse and dependence disorders. Prior to revision, the diagnosis of alcohol abuse required a pattern of pathological use lasting at least 1 month *and* impairment in social or occupational functioning due to alcohol. Tolerance or withdrawal symptoms *and* patterns of pathological use or impairment in social or occupational functioning were required for a diagnosis of alcohol dependence. Similar algorithms were used for dependence on and abuse of illicit drugs, with some variation from drug to drug.

The revisions to the DSM-III concept of dependence have been influenced by the Edwards and Gross Alcohol Dependence Syndrome (ADS), introduced over a decade ago.[7] The ADS, a set of seven criteria, allows for classifying the severity of alcohol dependence. The ADS distinguishes between alcohol dependence and alcohol-related impairment and predicts whether subsequent relapse is likely.

Like the ADS, dependence under the DSM-III-R system uses a multisymptom approach to diagnosing, requiring at least three of nine criteria to be positive. The essential feature of dependence as described by DSM-III-R is a "cluster of cognitive, behavioral, and physiologic symptoms that indicate that a person has impaired control of substance use and continues use despite adverse consequences." The diagnosis is dependent neither on occupational or social impairment nor on withdrawal or tolerance; even though clinicians may believe these symptoms to be more pathognomonic than the rest, the new diagnostic system recognizes all nine symptoms equally. DSM-III-R applies identical dependence criteria to all three categories of psychoactive substances (tobacco, alcohol, and drugs), which should allow for better communication among researchers and more meaningful and extensive comparisons to be made than was previously allowed.

The changes to the DSM-III system have been debated.[8–13] For example, removal of the requirement that tolerance or withdrawal symptoms be present is welcomed by some clinicians because it is expected to "widen the (DSM-III) net" for diagnosing substance dependence, resulting in earlier diagnosis and treatment.[8,9] However, others believe the new system is too inclusive. Rounsaville and colleagues tested the idea that DSM-III-R was too liberal by cross-checking the two systems. They found that diagnostic agreement between DSM-III and DSM-III-R dependence was highest when three or more positive symptoms out of nine was used as the threshold, rather than two or more, or four or more.[14] In addition, because the terms used in the duration criterion are imprecise, some feel this measure could be misinterpreted both by researchers and by respondents, ultimately leading to an increased chance for misclassifying disorders.

An important step in accepting a new nomenclature or adopting a unified theory of dependence is to develop structured interviews which can serve to test the new diagnostic criteria for reliability and acceptability in various cultures and discriminate illness among persons manifesting varying degrees of substance abuse and dependence. Interviews of this sort have been popular among both researchers and clinicians, providing a standardized format for questioning, thereby relieving the interviewer of relying on memory alone to ask questions necessary for making clinical diagnoses. Structured interviews also minimize the tendency for information bias which may arise when a certain line of questioning is pursued only among those persons thought to be at risk for substance abuse, while ignoring the same line of questioning among individuals perceived to be at lower risk. Additionally, standardized questions reduce the chance for multiple interpretations of one diagnostic criterion.

3. Structured Interviews with the Robins Influence

Despite the problems encountered in operationalizing concepts, it has been reported that there are approximately 180 questionnaires that assess drinking behavior[15] and an undetermined, but large, number of assessments to determine drug use.[16] The proliferation of such assessment tools reflects the difficulty and disagreement as how best to measure the simplest and most basic questions concerning substance use: how much and how often the substance is used.[1,2,16] Nearly all surveys and assessments contain questions about amounts, frequency, and duration of use; however, few are designed to assess diagnostic criteria for substance abuse and dependence disorders.

The Department of Psychiatry at Washington University School of Medicine has played a major role both in the development of diagnostic criteria and in their operationalization.[17,18] The tradition began with Eli Robins and the Department Interview. This interview was used for 20 years. It included a standard list of symptoms from multiple disorders and even made preemptive diagnoses, thus structuring the psychiatrist's diagnostic assessment.[19] The Department Interview later became the Renard Diagnostic Interview,[20] which assessed Feighner criteria, including severity of disorders.[21] Subsequently, Lee Robins and colleagues developed the NIMH Diagnostic Interview Schedule (DIS)[22]—an interview that operationalized criteria from the Research Diagnostic Criteria (RDC),[23] Feighner, and DSM-III diagnostic systems and could be used with community subjects by nonclinicians. This instrument was used in the Epidemiologic Catchment Area Survey to determine prevalence and incidence of psychiatric disorders among 20,000 household and institutional respondents from five U.S. metropolitan areas. The DIS has good reliability when results from nonclinicians are compared with those obtained by clinicians.[24] Results from studies originating in different countries show remarkably consistent prevalence rates of specific DIS disorders.[25] The DIS-III-R,[26] the latest version of the DIS, has been updated to meet the DSM-III-R criteria; similarly high reliability results are expected.

Recently, a new instrument has been developed by Drs. Robins, Cottler, and Babor at the request of the WHO/ADAMHA Task Force on Psychiatric Assessment Instruments. The development, begun in 1983, has benefited from the ideas of the Task Force, Dr. Jerome Jaffe, and staff at NIDA and NIAAA, including Drs. Pickens, Blaine, Chiarello, and Grant. This instrument, called the CIDI-SAM[27,28] (Composite International Diagnostic Interview Substance Abuse Module), is an expansion of the substance abuse sections of the CIDI. (The CIDI is an expanded version of the DIS, which also includes questions to assess Present State Examination criteria.[29]) The history of the SAM is detailed elsewhere, but briefly, the SAM, like the CIDI, is structured and precoded so that it can be administered by nonclinicians (who have undergone 1 week of training) and diagnoses can be scored by computer. The SAM covers substance abuse and dependence criteria according to Feighner, RDC, DSM-III, and DSM-III-R systems and the proposed criteria for ICD-10, which will enable nosological comparisons of dependence to be made across different cultures.

The SAM makes substance abuse and dependence diagnoses on both a lifetime and cross-sectional basis, for tobacco, alcohol, prescription psychoactive medications, and nine classes of illicit drugs. In addition, it ascertains data on specific withdrawal symptoms and their duration; specific physical, psychological, and social consequences from the use of psychoactive substances; age of onset and recency of each positive symptom; periods of abstention; and the severity and course of disorders.

The SAM underwent considerable pretesting as well as a test–retest study among 39 patients in treatment for alcohol and drug abuse in the summer of 1986. Cottler et al. report the SAM to have excellent reliability in this population.[30] Table I shows the values of the kappa statistic, which corrects for chance agreement, for the most common DSM-III and DSM-III-R substance use disorders in the sample: alcohol, cocaine, cannabis, and tobacco. The kappa values ranged from 0.65 to 0.92. Kappa values greater than 0.75 are generally considered to represent excellent agreement; values between

Table I. Reliability of CIDI Substance Abuse Module: Diagnoses ($N = 39$)

	Int.2 + A / – C	Int.2 – B / D	% Positive in either interview	K	95% Conf. int.	Y
Tobacco[a]						
DSM-III	23 / 0	2 / 14	64	0.89	(0.81–0.97)	0.88[c]
DSM-III-R	16 / 2	2 / 19	51	0.79	(0.68–0.91)	0.79
Alcohol[b]						
DSM-III	30 / 1	1 / 7	82	0.84	(0.75–0.94)	0.87
DSM-III-R—dependence	30 / 1	0 / 8	79	0.92	(0.86–0.99)	0.89[c]
DSM-III-R—dependence or abuse	30 / 1	0 / 8	79	0.92	(0.86–0.99)	0.89[c]
Cannabis[b]						
DSM-III	19 / 2	2 / 16	59	0.79	(0.68–0.91)	0.79
DSM-III-R—dependence	20 / 0	2 / 17	56	0.90	(0.82–0.98)	0.88[c]
DSM-III-R—dependence or abuse	22 / 1	1 / 15	62	0.89	(0.81–0.98)	0.90
Cocaine						
DSM-III—abuse vs. no abuse	11 / 1	3 / 24	38	0.77	(0.66–0.88)	0.81
DSM-III-R—dependence	7 / 1	3 / 28	28	0.71	(0.60–0.83)	0.78
DSM-III-R—dependence or abuse	7 / 1	4 / 27	31	0.65	(0.54–0.77)	0.75
Overall average				0.81		0.83
System averages						
DSM-III[b]				0.84		0.86
DSM-III-R[b]—dependence				0.75		0.79
DSM-III-R—dependence or abuse				0.82		0.91

[a]Dependence vs. no dependence.
[b]The following comparisons were made: DSM-III—abuse or dependence vs. neither; DSM-III-R—dependence vs. abuse or none *and* dependence or abuse vs. neither.
[c]Pseudo-bayesian estimate.

0.40 and 0.75 are considered to indicate fair to good agreement. The average kappa for DSM-III substance disorders was 0.84; for DSM-III-R dependence vs. abuse or none, it was 0.74; and for dependence or abuse vs. neither, 0.82. The item-by-item reliabilities ranged from fair to excellent.

We have archived no less than 20 different versions of the SAM since the first version of the interview was developed in 1983. After each version, we discussed the problems and need for revision and then rewrote and tested the emendations. Thus, we are in a position to describe the evolutionary process of the operationalization of drug and alcohol criteria. Also, since the test–retest reliability of the instrument has been shown to be very good, we are reasonably confident that our translation of the criteria is valid.

4. The Essentials of a Good Interview

Those who have been involved in constructing an interview that simultaneously serves multiple purposes have found the process to be lengthy and tedious. Robins offers 12 essentials of a good interview[31] (Table II). These essentials address areas ranging from the type of information gathered to the way the data are gathered. In spite of such a daunting task, those who are involved with developing and constructing diagnostic instruments should attempt to incorporate each of these elements into the final product.

In addition to Robins' specific criteria, we offer several other considerations that facilitate development of good survey instrumentation such as structure. One way of achieving structure is to provide closed-ended questions that require yes or no answers: categorical responses, such as "in the last month," "in the past year," or an actual number, such as the largest number of marijuana cigarettes smoked in a 24-hr period. Structure makes the answers easy to process for computer analysis.

Table II.   The Essentials of a Good Interview[a]

1. It should provide an accurate operationalization of multiple diagnostic systems.
2. Diagnostic coverage should be broad enough and specific enough to capture those who are ill.
3. It should be highly structured.
4. It should not allow for individual interpretations to be made.
5. Everyday impairments should not be classified as symptoms.
6. It should exclude physical origins of illness.
7. The questions should be easily understood by persons from all educational levels.
8. The language should be nonidiomatic.
9. The language should not be culture-specific.
10. The information obtained should not be dependent on record review.
11. The information should be obtainable in one sitting.
12. The interview should be acceptable to everyone.

[a]Source: Robins.[31]

Sometimes respondents have difficulty deciding how to answer a question that elicits only a yes or no answer. For example, when asked: "Have you ever felt dependent on drugs?" some respondents did not know what was meant by "dependent." This prompted us to add a definition of dependence to the question: "Have you ever felt dependent on drugs, or found that you were unable to keep from using them even though you wanted to?"

When asked: "Have you ever considered yourself an excessive drinker?" some respondents said they did not know how to answer the question because they had not thought so while they were drinking, but thought so *since* coming to treatment and *after* they stopped drinking. This response prompted us to provide an alternative category: not while drinking, but thinks so now. Although ethnographers and others involved in observational studies rely on the data from open-ended questions, most epidemiologists find that coding responses from open-ended questions is too tedious and the yield too inexact to use in operationalizing diagnostic criteria. For this reason, open-ended questions are avoided in the DIS, CIDI, and SAM.

Questions should have relevance for most of the respondents, otherwise the respondents may feel compelled to answer questions positively so as to make the interview less boring or may become annoyed at being asked about behaviors that do not pertain to them. For example, one of our early versions of the SAM required that anyone who had ever had an alcoholic beverage be asked all of the questions in the alcohol section, including questions about withdrawal symptoms and physical and emotional problems from the use of alcohol. Some respondents were irritated about being asked these questions. They thought we had misinterpreted their drinking history during earlier questions and often commented that some of the questions seemed unnecessary. A subsequent revision introduced an instruction to skip virtual nondrinkers out of the alcohol section. (Virtual nondrinkers were those who had never drunk at least once a month for six months or more *and* had never drunk more than four drinks in a day.)

We do not allow subsequent questions to be skipped once diagnostic criteria are met or once it is clear that the diagnosis will be negative. The use of early skipouts is disallowed so that epidemiological comparisons of symptoms can be made and so that there is flexibility on meeting criteria for different diagnostic systems. In addition, if the skipout after three positive symptoms were allowed and then the diagnostic threshold were raised to four or more symptoms, existing interviews could not be rescored using the stricter criteria. In the DIS, CIDI, and SAM, skipouts are allowed only when it is illogical for a subsequent question to be asked. The entire drug section is skipped if no drug has been used more than five times; additionally, specific questions about individual drugs are skipped if those drugs have not been used more than five times.

An additional consideration in design is the length of questions; short questions are better than long ones, but neither extreme is good. In our analysis of the SAM, we found that our questions had an average length of 19 words. Because lengthy questions might lead the respondent to misunderstand the meaning, we shortened SAM questions that had lower reliability *and* were longer than average.

Using value-laden terms is another threat to good question design. To assess "frequent intoxication when expected to fulfill major role obligations at work, school or home" (DSM-III-R dependence criterion A4), we might ask if the respondent had taken care of children while drunk. However, being "drunk" in the context of caregiving carries social and legal stigmas and many persons might deny this behavior. We decided to operationalize this criterion by asking the following: "Have you often taken care of children at a time when you were feeling the effects of alcohol?" This was easily understood by the alcoholics in our study. However, during the pretest of the DIS-III-R which used community subjects, we realized that this wording created a threshold that was too low, since anyone who had a glass of sherry while cooking dinner and also had children at home might answer this question positively. The wording was changed to "Have you often taken care of children at a time when you had drunk enough alcohol to make your speech thick or to make you unsteady on your feet?"

Inaccuracies in responses may be attributed to lying (a special concern with behaviors such as illicit substance use) and forgetting, but they may also be due to a poorly constructed question; hence, it is important to ask precisely what we mean to ask. Precision in choosing the words of a question becomes even more challenging when the diagnostic criteria are not clear in their meaning.

The imperative of precise questionnaire wording is further illustrated with the following example of assessing salience. To determine whether the DSM-III-R and ICD-10 criteria of salience were met, we asked respondents if they had ever given up important activities for substance use. If so, they were asked the following onset and recency question: "When was the (first/last) time you gave up activities for (DRUG)?"

Again, the pretest phase was very important because it revealed that some respondents were not sure how to answer this question. If a respondent had given up socializing in favor of using heroin 10 years ago and had not changed the behavior since, the interviewer would have coded both the onset and recency 10 years ago, because it had been that long since the last time the activity was given up. However, the recency would have been coded incorrectly; it should have been coded as "current." We changed the recency question to the following: "When was the last time your use of (DRUG) kept you from important activities?" The same response to this question would appropriately be scored as "currently."

Another concern is that of ensuring the correct use of the question for the diagnosis, that is, making certain that the computer program will correctly identify which questions are to be used to assess the criteria. The SAM, like the new DIS-III-R, includes labels in the margin adjacent to each question, which reference the diagnostic systems and criteria in the systems being assessed. This leaves no doubt in the investigator's mind about which criterion a particular question will serve. Labeling questions is tedious but is as important as writing questions in building a reliable operationalization of criteria. In fact, the process of writing computer algorithms and operationalizing criteria is symbiotic as well, because it sometimes reveals errors in the coverage of criteria. Errors are particularly likely when multiple diagnostic systems are being covered and a single question is asked to serve more than one system.

Further, the quality of the operationalization of criteria is probably enhanced when two or more measures, instead of one, assess the criteria. It seems obvious that criteria that rely on a single question will be less reliable than criteria that have several diagnostic questions. To the authors' knowledge, this issue has never been empirically tested.

Finally, we address the need for pretesting. It is one of the most time-consuming, yet worthwhile components of operationalization. Pretesting allows errors in skip instructions, wording, and coverage of criteria to be deleted and the lack of acceptability uncovered before the interview is circulated for widespread use. Many times the pretest subjects themselves have suggested revisions of questions or have helped to determine exclusionary situations.

5. The Evolution of Operationalizing Criteria

One example of the evolutionary process that a question undergoes from initial development to publication of the instrument is shown in Table III. The example illustrates four evolving approaches to operationalizing the DSM-III-R dependence criterion "preoccupation." The criterion does not state what a "great deal of time" is, so we define it loosely as a "period" and qualify it with the phrase "little time for anything else." Our first attempt underestimated the criterion and included only mental preoccupation. Our next attempt added the phrase "spent time looking forward to drinking." Because similar

Table III. The Evolution of Interview Questions

DSM-III-R dependence criterion "a great deal of time spent in activities necessary to get the substance, take the substance or recover from its effects"

1. Has there ever been a period when you had drinking on your mind so much that you had little time for anything else?
2. Has there ever been a period when you spent so much time looking forward to drinking or had drinking on your mind so much that you had little time for anything else?
3. Has there ever been a period when you spent so much time drinking or getting over drinking that you had little time for anything else?
4. Has there ever been a period when you spent so much time drinking alcohol or recovering from its effects that you had little time for anything else?

wording was used for the drug questions and was found to be more suitable for drug than alcohol abusers, it was reworded for drinking behavior. The revision was an improvement: "a period of spending so much time drinking or getting over drinking that there was little time for other activities." However, because "getting over drinking" was grammatically awkward and easily misunderstood, we revised the question again, opting for the more precise phrase "recovering from its [the alcohol's] effects." Additionally, the field test of the CIDI revealed concern over using the term "drinking"; to achieve cultural acceptability, the term was changed to "drinking alcohol."

One unique contribution of our SAM pilot study was to investigate why particular questions had poor reliability. A question that was unreliable because it was misunderstood could then be rewritten for clearer meaning. One week after the initial SAM interview, a retest interview was completed with a follow-up discrepancy interview. At the end of the second interview, the answers to predetermined questions from both SAM interviews were compared in the respondent's presence. If there were discrepancies, the respondent was asked to try to explain them. To help him, he was given a card listing possible explanations for discordant answers. A typical resolution went as follows: "You told me that you felt dependent on tobacco, but you told the first interviewer that you never felt this way. Could you tell me which answer is correct and why you might have given us two different answers?"

In our pilot study, there were 124 discrepancies in all. Respondents gave as their most common reasons for discordant answers: (1) information had been forgotten at the time of one of the interviews, (2) there was no known explanation for the discrepancy, (3) the question was misunderstood. This exercise was valuable to us because questions that were misunderstood were rewritten for better clarity.

6. Operationalization—What It Looks Like

Leon Gordis[32] states that epidemiologists should assure the quality of "raw" data so that the results generated from these data will also be of high quality. The way to achieve this, he states, is to subject the interview to peer review, include the instrument in journal articles for informational purposes, and, at the very least, describe the appropriate advantages and limitations attributed to its use.

The SAM has undergone considerable peer review among members of the WHO/ADAMHA Working Group. Because its length prohibits its publication here, we give the readers a sample of the questions used to assess DSM-III-R alcohol dependence in Table IV. The wording of questions on tobacco and drug use is often identical to that of the alcohol questions.

The DSM-III-R uses phrases such as "persistent," "frequent," and "often." To operationalize these terms, we used phrases such as "more than once" and

Table IV. Operationalization of DSM-III-R Dependence Criteria
According to the CIDI-SAM

A1. Substances often taken in larger amounts or over a longer period than the person intended.
Have you often ended up drinking much more than you expected to when you began, or over more days than you intended to?

A2. Persistent desire or one or more unsuccessful efforts to cut down or control substance use.
Have you more than once wanted to stop drinking but couldn't?
Did you make rules to control your drinking because you were having trouble limiting the amount you were drinking?

A3. A great deal of time spent in activities necessary to get the substance (e.g., theft), taking the substance (e.g., chain smoking), or recovering from its effects.
Has there ever been a period when you spent so much time drinking alcohol or recovering from its effects that you had little time for anything else?

A4. Frequent intoxication or withdrawal symptoms when expected to fulfill major role obligations at work, school, or home (e.g., does not go to work because of being hung over, goes to school or work "high," intoxicated while taking care of his or her children), or when substance use is physically hazardous (e.g., drives when intoxicated).
Did you neglect some of your usual responsibilities while you were on a binge or bender?
Has your drinking or being hung over often kept you from working or caring for your children?
Have you ever gotten into trouble driving because of drinking . . . like having an accident or being arrested for drunk driving?
Have you several times been high from drinking in a situation where it increased your chances of getting hurt . . . for instance, when driving a car or boat, using knives, machinery, or guns, crossing against traffic, climbing or swimming?
Have you ever accidentally injured yourself when you had been drinking, that is, had a bad fall or cut yourself with a knife, been hurt in a traffic accident, or anything like that?

A5. Important social, occupational, or recreational activities given up or reduced because of substance use.
Have you ever given up or greatly reduced important activities in order to drink . . . like sports, work, or associating with friends or relatives?

A6. Continued substance use despite knowledge of having a persistent or recurrent social, psychological, or physical problem that is caused or exacerbated by the use of the substance (e.g., keeps using heroin despite family arguments about it, cocaine-induced depression, or having an ulcer made worse by drinking).
Were there ever objections about your drinking from
a. your family
b. friends, your doctor, or your clergyman
c. your boss or people at work or at school
d. Did you ever get into fights while drinking?
e. Have the police stopped or arrested you or taken you to a treatment center because you were drinking?
Did you continue to drink (more than once) after having any of these problems?
There are several health problems that can result from long stretches of pretty heavy drinking. Did drinking ever cause you to have liver disease, yellow jaundice, give you stomach disease, or make you vomit blood, cause your feet to tingle or feel numb, give you memory problems even when you weren't drinking, or give you pancreatitis?

(*continued*)

Table IV. *(Continued)*

Did you continue to drink (more than once) knowing that drinking caused you to have a health problem or injury?

Have you continued to drink when you knew you had a serious physical illness that might be made worse by drinking?

Has alcohol ever caused you emotional or psychological problems such as feeling uninterested in things, depressed, paranoid, or caused you to have strange ideas?

Did you continue to drink (more than once) after you knew drinking caused these problems?

Have you ever continued to drink while taking medication you knew was dangerous to mix with alcohol?

A7. Marked tolerance: need for markedly increased amounts of the substance (i.e., at least a 50% increase) in order to achieve intoxication or desired effect, or markedly diminished effect with continued use of the same amount.

Did you ever get tolerant to alcohol, that is, you needed to drink a lot more in order to get an effect, or find that you could no longer get high on the amount you used to drink?

After you had been drinking for a while, did you find that you began to be able to drink a lot more before you would get drunk (before your speech got thick or you were unsteady on your feet)?

A8. Characteristic withdrawal symptoms.

People who cut down or stop drinking after drinking for a considerable time often have withdrawal symptoms. Common ones are the "shakes" (hands tremble), being unable to sleep, feeling anxious or depressed, sweating, heart beating fast, or the DTs, or seeing or hearing things that aren't there. Have you had any problems like that when you stopped or cut down on drinking?

A9. Substance often taken to relieve or avoid withdrawal symptoms.

Did you ever need a drink just after you had gotten up (that is, before breakfast)?

Did you take a drink right after you got up to keep from having a hangover or the shakes?

Have you ever taken a drink to keep from having withdrawal symptoms or to make them go away?

B. Some symptoms of the disturbance have persisted for at least 1 month, or have occurred repeatedly over a longer period of time.

Did you go on a binge several times or go on a binge that lasted a month or more?

Did your ability to drink more without feeling it last for a month or more?

Have you often ended up drinking much more than you expected to when you began, or over more days than you intended to?

Did you try to follow rules to control your drinking for a month or longer or make rules for yourself several times?

Did the period when you spent a lot of time drinking last a month or longer?

Did you give up or cut down on activities to drink for a month or more?

Have you often worked or taken care of children at a time when you had drunk enough alcohol to make your speech thick or to make you unsteady on your feet?

Have you had withdrawal symptoms several times?

Have you several times taken a drink to keep from having withdrawal symptoms?

Did you continue to drink (more than once) knowing that drinking caused you to have a health problem or injury?

Have you ever continued to drink when you knew you had a serious physical illness that might be made worse by drinking?

Have you ever continued to drink while taking medication you knew was dangerous to mix with alcohol?

Did you continue to drink (more than once) after you knew that drinking caused you psychological or emotional problems?

"several times." Criterion A6, "continued use despite problems," needed two questions—one to assess whether the behavior *ever* existed, and one to assess whether the behavior *continued* after knowledge of a problem.

Marked tolerance (A7) is defined in DSM-III-R as a "need for markedly increased amounts of a substance (at least a 50% increase)." The text of DSM-III-R states that "differences in tolerance for alcohol apply . . . ." We found no coherent way to operationalize the 50% increase.

To assess characteristic withdrawal symptoms for alcohol, one question was sufficient. We applied one list of withdrawal symptoms to all classes of drugs to standardize the questioning and allow comparisons to be made across all drug classes. Through systematic epidemiological surveillance we may be able to uncover additional symptoms of withdrawal not previously reported.

The duration and severity criteria contain words that are ill defined and vague. Some examples are "some," "persisted," "occurred repeatedly," "longer period of time," "few," and "many." We do not know how many "some" and "a few" are but chose a definition—such as more than one—so that scoring algorithms could be developed and diagnoses made. The chance for misclassification bias is evident. We suggest that investigators publish the algorithms that assess these criteria along with research results. Ultimately, the DSM-IV should strive for more precise terms.

7. Discussion

One of the first steps in accepting new nomenclature concerning substance abuse and dependence should be the operationalization of diagnostic criteria. Operationalization is simply defined by Babbie as the "specification of concepts."[33] It is the process of reducing or converting an abstract or concept—like salience, preoccupation with substances, or withdrawal—into an empirical indicator.

Babor et al. write "Continued efforts to operationalize key concepts in the alcohol (and drug) field would be a welcome development, inasmuch as it would lead to greater clarity in definitions and more informed debate over critical issues."[34] Besides the CIDI-SAM, CIDI, and DIS-III-R, several other instruments have recently been developed that assess DSM-III and/or DSM-III-R substance abuse and dependence criteria—Schuckit's structured diagnostic interview for identification of primary alcoholism—the Alcohol Research Center Intake Interview;[35] and Spitzer's Structured Clinical Interview for DSM-III-R (SCID). Working groups continue to meet in order to finalize the draft of the ICD-10 criteria; the DSM-IV Task Force is planning its course. These groups are working to achieve a more specific, precise, empirically based classification of drug and alcohol dependence.

Assessment tools can be generated to elicit subtypes of alcohol and drug dependence, discover genetic correlates, and test the multidimensionality of the dependence syndrome. But along with expanded interview modules and new assessments must come rational operationalization of the diagnostic criteria they hope to assess using guidelines such as those suggested here.

The WHO/ADAMHA CIDI-SAM appears to contain the essentials of a good interview. It includes criteria from multiple diagnostic systems, is highly structured, can be administered by nonclinicians, is computer-scored, and can be utilized in epidemiological and clinical studies. Currently, there are several studies underway to test the SAM's reliability and validity in various populations against other assessment tools. In the final analysis, the assessment tool is no better than the criteria on which it is based. One goal is that cross-cultural research will eventually produce a unified concept of dependence, a standardized system of diagnostic criteria, and one diagnostic interview acceptable to all.

ACKNOWLEDGMENTS. The authors wish to acknowledge the editorial assistance of Dr. Lee Robins and Becky Robinson. This research was supported in part by grants from the National Institute on Drug Abuse DA 05619-01, and DA 05585.

References

1. Robins LN: The epidemiology of drug use and abuse: Where are we now? in Robins LN (ed): *Studying Drug Abuse, Vol. 6.* New Brunswick, NJ, Rutgers University Press, 1985.
2. Kandel D: The measurement of "ever use" and "frequency–quantity" in drug use surveys. *National Inst Drug Abuse Res Monogr Series* 2:27–35, 1975.
3. Davidson R: Assessment of the alcohol dependence syndrome: A review of self-report screening questionnaires. *Br J Clin Psychol* 26:243–255, 1987.
4. Caetano R: When will we have a standard concept of alcohol dependence? *Br J Addiction* 82:601–605, 1987.
5. Robins LN: Diagnostic grammar and assessment: Translating criteria into questions, in Robins L and Barrett J (eds): *The Validity of Diagnosis.* New York, Raven Press, 1989.
6. American Psychiatric Association: *Diagnostic and Statistical Manual of Mental Disorders*, 3rd edition, revised. Washington DC, American Psychiatric Association, 1987.
7. Edwards G, Gross MM: Alcohol dependence: provisional description of a clinical syndrome, *Br Med J* 1:1058–1061, 1976.
8. Rounsaville BJ, Spitzer RL, Williams JBW: Proposed changes in DSM-III substance use disorders: description and rationale. *Am J Psychiatry* 143:463–468, 1987.
9. Caetano R: A commentary on the proposed changes in DSM-III concept of alcohol dependence. *Drug Alcohol Dependence* 19:345–355, 1987.
10. Segal BM: Letter to the editor. *Am J Psychiatry* 144:257–258, 1987.
11. Blackwell J: Letter to the editor. *Am J Psychiatry* 144:258, 1987.
12. Prado A. Letter to the editor. *Am J Psychiatry* 144:258, 1987.
13. Rounsaville BJ, Spitzer RL, Williams J: Dr. Rounsaville and colleagues reply. *Am J Psychiatry* 144:259, 1987.
14. Rounsaville BJ, Kosten T, Williams J, Spitzer RL: A field trial of DSM-III-R psychoactive substance dependence disorders. *Am J Psychiatry* 144:351–355, 1987.
15. Davidson R: Assessment of the alcohol dependence syndrome: A review of self-report screening questionnaires. *Br J Clin Psychol* 26:243–255, 1987.

16. Johnston LD: Techniques for reducing measurement error in surveys of drug use, in Robins L (ed): *Studying Drug Abuse, Vol. 6.* New Brunswick, NJ, Rutgers University Press, 1985.
17. Blashfield R, Feighner, et al: Invisible colleges and the Matthew effect. *Schizophrenia Bull* 8:1–5, 1982.
18. Robins LN, Helzer JE: Diagnosis and clinical assessment: The current state of psychiatry. *Annu Rev Psychol* 37:409–432, 1986.
19. Robins LN: The development and characteristics of the NIMH Diagnostic Interview Schedule, in Weissman MM, Myers JK, Ross CE (eds): *Community Surveys of Psychiatric Disorders.* New Brunswick, NJ, Rutgers University Press, 1986.
20. Helzer JE, Robins LN, Croughan JL, Welner A: The Renard Diagnostic Interview: Its reliability and procedural validity with physicians and lay interviewers. *Arch Gen Psychiatry* 38:393–398, 1981.
21. Feighner JP, Robins E, Guze SB, Woodruff RA, Winokur G: Diagnostic criteria for use in psychiatric research. *Arch Gen Psychiatry* 26:57–63, 1972.
22. Robins LN, Helzer JE, Croughan J, Ratcliff K: National Institute of Mental Health Diagnostic Interview Schedule: Its history, characteristics, and validity. *Arch Gen Psychiatry* 38:381–389, 1981.
23. Spitzer RL, Endicott J, Robins E: Research diagnostic criteria. *Arch Gen Psychiatry* 35:773–782, 1978.
24. Helzer JE, Spitznagel EL, McEvoy LM: The predictive validity of lay Diagnostic Interview Schedule diagnoses in the general population: A comparison with physician examiners. *Arch Gen Psychiatry* 44:1069–1044, 1987.
25. Helzer JE: Symptoms of dysthymia and depression. Presented at the World Psychiatric Association Regional Symposium, 1988.
26. Robins LN, Helzer JE, Cottler LB, Goldring E: *The Diagnostic Interview Schedule Revised*, St. Louis, 1988.
27. Robins LN, Cottler LB, Babor T: *The Composite International Diagnostic Interview Substance Abuse Module (CIDI-SAM)* St. Louis, 1983, revised 1984–1988.
28. Robins LN, et al: The CIDI-SAM: A new interview to assess substance abuse and dependence, manuscript in preparation.
29. Robins LN, Wing J, Wittchen HU, Helzer JE, Babor TF, Burke JD, Farmer A, Jablenski A, Pickens R, Regier DA, Sartorius N, Towle LH: The Composite International Diagnostic Interview (CIDI): An epidemiologic instrument suitable for use in conjunction with different diagnostic systems and in different cultures. *Arch Gen Psychiatry* 45:1069–1077, 1988.
30. Cottler LB, Robins LN, Helzer JE: Reliability of the CIDI-SAM—a comprehensive substance interview. *British Journal of Addiction* 84:801–814, 1989.
31. Robins LN: Composing the CIDI: A collaboration with the WHO/ADAMHA. Presented at the Department of Psychiatry Research Seminar, St. Louis, 1988.
32. Gordis L: Assuring the quality of questionnaire data in epidemiologic research. *Am J Epidemiol* 109:21–24, 1979.
33. Babbie ER: *Survey Research Methods.* Belmont, Wadsworth, 1973.
34. Babor TF, Lauerman RJ, Cooney NL: In search of the alcohol dependence syndrome: A cross-national study of its structure and validity, in Paakkanen P, Sulkunen P (eds): *Cultural Studies of Drinking and Drinking Practices.* Helsinki, Social Research Institute on Alcohol Studies, 1987.
35. Schuckit MA, Irwin M, Howard T, Smith T: A structured diagnostic interview for identification of primary alcoholism: A preliminary evaluation. *J Stud Alcohol* 49:93–99, 1988.

4

From Basic Concepts to Clinical Reality

Unresolved Issues in the Diagnosis of Dependence

Thomas F. Babor, Barbara Orrok, Neil Liebowitz, Ronald Salomon, and Joseph Brown

Abstract. This chapter discusses clinical and conceptual issues pertaining to the diagnosis of alcohol and drug dependence. Emphasis is given to the difficulties involved in moving from diagnostic concepts, such as those contained in the major psychiatric classification systems, to the clinical situation where diagnostic decisions are made. To illustrate how diagnostic concepts approximate clinical reality, a set of case histories is used to organize a discussion of unresolved issues in the diagnosis of dependence. These issues include the putative syndrome nature of dependence, the problem of diagnosing polysubstance use, the primary–secondary distinction, the presence of other psychopathology, and the use of multiaxial evaluation.

1. Introduction

Nosology is among the most maligned and neglected areas of addiction studies. Classification or nosology is the process of grouping individuals into categories representing specific substance use disorders on the basis of some shared characteristics. The precise attributes used to classify a sick person as having a substance use disorder are called diagnostic criteria. The obvious importance of diagnostic criteria derives from their usefulness in making clinical decisions, estimating disease prevalence, understanding etiology, and planning treatment. This chapter discusses clinical and conceptual issues pertaining to the diagnosis of alcohol and drug dependence, giving particular emphasis to the difficulties involved in moving from diagnostic concepts, such as those contained in the major psychiatric classification systems,[1–3] to

Thomas F. Babor, Barbara Orrok, Neil Liebowitz, Ronald Salomon, and Joseph Brown • Department of Psychiatry, University of Connecticut School of Medicine, Farmington, Connecticut 06032.

the clinical situation where diagnostic decisions must be made and treatment planning must be conducted. To the extent that the interface between concepts and clinical reality takes place in the context of diagnostic systems (e.g., DSM's "multiaxial" system), this chapter discusses how these systems fit representative patients. To achieve this objective, each set of basic concepts and clinical issues is introduced by a case history obtained from the authors' records or experience.

Alcoholism and drug addiction have been variously defined as medical diseases, mental disorders, behavioral conditions, and, in some cases, as the symptom of an underlying mental disorder.[4] The intent of many of these definitions is to permit the classification of alcoholism and drug dependence within standard nomenclatures such as the *International Classification of Diseases* (ICD) or the *Diagnostic and Statistical Manual of Mental Disorders* (DSM) of the American Psychiatric Association. In the past 20 years several distinct traditions have emerged among psychiatrists and psychologists occupied with the development of definitions and diagnostic criteria. Two of the most influential approaches have been associated with the World Health Organization, on the one hand, and the American Psychiatric Association, on the other.

The ninth edition of the *International Classification of Diseases* (ICD-9) is the official classification system of the World Health Organization.[5] With the increasing recognition of the international dimensions of problems associated with psychoactive substance use, the need for a common frame of reference for communication and statistical reporting has taken on added significance. Recent developments in the revision of the ICD section on psychoactive substance use are reflective of this need. Continuing a programmatic effort to join expert opinion with cross-cultural clinical experience, the Mental Health Division of WHO has refined the concept of alcohol and drug dependence in a way that permits classification of different substances according to an identical set of criteria.[3,6]

The second major trend in the area of formal diagnostic criteria has emerged in the past 20 years in the United States. Developed primarily by a group of researchers affiliated with the Washington University School of Medicine, this "research diagnostic" approach has strongly influenced the most recent classification of substance use disorders adopted by the American Psychiatric Association[2] in the revised third edition of its *Diagnostic and Statistical Manual* (DSM-III-R). As part of the APA's ongoing program of work on nomenclature and classification, a set of changes has recently been made to the entire Substance Use Disorders section of DSM-III.[7] The modification of criteria for dependence aims to remedy some of the shortcomings noted in DSM-III.[1] The most important changes involve adopting a dimensional model of dependence that closely resembles the WHO alcohol dependence syndrome concept.[6] Significantly, the medical and social consequences of both acute and chronic intoxication are not among the primary diagnostic criteria. These do, however, enter into the diagnosis of substance abuse in DSM-III-R, which is now defined as continued use despite persistent social, occupational, psychological, or physical problems that are caused or exacerbated by substance use. Like DSM-III, DSM-III-R proposes five axes to permit a more comprehensive evaluation of the individual's condition.

In this chapter, a number of issues are raised that are of potential importance for enhancing the clinical utility of these revised diagnostic systems. These issues include the applicability of the new dependence criteria to the classification of complex patterns of substance use, the utility of distinguishing between primary and secondary substance use disorders, the importance of considering other psychopathology that may be either antecedent or consequent to substance use, and the merits of multiaxial classification.

2. The Concept of Dependence

Case 1: John B.

John B., a 33-year-old white man, died of acute toxicity from cocaine and heroin in 1982. Born in Wheaton, Illinois to immigrant parents, he indicated no history of psychiatric or personality disorder before the onset of drug use at age 19. He began experimenting with marijuana, hallucinogens, and barbiturates as a college student, occasionally selling marijuana to earn extra money. After college he was employed in Chicago as an actor and comedian, later moving to New York at age 24 to work in improvisational theater productions. When a friend gave him cocaine during a rehearsal, this quickly became his drug of choice. Although most of the cast used drugs regularly, the manager and fellow–actors began to criticize John for getting high before performances. At this time he began to use methaqualone as an antidote to cocaine, and he began to improvise drug-related themes in his comedy routines.

At age 26 John B. was hired as a cast member for a new live television comedy program. The increased income allowed him to afford an almost daily supply of cocaine, which had become an integral part of his life. Not only did he consume larger amounts than his friends, he also tended to use alcohol, marijuana, and methaqualone along with cocaine in the course of long binges that lasted up to 3 days. Although his wife and friends continued to complain about his drug use, he claimed that drugs were essential to his professional life by making him funny, intense, driven, and keyed up for performances. During this period he made repeated attempts to cut down or stop his cocaine use. He manifested a high degree of tolerance, being capable of snorting up to a gram of cocaine at one time. When he was finally persuaded to see a psychiatrist, the medical record showed that he smoked three packs of cigarettes per day, used alcohol and diazepam occasionally, used mescaline and LSD regularly, smoked marijuana four times a week, and felt dependent on methaqualone and cocaine.

When psychiatric consultation failed to change his drug use, John B.'s life became progressively involved in the drug subculture connected with the New York and Los Angeles entertainment industries. He began to organize almost every aspect of his personal and professional life around the acquisition and use of drugs. Although a bodyguard who was hired by his wife succeeded in limiting his access to drugs for almost a year, intense cravings for cocaine eventually led to a relapse with the rapid reinstatement of many of the behaviors, symptoms, and consequences that had characterized his drug use previously. In late 1982 he began associating with a female heroin addict who supplied him with cocaine and provided him with alternating injections of heroin and cocaine over a period of several weeks. On the morning of March 5, 1982, he died of respiratory arrest associated with a series of combined doses of cocaine and heroin.

The short life and fast times of John B., detailed in Bob Woodward's 1984 biography[8] of the popular comedian John Belushi, provide ample evidence of an interrelated syndrome of behavioral, psychological, and physical symptoms that constitute the new criteria for dependence in the proposed tenth revision of the *International Classification of Diseases,*[3] and in the revised third edition of the American Psychiatric Association's *Diagnostic and Statistical Manual.*[2] Central to the emerging approach to the classification of alcohol and drug dependence is the concept of a dependence syndrome that is distinguished from disabilities caused by substance use.[6] The dependence syndrome is seen as an interrelated cluster of cognitive, behavioral, and physiological symptoms. A diagnosis of dependence in the proposed ICD-10 system is made if three or more of the following have been experienced or exhibited at some time in the previous 12 months: (1) a withdrawal state; (2) substance use with the intention of relieving withdrawal symptoms and with awareness that this strategy is effective; (3) an impaired personal capacity to control the onset, termination, or level of use; (4) a narrowing of the personal repertoire of patterns of use, e.g., a tendency to use the substance in the same way on weekdays and weekends, regardless of the social constraints; (5) progressive neglect of alternative pleasures or interests in favor of substance use; (6) persistence of use despite clear evidence of overtly harmful consequences. DSM-III-R uses a similar set of criteria to diagnose dependence.

In the months before his death, John B. exhibited practically every characteristic of the drug dependence syndrome as defined in ICD-10 and DSM-III-R. There was a progressive narrowing of his interests around drug use over a period of 4 years, with a gradual stereotyping of the timing and rituals associated with the substances he used most frequently. He would go to great extremes to satisfy intense cravings for cocaine and other drugs. If he did not have a ready supply of cocaine, he would search the streets of New York and Los Angeles until he could buy or borrow some. Once he had initiated an episode of drug use, he would often stay intoxicated for days, unable or unwilling to stop until he collapsed. Over the years he built up a high tolerance for barbiturates and cocaine; often experienced irritability, dysphoria, nausea, and other withdrawal symptoms when he stopped; and frequently used drugs in direct response to these symptoms. As tolerance and physical dependence developed, his life became progressively centered around drug use. This was reflected in his constant preoccupation with drugs, his neglect of people and activities that were not related to drug use, and his persistence in drug taking despite numerous instances of social disapproval, work problems, and medical complications (e.g., a perforated nasal septum). The mutually reinforcing nature of this process is suggested by the cooccurrence of many of these dependence features. Changes in internal states, interpreted as cravings, precipitated drug-seeking behavior and compulsive use, which continued despite attempts by John B. and others to stop or at least moderate his drug use.

According to the new dependence model described in ICD-10 and DSM-III-R, a complete description of an individual's substance-related pathology must include the nature and severity of dependence, the kinds and degrees of disability, and the personal and environmental factors that influence the substance use. This model departs significantly from the older binary classification schemes by emphasizing that both dependence and related disabilities exist in degrees rather than in an all-or-none state. The notion of a generic drug dependence syndrome that applies to all psychoactive substances makes it possible to compare different drugs of abuse along the same dimensions of symptomatology.

Following Edwards'[9] formulation of the dependence syndrome, it is important to distinguish between the natural history of dependence and the roles drug users assume and play as they become socialized into the drug subculture. Natural history refers to the sequential development over time of biological and psychophysiological responses to psychoactive substances in relation to a variety of body systems. These processes include the development of metabolic and physiological tolerance, as well as the adaptive mechanisms that are reflected in drug-specific abstinence syndromes. In contrast to the natural history of drug dependence, there are also behavioral and psychosocial changes that characterize the individual's personality, self-concept, and interpersonal relations. These aspects of the drug use career result in the individual's self-identification as a member of a drug subculture, and are manifested in the learning of prescribed behaviors and roles. In John B.'s case, the natural history of dependence developed in parallel with his drug use career, both of which culminated in an overdose that many of his close friends considered inevitable.

3. Polysubstance Use

Case 2: Joe H.

Joe H., a 41-year-old single man with a 20-year history of multiple and polysubstance use, was interviewed about his drug use career. Data were collected for two periods: a self-defined "worst period" 8 years prior to interview, and the most recent period that led to treatment. During the worst period, the patient reported daily use of alcohol and cannabis and almost daily use of opiates (heroin) and cocaine. This period was also characterized by irregular use of sedatives (Valium and Tranxene) for the purpose of sleep induction following cocaine use and use of nitrous oxide on a monthly basis. Much of the cannabis use during this period was described as an attempt to manage the effects of cocaine, and Valium was used to come down from cocaine.

Alcohol use during this period was a stimulus for cannabis use, which in turn led to heroin or cocaine use, depending on availability. The more recent period recorded a diminution in substance use, with opiates (in the form of methadone maintenance and heroin) being used on an almost daily basis. There was a complete cessation of alcohol and cannabis use after a recent hospitalization at an alcohol treatment program, but cocaine use continued on a weekly basis, and sedative use increased. The patient reported use of three or more substances simultaneously on a daily basis in the worst period and on a weekly basis in the latter period.

The clinician with even cursory experience in treating substance use disorders knows just how common the preceding case history is. Rare is the case where a single class of substance is used exclusively. The increased availability of illegal drugs, in conjunction with the aging of persons who came to adulthood during the drug epidemic of the 1960s, has resulted in a dramatic change in the clinical profile of patients treated within the alcohol and drug rehabilitation network. Even among the generally older veterans serviced within the Veterans Administration medical system, the purely alcohol-dependent patient is becoming an anomaly. Among the 188 clients identified as primarily alcoholics within the Treatment Outcome Prospective Study (TOPS),[10] 63.1% reported weekly or greater marijuana use, 27.3% reported a similar frequency of amphetamine use, and 18.3% used minor tranquilizers at least once a week. Of clients identified as primarily drug abusers, at least 50% reported weekly or greater alcohol use. Missing in the TOPS data is discussion of simultaneous polysubstance use, where three or more substances are used within a single consumption period.

With the advent of criterion-based diagnostic schemes such as the DSM-III, the existence of multiple- and polysubstance users has been recognized. The DSM-III-R diagnostic schema has refined the means by which polysubstance use is classified. Specifically, rather than relying on only three categories of polysubstance abuse or dependence as utilized in DSM-III, DSM-III-R permits a diagnosis of polysubstance dependence, where three or more classes of substances are used in such a way as to meet dependency criteria when all substances are considered together and none meet criteria alone. As in the earlier DSM-III, multiple dependency diagnoses are also permissible provided each class of substance meets the criteria for dependence. Within DSM-III-R there is also the recognition of multiple substance abuse, where more than one class of substance is abused, if this coincidental use does not meet the criteria for polysubstance dependence. In such a case, multiple diagnoses of abuse are made, one for each class of substance.

Lacking from the DSM-III-R, however, is the companion diagnosis of polysubstance abuse, where neither polysubstance dependence nor multiple individual abuse diagnoses are appropriate. This deficiency results in a less than exhaustive or mutually exclusive diagnostic schema. It is possible that a pattern of polysubstance use might be a precursor to later polysubstance dependence, multiple abuse, or even multiple dependence. It would be logical to assume that use of many substances would carry with it a greater risk of eventual dependence on at least one substance than would use of a single substance. If this were indeed true, then a polysubstance abuse diagnosis might serve as an early indicator of high risk for any future dependence. A polysubstance abuse concept might therefore play an important role in targeting early interventions.

4. The Primary–Secondary Distinction

4.1. Case 3: Allen T.

Allen T. served in Vietnam with the U.S. Navy from 1966 to 1968. He frequently handled dead bodies and Agent Orange, two symbols of the Vietnam experience. He received a number of decorations for service and valor. In 1983 he presented for hospital care, describing multiple somatic symptoms.

Prior to the service, Allen T. was among the top students in his high-school class. He was the youngest of four boys in a tightly knit family. His family history shows no alcohol abuse, substance use disorder, or psychopathology. After returning from Vietnam, Allen T. married and had two children. Retrospectively, post-traumatic stress disorder (PTSD) was probably present at this time, but was masked by substance abuse. He worked odd jobs and increasingly resorted to alcohol to cope with financial, social, and somatic problems. He was never violent at home; instead he resorted to long, isolative binges. His wife divorced him, and he remarried. He had been totally unable to work for 3 years after his knee was dislocated in a car accident. This required narcotic analgesia and two surgical corrections, gradually restoring leg function. However, he remained addicted to narcotics as well as alcohol and continued the marijuana use begun in Vietnam. Now diagnosed as PTSD, his symptoms of depression and isolative behavior worsened.

Allen T. refused psychiatric hospitalization or medical detoxification. Instead, he opted for a guided outpatient treatment. Chlordiazepoxide was given with frequent supportive visits, and he began to maintain abstinence for several weeks at a time. The motivational malaise and depression worsened. Desipramine therapy was initiated. Lithium was added after the patient showed little change in his depression, even after stopping narcotic use. Slight changes in his depression were noticeable. He drank in bars instead of alone and allowed his second wife to participate in some therapy visits. He brought his two young sons in for evaluation owing to his concerns about their responses to him and his illness. Finally, he agreed to inpatient rehabilitation treatment for alcohol dependence. Lithium was discontinued, with no loss in the moderate benefit to depression and anxiety symptoms. The patient's acquiescence to the PTSD diagnosis and acceptance of an inpatient treatment program have been the latest milestones in his 20-year history of PTSD.

4.2. Case 4: George B.

George B. was seen by the psychiatric consultation service at his first hospitalization, when he was 47 years old. He began drinking when he was 12, and by 14 found a way to get "high" every weekend. His father and two older brothers also drank frequently. Though his mother frowned on the habit, her own father and three brothers had been alcoholics until their premature deaths.

George B. smiled throughout the initial diagnostic interview and was affable and pleasant. He denied that his daily intake, which he estimated as "less than a fifth," was a real problem. He felt that it was not excessive, because there were periods when he drank 2 qt daily for a week. He wondered how his wife put up with him at those times.

George B. worked at a desk job, drinking only "when necessary" at his place of employment. Drinking helped him "get through meetings." He liked the people he worked with except his supervisor, whom he described as "stuffed." When told that he should stay for detoxification and rehabilitation treatment, he seemed shocked. He tried to joke, saying, "Who'd I kill?" He waved off the interviewer, saying that when he thought there was a problem, he would come back. He also insisted that if he wanted to, he could stop drinking at any time.

Primary vs. secondary alcohol or drug dependence is an evolving notion first formulated in the 19th century.[11] It is based on observations that there appear to be two types of substance use disorder. In recent formulations of alcohol dependence, for example, the following types have been differentiated: (1) a primary form where substance abuse is not preceded by identifiable personality problems or psychiatric disorder; and (2) a secondary form that manifests after the onset of other psychiatric problems, such as depression and antisocial personality disorder.[12] Research attempting to elucidate the etiology of secondary alcoholism, while concentrating mainly on antecedent psychopathology, has suggested that such vulnerability factors as familial history of alcoholism and antisocial personality, minimal brain dysfunction, conduct disorder, aggressiveness, shyness, and hyperactivity may also contribute to a distinct form of substance abuse.[13–15]

George B. is clearly an example of primary alcoholism. Allen T.'s illness is "secondary" in this scheme, not only because of his other "primary" disorder, but because his family history is devoid of alcoholism, his abuse began later in life, and his alcohol intake never became extreme. Identification of alcohol and substance abuse disorders in patients such as Allen T. is frequently one of the easier tasks encountered in their treatment. Family, friends, and employees will usually pressure the patient to seek help when drinking patterns become harmful or disruptive. The diagnosis of an underlying psychiatric disorder (commonly depression, bipolar disease, panic states, other substance abuse, or personality disorder) is more difficult.[16,17] In Allen T.'s case, the anxieties related to PTSD were presumably "self-medicated" with alcohol. Despite the best intentions of the patient, who clearly stated a wish to resume a normal life, his focus on alcohol abuse as "his problem" rendered the PTSD symptoms unrecognizable to himself and his early therapists. The epiphenomena of substance abuse (e.g., intoxication, withdrawal syndromes, craving, personality regression, denial, and disastrous life consequences) frequently alter the symptom severity of other diagnosable entities. Research has shown that codiagnoses are common. The primary–secondary distinction is evolving in step with a better understanding of psychiatric epidemiology and treatment outcome research.[16–21]

Brown and Schuckit's[18] definition of secondary alcoholism depends on a retrospectively demonstrable, preexisting major psychiatric diagnosis. This follows closely a medical model for the primary/secondary distinction: renal failure is not diagnosed as "primary" because of its severity, but rather because of an absence of other etiological causes. What remains unclear is whether, as in internal medicine, the patient can have two "primary" disorders. Though some polydiagnosable patients may have clearly interdependent relationships between their syndromes, others may not. The notion of codiagnosis avoids this issue.

The high prevalence of codiagnosed illness in alcoholic men and women is well documented. Most frequently found are depression, drug abuse, and antisocial personality. Codiagnosis in the Epidemiologic Catchment Area study[22] was common among alcoholics. Most significant were findings of antisocial personality, other substance use, and mania. All three of these diagnoses have complex relationships to alcohol dependence, and in most of these patients the alcoholism has a later onset. Does this make alcoholism simply "secondary" and diagnosable as a part of the "primary" disorder? Will this notion account for all of the etiological data? Will third-party reimbursement be affected by this primary/secondary distinction? If a "primary" diagnosis is missed, will the "secondary" alcoholic be treatable? These questions remain unanswered, but their answers might help us understand the relationships among psychiatric diagnoses. The importance of improving diagnostic accuracy is pointedly shown by the high frequency of suicide attempts among alcoholics with multiple psychiatric diagnoses.[16,19]

In the final analysis, the neurochemical pathways involved in these coexisting syndromes may provide a clearer basis for defining primary/secondary distinctions. Evidence for independent pathways may be found relating to different aspects within the alcoholism picture. Only when we can more clearly delineate biological insults to these systems will we know, with some reasonable certainty, what makes alcohol dependence primary.

5. Other Psychopathology

5.1. Case 5: Gerald A.

Gerald A., a 39-year-old, separated man, presented to the emergency room for severe depression and suicidal ideation. He stated that he had abused alcohol since age 12 and soon afterward began using a variety of substances, including inhalable solvents, cocaine, and marijuana. He did well in school despite his drug use. He attended college, majoring in business. In college his preferred drug was alcohol, with only episodic use of cocaine and marijuana. He was able to sustain a job in sales and to have romantic relationships despite almost daily consumption of one-fifth gallon of spirits.

One month prior to hospital admission, Gerald A.'s wife of 5 years told him to leave, in part because of his alcohol abuse. He moved out and lived on a boat. His alcohol intake increased. After falling overboard in a drunken stupor and nearly drowning, he decided to enter inpatient treatment for detoxification and rehabilitation for alcohol dependence.

During the first few days in treatment Gerald A. was detoxified with benzodiazepines and remained withdrawn, depressed, and irritable. On the third hospital day cigarette burns were noted on his wrists. He explained this self-mutilatory behavior as an attempt to distract himself from his intensive cravings for alcohol. This was a relatively new behavior he discovered while living on his boat the previous month.

Gerald A. was promptly transferred to the Psychiatry Service, where he received chlorpromazine for agitation. Consideration was given to a lithium trial to control "mood swings." After less than a week on the Psychiatry Service, the patient was interviewed at case conference after refusing to take more neuroleptic. He revealed that his alcohol consumption had been relatively constant over the past 20 years, unaffected by his changes in mood. There was a significant history of affective symptoms, but there was never a period of abstinence lasting more than a few days. In fact, the current 9 days in hospital was the longest period of sobriety in many years. His mood had improved and he asked to be transferred back to the alcohol rehabilitation service.

5.2. Case 6: Betty B.

Betty B., a 45-year-old divorced woman, was admitted to the same alcohol rehabilitation service. Although presently unemployed, she had earned a Ph.D. and had worked full-time in a number of professional positions. She had a history of episodic heavy alcohol consumption which resulted in blackouts and several arrests for driving under the influence of alcohol. She was admitted twice in the past year for alcohol detoxification at a state hospital and spent one night in state prison for disorderly conduct. She stated that she suffered from extreme anxiety symptoms for which she had to drink or take several benzodiazepines in order to attend meetings at work. On the treatment unit she demonstrated mood lability and agitation. She left early against medical advice, with a diagnosis of alcohol dependence and borderline personality disorder.

Betty B. subsequently moved to another state to take a new job near her parents, but had similar problems. She reported intoxicated and hostile to a staff meeting at her new job and was fired. She was brought to a psychiatric hospital on the insistence of her family, where a detailed history revealed that her alcohol consumption increased during periods of hyperactivity, which included spending sprees and irritability. Her mother suffered from similar symptoms and also abused alcohol. Her mood was labile and she had not slept during the first three nights of hospitalization. These symptoms persisted despite detoxification. She was begun on lithium with the diagnosis of bipolar disorder, mixed type.

The patient has since returned to her home state and has remained on lithium. She denies any desire to drink and has been abstinent for over 2 years without the support of alcohol treatment but in psychiatric care. She has begun a new profession for which she is gaining recognition. She has expressed anger that her illness was not recognized and treated earlier, prior to the massive disruption in her life. She now reaches out to other patients to encourage their compliance with treatment.

These two cases represent patients who meet criteria for both a psychiatric and a substance use disorder. There have been several approaches to deal with the problem of classifying the dually diagnosed patient. One approach, as noted in the previous section, has been to historically identify the disorder that preceded the other and label that one primary. Obtaining an accurate history is difficult and may require family informational sources.[23] This approach does not allow for the development of late-onset psychiatric disorders. A heuristic model identifying transient and persistent symptom states has been proposed by Kranzler and Liebowitz.[24]

Case histories 5 and 6 illustrate descriptively the two symptom states in which substance-abusing patients may present psychiatric symptoms. The first, termed the transient state (Case 5), includes symptoms lasting for days or, at most, a few weeks. The intensity of the symptoms may be high, but it is not sustained. Patients may have a low-grade depressive or anxiety state with brief periods of exacerbation. Symptoms may be secondary to withdrawal or a reaction to psychosocial stressors that arose as a consequence of substance use. Treatment of the withdrawal reaction or simply the passage of time with continued abstinence will, by definition, result in resolution of these symptoms. Sometimes the transient nature of the symptoms is not so apparent because the individual does not allow a long enough period of sobriety to occur.

In contrast, Case 6 illustrates the persistent symptom state, which includes conditions for which psychiatrists are most often consulted. Symptoms may be intense and last periods of weeks to months. Although there may be diurnal variation or brief periods of decreased intensity, there is less variability in these symptoms than in the transient state. Untreated these states are much less likely to resolve spontaneously. Rather, they may become chronic with greater resultant morbidity and mortality.

Gerald A. (Case 5) is a complex case of a patient who had transient affective symptoms in relation to alcohol abuse. The transient nature of the symptoms was obscured by the lack of a sober period until the current hospitalization. The symptoms, however, were dramatic and had met criteria for an affective illness, leading the psychiatry staff to consider long-term treatment with lithium. However, the evident recent clinical improvement after detoxification suggested that the symptoms may have been only transiently drug induced.

The case of Betty B. (Case 6) represents a fairly clear example of the self-medication model of drug abuse. Betty B. manifested persistent psychiatric symptoms even during periods of abstinence and gave a history of episodic abuse coincident with exacerbation of psychiatric symptoms in an effort to ameliorate them. Had she remained under observation long enough during the original hospitalization, her underlying psychiatric disorder might have been recognized and treated.

As mentioned in the preceding section, data from the Epidemiologic Catchment Area study revealed substantial prevalence of substance use disorders and psychiatric illness in the general population.[25] Studies of the comorbidity of substance use and psychiatric disorders in both clinical samples and population surveys reveal morbid risks that are more than additive.[22] Our current nosology has addressed this only in a descriptive fashion.

The DSM-III-R[2] and the proposed ICD-10[3] incorporate a hierarchical system of diagnosing patients with more than one possible diagnosis. This is generally in the form of exclusionary criteria. For example, in considering a diagnosis of manic episode in the DSM-III-R, criterion F states: "It cannot be established that an organic factor initiated and maintained the disturbance" (p. 217). The ICD-10 is not so explicit, allowing for multiple diagnoses but suggesting the clinician identify the "main diagnosis" as that which is most relevant to the purpose for which the diagnoses are being collected.[3] Numerical priority, however, is given to the organic disorders. The proposed ICD-10 makes provision for a diagnosis of drug- or alcohol-induced residual state, subtypes of affective state, and late-onset, drug-induced psychotic disorder. The difficulty in these formulations is determination of whether the abused substance was etiological in the course of the psychiatric illness.

In clinical practice patients present with a spectrum of illness comorbidity. This population includes patients who seemingly have drug dependence as well as a sustained mental illness, i.e., dual diagnosis. The relationship between the substance abuse and major psychiatric illness appears to be bidirectional, with each affecting the other in one or more of the following ways: (1) a causal manner, (2) a predispositional relationship, or (3) in a way in which one serves to exacerbate the other. For example, in a 2.5-year follow-up study of opiate addicts, persistence of affective symptoms was associated with relapse in substance abuse.[26] This indicated that for addicts with affective symptoms each condition exacerbated the other.

Most of the commonly abused substances, including alcohol, opiates, sedatives, and stimulants, have been found to have negative effects on mood and anxiety in acute intoxication, chronic use, and withdrawal. These effects frequently are indistinguishable from the endogenous psychiatric syndromes except that most patients improve with abstinence. There is a subpopulation that has persistent symptoms, which left untreated increase the rapidity of relapse to substance use.[26] Similar conclusions can be drawn from patients presenting with drug abuse and psychosis. Tsuang et al.[17] noted that patients with drug abuse and psychotic symptoms of 6 months' or longer duration more closely resemble patients with schizophrenia in terms of family history of mental illness and course of outcome. In contrast, patients who presented with psychotic symptoms of less than 6 months' duration had a profile closer to the nonpsychotic drug-abusing population. A 10-year follow-up study further supported this finding.[27] Here again is an example of the psychiatric and substance use disorders interacting with each other but differently in different subpopulations.

In summary, current nosologic systems encourage evaluation of organic pathology, including substance abuse, prior to making a diagnosis of another major psychiatric syndrome. However, they do not address the interactional complexity of dually diagnosed individuals.

6. Use of the Multiaxial System

One of the hallmarks of descriptive psychiatry, as expressed in DSM and ICD, is the use of the multiaxial system.[28] The axes have been developed in accordance with the biopsychosocial model of psychiatry, to make diagnosis more comprehensive and clinically useful. The axes attempt to reliably and validly define dimensions of symptomatalogy. Inclusion and exclusion criteria help to standardize diagnosis. There have been difficulties in formulating criteria, which are not easily operationalized, and in using clinical judgment in diagnostic evaluation.[29]

Case 7: Alex B.

Alex B., a 61-year-old, white, married, childless, Ivy League graduate, combat veteran, unemployed for many years, was treated for alcoholism and bipolar illness. In outpatient treatment he received medication, and he and his wife were seen in couple's therapy. Their 35-year marriage involved mutual drinking and moderate physical abuse, both of which had increased since Mrs. B.'s retirement. The couple also had a history of debts to liquor stores, although they considered themselves to be misunderstood American gentry, unjustly rejected by other families. Unable to stay sober for more than a month at a time, Alex B. typically would stop his medication, become manic, start drinking, and get admitted to either the general psychiatry or alcohol service. The usual precipitant was marital conflict. His most recent alcohol admission came at the insistence of the couple's therapist.

On the unit, Alex B. responded well to cessation of alcohol and reinstatement of medication. He became an engaging, eloquent man, highly respected by his peers for his intelligence and temperament. Almost secretly, he called his wife at least twice daily, despite making plans to separate from her until both could attain some degree of stable sobriety. A couple's meeting was arranged with the alcohol counselor and family therapist. After some initial verbal abuse of the therapists from Mrs. B., Alex B. precipitously announced his plans to leave his wife. She was unconsolable; her verbal abuse and threats escalated, and she revealed that Alex B. had come home on his pass, a strict violation of his treatment contract, which was grounds for discharge.

Alex B. was discharged home and remained in touch with the alcohol program for several weeks. Staff surmised that if he stopped drinking, Mrs. B. would kill herself.

This case contains typical ingredients of chronic alcoholism in extreme form. As noted earlier, the interaction between substance use and other psychiatric disorders is not uncommon and can be quite disabling. Alex B.'s DSM-III-R multiaxial diagnoses are summarized in Table I.

Alcoholism, almost by definition, is associated with general decline in psychosocial and biological function.[4] Addiction without associated global dysfunction is often not considered a problem that requires diagnosis or treatment. Social and religious efforts to combat alcoholism predate medical intervention. The most strenuous efforts to eradicate alcoholism have been

Table I. Multiaxial Diagnostic Evaluation of Alex B.

Axis I. Clinical syndromes and conditions not attributable to a mental disorder
   303.90 Alcohol Dependence—Severe
   296.40 Bipolar Disorder, Manic
   V61.10 Marital Problem
Axis II. Developmental disorders and personality disorders
   799.90 Deferred (dependent and passive aggressive traits)
Axis III. Physical disorder or conditions
   None
Axis IV. Psychosocial stressors that contribute to present disorder
   Unemployment, retirement, continued drinking by both spouses, marital discord, physical abuse. (Severity: 3—moderate, predominantly enduring circumstances)
Axis V. Global assessment of functioning
   On admission: 30
   Highest functioning past year: 40

based on the recognition of its social, not necessarily medical, consequences. The Temperance Movement, perhaps the most systematic and successful attempt to eliminate alcoholism, was based substantially on the social and economic devastation brought about by excessive use of alcohol.[30] Contemporary efforts, such as Alcoholics Anonymous and employee assistance programs, emphasize fellowship and improved social, familial, and occupational function. The resulting improvement in self-esteem and quality of life are rewards for sobriety. Medical intervention for alcoholism aims at treating the medical sequelae of alcoholism. Psychiatric interventions are often targeted at identifying and treating other psychiatric illnesses that precipitate alcohol abuse and at teaching techniques to understand dependence and prevent relapse. Most treatment providers believe that medical and psychiatric interventions work best when coupled with the social emphasis provided by mutual-help groups such as Alcoholics Anonymous.

Social and familial disruption as well as significant decline in occupational function are commonly seen in alcohol dependence. As dependence progresses, the alcoholic's behavioral, intellectual, and emotional life becomes focused on the pursuit of alcohol and intoxication. Friends and family are neglected. Job performance becomes erratic. In some cases, friends and family abandon the drinker. Sometimes their relationships become cemented in dysfunctional, mutually reinforcing patterns.

Exacerbation of coexisting medical or psychological problems is frequent in alcoholism. Continued drinking in the face of aggravating other illnesses is often used to identify alcohol dependence.[2] The use of alcohol as a self-administered medication for affective disorder, anxiety, and somatic symptoms is thought to be widespread. A frequent consequence of this self-medication is the development of dependence. Another frequent complication is a rebound effect of increased psychiatric symptoms, either from intoxication or from withdrawal. A downward spiral develops as the psychiatric and dependence syndromes become mutually reinforcing.

Alex B.'s case illustrates many of these points and suggests the potential usefulness of applying the multiaxial diagnostic system to substance use disorders. In recognition that there are different aspects of mental disorder, a number of axial diagnostic systems have been proposed over the years. Each axial system includes a series of dimensions that its creators find useful in describing psychiatric conditions.

The biopsychosocial model of psychiatry is the basis for the axes used in DSM and ICD.[28] The international popularity of DSM-III attests to the usefulness of operationalizing the biopsychosocial model and to the ascendancy of descriptive psychiatry. The revised diagnostic scheme, DSM-III-R, is likely to be equally successful. The five axes describe signs and symptoms classically associated with different types of mental disorder as well as associated physical conditions, precipitating stressors, and recent and general level of functioning. Each axis is evaluated separately, but when taken together, they have the potential to describe the illness, its effect on the patient, and the vulnerability of the patient to stressors and symptoms. A carefully prepared, multiaxial diagnosis provides a thumbnail sketch of the patient which can be used to plan and evaluate clinical intervention as well as research.

Descriptive psychiatry as applied by DSM does not attempt to link diagnosis with etiology except in clearly defined physiological cases, such as certain dementias. This does not mean that descriptive psychiatry is atheoretical. Nor is it apolitical. The use of inclusion and exclusion criteria helps to standardize diagnosis and to make it more reliable and valid.

Rating scales help to standardize severity of illness. However, the choice of criteria and of diagnoses to be assigned psychiatric significance has become increasingly important with increasing use of DSM. These assignments have involved a great deal of negotiation in the international community. In the United States, assignment of DSM diagnoses has come to influence economic reimbursement for treatment. This has put pressure on the diagnostic system to define mental illness. A final comprehensive series of diagnostic criteria has not yet been set. The infinitely complicated nature of the brain and its diseases creates difficulties in formulating criteria that can be easily operationalized. No matter how precise descriptive criteria become, an imprecise arena requiring clinical judgment in diagnostic evaluation will always remain.

As with other psychiatric disorders, a brief but often vivid description of the substance abuser's predicament can be provided with thoughtful use of the DSM multiaxial system. Alex B.'s case can be used to highlight some advantages of using multiaxial diagnosis to define the extent of disorder, to suggest course of treatment, and to assign prognosis.

As noted earlier, alcoholism can be a cause or a result of affective or other Axis I diagnoses. For Alex B., alcoholism and bipolar illness seemed to be inseparable and mutually reinforcing. However, Alex B.'s marital problem was a force at least as potent as his dependence and affective disorder in maintaining his level of function. Marital discord is widely recognized as both an etiological factor and an outcome in alcoholism. Both the professional and the self-help treatment communities stress the importance of the family's contributions to maintaining sobriety or drinking behavior.

The DSM-III-R multiaxial system provides several options to specify relevant circumstances that influence the course of psychiatric illness. These are frequently overlooked. With Alex B., as with many alcoholics, the "V" codes can be used to draw attention to associated factors that are central to maintaining drinking behaviors. All but one are coded on Axis I. Similar codes have been adapted from the ICD-9-CM in the "Supplementary Classification of Factors Influencing Health Status and Contact with Health Services."[5] The V code may identify the most important focus for treatment. V-code conditions likely to be found in active alcoholism and associated with relapse include academic problems, adult antisocial behavior, noncompliance with medical treatment, occupational problems, and parent–child problems. Identification of these factors can aid the clinician in directing treatment, in both acute and chronic settings.

Alex B.'s Axis II diagnosis was slightly more controversial, in light of the Axis I diagnoses. While drinking and being engaged in the destructive relationship with his wife, Alex B. met many of the criteria for dependent and passive–aggressive personality disorders. Much of this disappeared during his brief admission, leaving staff uncomfortable about making a baseline Axis II diagnosis. Anecdotally, Axis II diagnoses often change between periods of active drinking and sobriety.

In this case, there is no Axis III diagnosis. However, Axis III can highlight medical sequelae of alcohol dependence and draw attention to advanced or life-threatening disease. Other medical illnesses that may be psychological stressors or may provide contraindications for pharmacotherapy are also listed on this axis. Axis III can be helpful in assessing stage of illness and prognosis.

Axis IV, which identifies severity of psychosocial stressors, gives another option to specify circumstances influencing the course of illness. It, too, can be helpful in developing a prognosis and designing treatment. It gives information about the patient's current life-style and also about vulnerability to stressors. An alcoholic who relapses under conditions of mild stress carries a poorer prognosis than one who relapses only under catastrophic conditions. The brief description of stressors may alert the clinician to the life-style factors that maintain sobriety. A brief listing of stressors, including an indication of whether the nature of the stressor is acute or chronic, is followed by an overall estimate of level of stress.

Axis V, the Global Assessment of Functioning Scale, describes the extent of psychological and social impairment. This can be used to estimate prognosis and identify long-term treatment needs.

The multiaxial system does not solve all problems of diagnosis. Despite efforts to clarify the cutoff points for abuse and dependence, there are still gray areas. The primary–secondary distinction may never be known in all cases of psychiatric comorbidity. Descriptive psychiatry does not assign etiologies, because at this time, etiologies are largely unknown. However, careful use of the DSM axes can provide a brief, but thorough sketch of the alcoholic which can be useful in planning treatment.

7. Conclusion

The cases presented and discussed in this chapter provide ample testimony to the complexity of diagnosing substance use disorders in the clinical setting and the variety of associated features that must be taken into account to understand and manage persons who are dependent. Advances have been made in the conceptualization of dependence, the formulation of diagnostic criteria, and the development of interview procedures to operationalize concepts. Nevertheless, a number of unresolved issues remain.

At a fundamental level, the difficulties of diagnosing alcohol and drug disorders are related to the applicability of the disease concept and the medical model to psychoactive substance use. The medical model is a way of viewing a patient's *dis-ease* as *disease,* although critics have viewed it more in terms of psychiatrists' attempt to establish medical hegemony over psychological phenomena by equating behavior disorder with underlying physical causes. In addition to the biological disease model of substance use disorders, psychiatrists have also incorporated psychological disease models into clinical practice. The psychoanalytic model is the clearest example of this. Less theoretical psychodynamic approaches, such as those illustrated by the primary–secondary distinction, have also been influential. While psychiatrists have assumed primary responsibility for the management of substance use disorders in this country, psychologists, despite their skepticism of the disease concept, have found the medical model compatible with their emphasis on psychological and environmental interventions.

Other objections that have been raised to the medical model of dependence, as represented in the nomenclature and classification systems, are that the labeling of persons as alcohol or drug dependent creates psychological stigma, provides substance users with a socially accepted excuse for their behavior, and acts as an impediment to the individual's ability to change without medical management. Although these are provocative notions that have gained some degree of acceptance in psychology and sociology, there is little evidence to support them. Despite the philosophical and political objections that have been advanced, these have had little influence on the continued integration of dependence concepts within the medical nomenclatures and psychiatric classification systems.

Nevertheless, the adoption of a generic dependence syndrome concept as the basis for national and international classifications of psychoactive substances is an invitation to conduct research that will evaluate the major assumptions of this model. That research should determine the independence of substance-related problems from the dependence elements themselves, the actual coherence of dependence symptoms into a clinical syndrome, and the generalizability of the dependence concept across drugs and across cultural groups. To the extent that consistency is found across disparate samples of alcoholics and users of other substances in different cultures, the case for a universal dependence syndrome would be strengthened. Since cultural context is an important determinant of both substance use patterns and related consequences, an organizing principle that has cross-cultural applicability is desirable, especially in the context of ICD.

Another set of unresolved issues concerns the practical problems of diagnosing alcohol and drug dependence. As the case histories in this chapter illustrate, the process of conducting a clinical interview, mental status examination, and psychiatric history in order to arrive at a multiaxial evaluation of the patient is complex and difficult. Factors that influence this process are the skills of the clinician, the physical and mental condition of the patient, the amount of time devoted to the evaluation, the rapport established with the patient, and patients' perception of the situation as threatening or in their own best interest. A major question for future consideration in the development of diagnostic procedures is the extent to which current concepts can be translated into effective clinical practice. For example, how valid is the procedure of making DSM-III-R substance use diagnoses on the basis of a single clinical interview? Intake personnel at treatment facilities often rely on single interviews to determine diagnoses. The complex histories of the patients reviewed in this chapter suggest that important clinical information becomes available only after prolonged observation and history taking.

Finally, this chapter highlights a number of variables that color the clinical picture in complex ways. Polysubstance use makes it more difficult to classify substance use disorders according to individual drugs. Other mental and physical disorders, which may be either primary or secondary to substance use, further complicate the diagnostic task. Three descriptive models that attempt to deal with this complexity are discussed: primary–secondary, transient–persistent states, and biopsychosocial. Conducting the evaluation along multiple dimensions of the multiaxial schema provides valuable insights into the underlying dynamics of substance use disorders, primarily because personality factors, developmental disorders, and psychosocial stressors all affect natural history and prognosis.

ACKNOWLEDGMENTS. The writing of this chapter was supported in part by grants from the National Institute on Alcohol Abuse and Alcoholism (AA07290, AA03510, and AA06558).

References

1. American Psychiatric Association: *Diagnostic and Statistical Manual of Mental Disorders*, 3rd edition. Washington, DC, APA, 1980.
2. American Psychiatric Association: *Diagnostic and Statistical Manual of Mental Disorders*, 3rd edition, revised. Washington, DC, APA, 1987.
3. World Health Organization: *I.C.D. 10, 1988*, Draft of Chapter V, Categories F00–F99, Mental, behavioral and developmental disorders: Clinical descriptions and diagnostic guidelines. Geneva, World Health Organization, 1988.
4. Babor TF, Kranzler HR, Kadden RM: Issues in the definition and diagnosis of alcoholism: Implications for a reformulation. *Progress Neuro-Psychopharmacol Biol Psychiatry* 10:113–128, 1986.
5. World Health Organization: *International Classification of Disease*, rev. 9. Geneva, World Health Organization, 1978.
6. Edwards G, Arif A, Hodgson R: Nomenclature and classification of drug- and alcohol-related problems: A WHO memorandum. *Bull WHO* 59:225–242, 1981.
7. Rounsaville BJ, Spitzer RL, Williams JBW: Proposed changes in the DSM-III substance use disorders: Description and rationale. *Am J Psychiatry* 143:463–468, 1986.
8. Woodward R: *Wired: The Short Life and Fast Times of John Belushi.* New York, Simon & Schuster, 1984.

9. Edwards G: Drinking in longitudinal perspective: Career and natural history. *Br J Addiction* 79:175–182, 1984.
10. Bray RM, Hubbard RL, Valley RJ, Cavanaugh ER, Craddock SG, Collino JJ, Schlenger WE, Allison M: Characteristics, behaviors, and intreatment outcomes 1979—TOPS admission cohort. Research Triangle Park, NC, Center for the Study of Social behavior: Research Triangle Institute Projects 230-1500 and 234-1901.
11. Babor TF, Dolinsky ZS: Alcoholic typologies: Historical evolution and empirical evaluation of some common classification schemes, in Rose, RM, Barrett, JE (eds): *Alcoholism: Origins and Outcome.* New York, Raven Press, 1988.
12. Meyer RE, Babor TF, Mirkin PM: Typologies in alcoholism: An overview. *Int J Addict* 18(2):235–249, 1983.
13. Tarter RE, McBride H, Buonpane N, and Schneider D: Differentiation of alcoholics; childhood history of minimal brain dysfunction, family history, and drinking pattern. *Arch Gen Psychiatry* 34:761–768, 1977.
14. Alterman AL, Petrarulo E, Tarter R, Edwards KL: Hyperactivity and alcoholism: Familial and behavioral correlates. *Addict Behav* 7:413–421, 1982.
15. Kellam SG, Ensminger PE, Simon MD: Mental health in first grade and teenage drug, alcohol, and cigarette use. *Drug Alcohol Dependence* 5(4):273–304, 1980.
16. Helzer JE, Przybeck TR: The co-occurrence of alcoholism with other psychiatric disorders in the general population and its impact on treatment. *J Stud Alcohol* 49:219–224, 1988.
17. Tsuang MT, Simpson JC, Kronfol Z: Subtypes of drug abuse with psychosis. *Arch Gen Psychiatry* 39:141–147, 1982.
18. Brown SA, Schuckit M: Changes in depression among abstinent alcoholics. *J Stud Alcohol* 49:412–417, 1988.
19. Hesselbrock M, Hesselbrock V, Syzmanski K, Weideman, M: Suicide attempts and alcoholism. *J Stud Alcohol* 49:436–442, 1988.
20. Penick EG, Powell BJ, Liskow BI, Jackson JO, Nickel EJ: The stability of coexisting psychiatric syndromes in alcoholic men after one year. *J Stud Alcohol* 49:395–405, 1988.
21. Rounsaville BJ, Dolinsky ZS, Babor TF, Meyer RE: Psychopathology as a predictor of treatment outcome in alcoholics. *Arch Gen Psychiatry* 44:505–513, 1987.
22. Robins LN, Helzer JB, Przybeck TR: Epidemiological perspective on alcoholism: ECA data, in Rose RM, Barrett JE (eds): *Alcoholism: Origins and Outcome.* New York, Raven Press, 1988.
23. Schuckit M: The clinical implications of primary diagnostic groups among alcoholics. *Arch Gen Psychiatry* 42:1043–1049, 1985.
24. Kranzler H, Liebowitz N: Anxiety and depression in substance abuse: Clinical implications. *Med Clin North Am* 72:867–885, 1988.
25. Myers JK, Weissman MN, Tischler GL, Holzer CE, Leaf PJ, Ovaschel H, Anthony JC, Boyd JH, Burke JD, Kramer M, Stoltzman R: Six-month prevalence of psychiatric disorders in three communities. *Arch Gen Psychiatry* 41:959–967, 1984.
26. Kosten T, Rounsaville B, Kleber H: A 2.5 year follow-up of depression, life crises and treatment effects on abstinence among opioid addicts. *Arch Gen Psychiatry* 43:733–738, 1986.
27. Perkins K, Simpson J, Tsuang M: Ten-year follow-up of drug abusers with acute or chronic psychosis. *Hosp Community Psychiatry* 37:481–484, 1986.
28. Strauss JS: A comprehensive approach to psychiatric diagnosis. *Am J Psychiatry* 132:1193–1197, 1975.
29. Tischler GL: Evaluation of DSM-III, in Kaplan HI, Sadock BJ (eds): *Comprehensive Textbook of Psychiatry,* 4th edition. Baltimore, Williams and Wilkins, 1985, pp. 617–621.
30. Babor TF, Rosenkrantz BG: Public health, public morals and public order: Social science and liquor control in Massachusetts: 1880–1916, in Barrows S, Room R (eds.): *The Social History of Alcohol: Drinking and Culture in Modern Society.* Berkeley, University of California Press, in press.

Social Deviancy and Alcohol Dependence

Alfonso Paredes, Section Editor

Complex clinical syndromes such as the addictive disorders may be explained at various levels. Each of these levels is the domain of a particular science with its own descriptive language and methodology. Explanations at lower levels, such as the molecular, biochemical, and physiological, are more amenable to quantification and to the application of mathematical models. Investigators who assume that causality rises from the lowest hierarchical levels of knowledge to the higher appreciate these approaches. This is reflected by the current enthusiasm for genetic, biochemical, and physiological explanations and the wariness with explanations that attempt to reach higher levels of understanding. Some investigators feel it may be possible to account for the signs and symptoms of alcoholism and related personality traits in terms of underlying pathophysiological mechanisms involving neural systems with modulators such as dopamine, serotonin, and epinephrine. It is also emphasized that different fields of research may contribute important information.[1]

Higher-level explanations at the behavioral or social levels work with perhaps less reliably quantified data; however, these data offer variables highly predictive of relevant features of alcohol and drug use and the addictive disorders. Eventually explanatory models will have to be constructed that incorporate horizontal explanations deriving from particular sciences into vertical constructs that use information from all relevant hierarchical levels of knowledge.[2]

This section is concerned with the role of social factors in alcohol dependence and other substance addictions. Through the various chapters it will become increasingly evident why in discussions on alcohol dependence it is important to consider other drug dependencies. By the same token, analyses of drug dependence require a review of the implications of alcohol use. Ado-

Alfonso Paredes • Brentwood Division, West Los Angeles VA Medical Center, and Department of Psychiatry, School of Medicine, University of California–Los Angeles, Los Angeles, California 90073.

lescent as well as adult behavior is covered in the following chapters. This provides a longitudinal perspective which should give a more accurate view of the nature of addictive disorders.

In the first chapter, Kathleen K. Bucholz examines the correlates of alcohol use and alcohol problems in adolescence. She points out that there is considerable consensus in the literature regarding the relevant correlates regardless of the populations investigated. Certain demographic, social, and psychiatric variables are consistently associated with alcohol use among adolescents. Particular factors are age, ethnicity, religion, parental attributes, and peer influences. Bucholz also reviews the role of peer group influence. An association between peers who drink and alcohol consumption in adolescents has been found. However, she points out that it is not clear whether adolescents seek involvement with drug-using peers because they intend to use the drug. Research on adolescence has established that alcohol use precedes exposure to other illicit substances (see Chapter 5). This is an important aspect to examine since understanding of the correlates of adolescent alcohol use will help us to understand other drug use.

Kazuo Yamaguchi, author of the chapter on drug use and its social covariates from adolescence to young adulthood, points out that sociodemographic and contextual variables, such as the youth's age, age at the onset of drug use, family and work roles, and the influence of significant others, correlate in specific ways with drug use. The period of transition from adolescence to young adulthood is a critical time during which the risk of initiating the use of drugs such as marijuana is high. Early exposure to drugs predicts a longer period of lifetime use and increases the probabilities of progression in their use. Current and former marijuana habit increases the probabilities of becoming a consumer of other illicit drugs. Yamaguchi makes interesting observations on the progression from marijuana to other drugs. Drinking of alcoholic beverages, as indicated earlier, plays a significant role. Youths who postpone the onset of alcohol drinking are at a lesser risk of initiating the use of drugs such as marijuana (see Chapter 8).

Several interactions have been observed between marijuana use and other social behaviors. For example, current use of marijuana postpones the timing of marriage and reduces the probability of getting married. Current marijuana use during marriage is associated with a postponement of parenthood and reduces the probabilities of becoming a parent. Parenthood after marriage increases the probability of discontinuing the marijuana habit.

Certain sexual and reproductive behaviors are associated with illicit drug use. Users are more likely to undergo an abortion and less likely to have children after marriage. It is apparent that there is incompatibility between marijuana use and conventional adult family roles.

Health professionals working daily with problems of alcohol or drug dependence, observe that patients under their care often report using more than one addicting drug. Empirical data support this impression. Yih-Ing

Hser and associates, in their chapter on the longitudinal patterns of alcohol use by narcotics addicts, note that use of alcohol and drugs may be concurrent or alternating. Their research with opiate addicts describes periods of alcohol abuse during abstinence from opiates alternating with periods of opiate use. Some patients continue to drink excessively while on opiates, thus exhibiting a concurrent abuse pattern. A drug may be consumed during periods of abstinence from other drugs or concurrently with other drugs to enhance effects, to counteract undesirable effects, or to substitute for the preferred drugs that may not be available or are difficult to procure. Hser's longitudinal perspectives derive from follow-up studies of opiate addicts covering a period of more than 20 years. This follow-up provides a good picture of the addiction phenomena. Only a relatively small proportion of the patients investigated were able to achieve a drug-free life-style. Alcohol and drug addiction emerge as chronic and progressive disorders. For example, drinking assessed at the time of the first and the second interview several years later showed greater levels of consumption at the time of the last assessment (see Chapter 7).

Stanley W. Sadava, who authors the chapter on problem drinking and alcohol problems, is impressed by the fact that among normal-population drinkers the incidence and intensity of alcohol-related problems are only modestly related to the level of alcohol consumption. This is used as a point of departure to examine the factors that may contribute to the differential vulnerability to problems among drinkers. He points out that we must widen research on the circle of covariation beyond alcohol-specific factors.[3] He appears to be strongly influenced by Jessor, who felt that becoming a drinker is an integral part of the process of adolescent development. Abstainers differ from youth who drink in a number of characteristics reflecting a pattern of conventionality, i.e., greater value on achievement or successful performance in school setting, less value on independence relative to achievement, greater intolerance of deviant behavior, greater religiosity, greater involvement with parents and friends whose outlook is similar to that of the parents, fewer friends who drink and friends who approve less of drinking, and greater involvement with church and concern with grades in school, while there is less involvement in general transgression. This pattern of conventionality tends to erode with time irrespective of drinking status or drug use.[4]

Proneness to the use of drugs such as marijuana also results from the existence of a coherent and integrated pattern of specific psychosocial attributes within the personality, the perceived environment, and other behavior systems. Concerning personality, those at risk place greater value on independence than on academic achievement. They have lower expectations for academic achievement, greater tolerance of deviance, and less religiosity. In the area of the perceived environment system, there is less compatibility between the adolescent's two major reference groups, parents and friends, less influence of parents relative to friends, and greater approval for peers who serve as models for marijuana use and other problem behaviors. In the behavior system, there is greater actual involvement in other problem behaviors and less participation in conventional activities.[5]

Sadava asserts that a set of behaviors including cigarette smoking, drinking alcoholic beverages, illicit drug use, certain forms of political activism, illegal or delinquent behaviors, and precocious sexual involvement correlate negatively with conventional behaviors such as church and school attendance. Behaviors such as low abidance for the law, criminal activities, early sexual involvement, and low academic performance correlate positively with teenage multiple drug use. Drinking and illicit drug use are therefore considered just some elements within a matrix of related behaviors.[3]

Developmental features of the nuclear family are mentioned by the section's authors. These affect not only the tendency to alcohol problems and their consequences, but also the evolution of drinking behavior. Characteristics such as poor relationships between parents are significantly associated with increased alcohol consumption. A developmental factor impacting on substance abuse is parental loss, whether through death, desertion, marital breakup, or inability of parents to relate emotionally to their children. Dysfunctional parental—marital behavior predicts a greater probability of drug involvement by the offspring in the use of illicit drugs. Progression from marijuana use to other drugs is also to a great extent related to dysfunctional marital–parental behaviors. This is confirmed by a body of research that has amply documented that social interaction within the family during childhood and adolescence plays a major role in determining the mental health of individuals.[6]

I have presented highlights from the chapters of this section. Eventually we may have to frame this information within a conceptual framework. Talcott Parsons[3] has proposed that social systems consist of networks of interactive relationships in which the members of a system orient their actions according to certain value standards. Membership in such collectivities is characterized by patterns of solidarity obligations that conform with defined cultural expectations. Alienative experiences, such as severe conflict during critical periods of development, may lead to movement within a conformity—deviancy dimension. Deviancy, a probable result, is a tendency to behave in contraversion with one or more institutionalized normative patterns. Some elements of this behavior are rebelliousness and withdrawal. Drinking and the use of illicit drugs are just a few among this range of behaviors identified as problem behaviors.

Preventive as well as therapeutic interventions to promote movement toward the conventional pole will require the design of schedules of resocialization to reduce alienative need dispositions and help the person to move in the expected direction within the conformity–deviancy dimension. Development of a pattern of solidarity obligations close to the conformity pole would have to be encouraged. Rational interventions will not be functional if they are focused on only a few problematic behaviors, such as drinking or drug use, which occupy just a segment of the total drinking pattern. Furthermore, drinking and drug use are corporate behaviors that require the cooperation and participation of members of particular subsystems.

Design of successful intervention models remains a challenge. The data presented suggest that research on the broad interactions between social variables and alcohol and drugs is a fruitful avenue to follow in our investigations. Building of such a database is required before we can create successful intervention models.

References

1. Cloninger CR: Neurogenetic adaptive mechanisms in alcoholism. *Science* 236:410–415, 1987.
2. Blois MS: Medicine and the nature of vertical reasoning. *N Engl J Med* 318:847–851, 1988.
3. Parsons T: *The Social System*. New York, Free Press, 1951.
4. Jessor R, Jessor SL: Adolescent development and the onset of drinking. *J Stud Alcohol* 36:27–51, 1975.
5. Jessor R, Chase JA, Donovan JE: Psychosocial correlates of marijuana use and problem drinking in a national sample of adolescents. *Am J Public Health* 70:604–613, 1980.
6. Bowlby J: Developmental psychiatry comes of age. *Am J Psychiatry* 145:1–10, 1988.

A Review of Correlates of Alcohol Use and Alcohol Problems in Adolescence

Kathleen K. Bucholz

Abstract. The literature on correlates of adolescent alcohol use has generally identified similar correlates, despite differences in types of populations studied, definitions of both alcohol use and potential correlates, and time periods over which use is assessed. Still at issue, however, is the relative importance of each correlate. This chapter summarizes the principal findings from recent literature about demographic, social, and psychiatric correlates of adolescent alcohol use. Given that part of an effective national antidrug policy will be curbing society's appetite for drugs, which begins in adolescence and in which alcohol plays a large role, it is a propitious time to call for more intensive inquiry into the mechanisms underlying the above-identified correlates of adolescent alcohol use.

1. Introduction

Research on stages of adolescent drug use has established that alcohol use precedes use of illicit substances.[1] Therefore, understanding the correlates of adolescent alcohol use is important. If the stages represent a causal chain, reducing exposure to alcohol use by capitalizing on what is known about adolescent alcohol users would induce a reduction in use of illicit substances.

There is little controversy over correlates of adolescent alcohol use. The few disagreements concern not the correlates themselves, but the relative importance of each among all that are related to adolescent alcohol use. Research findings have generally identified the same correlates, regardless of the type of adolescent population being studied, definitions of alcohol use, time periods over which use is assessed, and ways in which potential correlates are defined. Indeed, the consistent pattern of correlates that has emerged

Kathleen K. Bucholz • Department of Psychiatry, The Jewish Hospital at Washington University School of Medicine, St. Louis, Missouri 63110.

despite the above-noted differences is a strength of this literature. A recent dividend accruing from the consistency of findings is that attention may now be given to theoretical explanations for adolescent alcohol and other psychoactive substance use, a research endeavor that, up to now with few exceptions,[2,3] has been largely overlooked.

Adolescent populations that have been studied include those from the United States as a whole,[4-8] specific states and provinces,[2,9-11] rural areas,[12,13] specific cities,[14] and specific schools and treatment facilities.[15-18] Definitions of alcohol use have ranged from simple overall frequency of drinking,[5,12] quantity of alcohol consumed linked with frequency of drinking occurrences,[10,11,13,16,19] quantity–frequency together with negative consequences experienced,[4,6,20] to outright substance abuse and/or dependence based on specific diagnostic criteria.[18] Time periods over which alcohol use is assessed have ranged from lifetime use[8] to use during the last 7 days.[16] Other correlates examined include socioeconomic status, parental and peer influences, school achievement, personality characteristics, general deviant behavior, and others, but many of these are not defined in the same way across studies, complicating comparability. For example, some of the ways in which peer influences, which have been strongly linked to alcohol use, have been measured include friends' approval of drinking,[4] parents' approval of friends,[5] friends' drug use,[21] and proportion of friends who get drunk on a weekly basis.[10]

The present task is to provide in a capsule the principal findings from the recent literature (since 1978) about the demographic, social, and newly emerging psychiatric correlates of adolescent alcohol use and problem use. Two excellent reviews of the literature with rich details about relevant literature published prior to 1978 are available to which readers are referred.[6,22] In general, the literature reviewed here reflects those studies using large, representative samples of adolescents. Most of the studies covered here report univariate or bivariate results. Relatively few have carried out multivariable analyses to assess the relative contribution of a number of potential influences. Furthermore, of the studies conducting multivariable analyses, results are often reported for groups of variables, and not for each correlate separately, so that the contributions of an individual variable from both univariate and multivariable perspectives are not always available. Thus, the present summary reflects principally the univariate relationships that have been found, but, wherever possible, also presents evidence about whether the relationships persist in a multivariable framework.

Discussion of correlates is organized into the following categories, based on the review by Blane and Hewitt[22]: demographic (e.g., age, gender, ethnicity, religion, socioeconomic status); parental attributes (e.g., parental relationships, parental attitudes toward drinking, and drinking behavior); peer influences (e.g., attitudes, actual drinking behavior, and group membership); personality and personal values (e.g., subscription to traditional values such as doing well in school and religion and personal characteristics, such as, sense of alienation, degree of self-esteem); and last, psychiatric correlates, including general deviant behavior and depressive symptomatology.

2. Demographic Correlates

2.1. Age

Without exception, studies have found that alcohol users, heavy drinkers, and problem drinkers were older than abstainers, nonheavy users, and nonproblem drinkers. Lowman,[23] summarizing findings from a large national study,[6] reported sharp increases in weekly drinking and heavy drinking between tenth and twelfth grades. Donovan and Jessor[4] found that problem drinkers, whether defined by frequency of drunkenness in the last year, number of negative consequences, or both, were significantly older than nonproblem drinkers. Multivariable analyses established that older age was both a significant discriminator between abstainers and drinkers as well as a significant predictor of absolute alcohol consumed per day.[10]

2.2. Gender

Most studies report that males were more likely than females to be drinkers, heavy drinkers, and problem drinkers. Gender differences were especially apparent in the heavy drinking category. For example, Lowman[23] reported that 33% of boys, compared to 21% of girls, drank on a weekly basis, but 21% of boys, compared to only 9% of girls, were classified as weekly heavy drinkers. Similarly, Zucker and Harford[7] found the sharpest gender differences in the heavy drinking categories, where more than twice as many boys as girls were heavy drinkers. Rates of problem drinking among boys exceeded those among girls (23% vs. 15%).[4] One exception to these findings was a survey of Canadian adolescents,[11] in which more girls than boys aged 14–16 reported regular use of most psychoactive substances, including alcohol. However, the inferred abstention rate among boys (46%) was considerably higher than that reported in other studies, suggesting that this may not be a typical group of boys. In studies using multivariable analyses, males were more likely than females to be drinkers than abstainers and had higher average daily alcohol consumption.[10]

2.3. Ethnicity

Studies have shown that white adolescents have the greatest prevalence of alcohol use, heavy use, and problem drinking.[7,8,23,26] Black adolescents were more likely than white adolescents to be nondrinkers and in general have rates of other drinking levels much lower than those of whites, particularly for heavy drinking. For example, ratios of white to black rates show a steady increase from any lifetime use, monthly use, weekly use, to weekly heavy use[23]: 1.07, 1.35, 1.58, and 4.0, respectively. In addition, fewer black adolescents were classified as alcohol misusers.[24] Others have reported similar findings.[7] One reservation is that these findings may not accurately reflect rates in all black adolescents, since only enrolled student populations and not dropouts (many of whom are black) are studied. However, mitigating this objection is that similar observations about the lower prevalences of drinking among blacks have been made in adult populations.[25]

Black adolescents have also been found to consume significantly less alcohol per day than white adolescents. However, Asian, not white, adolescents had the highest amounts of daily alcohol consumption.[10,26] However, mean number of alcohol-related problems per ounce of alcohol consumed was highest among male and female black adolescents.[26] These findings mirror observations from studies in adult populations.[25]

2.4. Religion

Adolescents from Catholic families were more likely to be both drinkers and heavier drinkers than their Protestant peers.[7,24] Even though a higher proportion of Jewish adolescents were drinkers compared to their Christian peers, some studies have reported lower rates of heavy or problem drinking among Jewish, compared to non-Jewish, adolescents.[22] A recent study[7] did not corroborate this finding, but the extremely small sample of Jewish adolescents in the study suggests that these findings ought to be interpreted cautiously. It is a well-established finding of adult alcohol research, however, that Jews have uncommonly low rates of alcoholism and of problem drinking.[25]

2.5. Socioeconomic Status

Socioeconomic status is perhaps one area in which the literature is equivocal. Complicating generalizations of findings regarding socioeconomic status are the variety of ways in which socioeconomic status has been measured. Most common include parental educational level, family income, occupational status of father and/or mother, or some combination of these. Of five studies published since 1978 in which parental educational level was assessed, there were four significant associations (two positive, two negative) and one nonsignificant association. The positive associations included one with number of times intoxicated in the last year[21] and the other with any alcohol use in the last year.[8] The two negative associations included one with heavy drinking[7] and one with problem drinking (but males only).[4] Finally, regular alcohol use was not significantly associated with parental education.[11] In two studies carried out in different geographical settings, family income was not significantly related to alcohol use.[11,12] However, another study found that subjects' own earned income was positively related to alcohol consumption.[15] Mother's high occupational level was positively associated with both amount usually consumed and heavy drinking[13] and with substance abuse in general.[18] Few studies conducted multivariable analyses; those that did generally found weak relationships between socioeconomic status and alcohol use, once other factors were taken into account.[13,21]

3. Parental Attributes

Parental drinking behavior, parental attitudes toward alcohol, and, less typically, quality of parental associations (both parent-to-parent and parent-to-child) are the most commonly studied family influences on adolescent drinking behavior. Blane and Hewitt[22] noted other factors that have been studied including family size, birth order, and family structure, but these have not been prominent in recent publications. Usually, information about parental characteristics is based on adolescent report; parents are rarely queried independently.

Of the three potential influences, drinking behavior of parents would be expected to exert the most effect on adolescent drinking, since parents serve as models for children. In general, this expectation is confirmed. Donovan and Jessor[4] reported, in univariate analyses, that female problem drinkers saw more parental models for drinking than did nonproblem drinkers. Rachal et al.[6] found that over half the adolescents whose parents did not drink, compared to only 12% of those with at least one regularly drinking parent, abstained. At the other end of the drinking spectrum, the proportion of heavy drinkers was greater among those with at least one regularly drinking parent, compared to those whose parents did not drink. Schwartz et al.[17] reported that adolescents in the high-alcohol-use group were significantly more likely to report that a family member drank alcohol daily than those in the low-use group. Brook et al.[27] reported a significant positive association between paternal alcohol use and initiation of alcohol use. Alcoholism in first-degree relatives was more common among substance abusers than nonabusers; it was present in 35% of abusers, compared to 20% and 13% of users and low users, respectively.[18]

In a complex path-modeling process, Hansen et al.[16] found that adults' alcohol use had only a weak influence on adolescents' alcohol use. However, several methodological considerations merit attention; the construct was not specific to parents and did not ascertain either regularity or quantity of use. Moreover, the students were very young adolescents, perhaps not comparable to other studies with older high-school students. Other studies using multivariable analyses have often grouped parental drinking behavior with other variables representing "perceived environment." The overall effect of this group of variables has often been significant, but the grouping has prevented a separate assessment of parental drinking behavior.[4,19]

Still other studies have assessed the effect of perceived approval of parents toward adolescent drinking. The findings are as one would expect. In studies measuring perceived parental approval of drinking,[4,6,10] more of the heavier drinkers reported parental approval of drinking than those who were not heavy drinkers. Furthermore, the effect of parental approval persisted in multivariable analyses, in which students whose parents approved of adolescents drinking had much higher daily alcohol consumption than those whose parents disapproved.[10]

Less often studied, poor quality of family relationships (e.g., parent–child interactions, parent-to-parent relationship) is also associated with adolescent drinking behavior. A recent study[12] found that poor relationships between parents significantly increased the frequency of adolescent alcohol consumption.

4. Peer Influences

Peer influences on adolescent drinking have received considerable attention, although there have been only a few studies to consider peer influence as one of a variety of influences on adolescent drinking, thereby permitting an assessment of how important these influences are.[2,4,10,16,27] As Blane and Hewitt[22] noted, some researchers view adolescent drinking as a function of peer groups, while others argue that parental influence intercedes with, and may even moderate, peer influence. The types of influences that have been studied include peer pressure to drink, peer attitudes toward alcohol use, and use of alcohol by peers. As with measures of parental attributes, peer measures are based on self-reports by adolescents about their friends' attitudes, alcohol use, and pressuring them to drink. Studies have linked these influences to adolescent drinking, heavy drinking, and problem drinking.

Rachal et al.[6] noted that peer pressure to drink has been found to have a weak relationship with adolescent drinking levels, particularly in comparison to the effects of peer attitudes toward alcohol use and peer drinking behavior. This assertion was based on the fact that adolescents have rarely cited as primary reasons for drinking either gaining peer acceptance or avoiding peer derision. Donovan and Jessor[4] reported that while univariate analysis established that problem drinkers saw more pressure for drinking than non-problem drinkers, both friends' approval of, and models for, drinking behavior were stronger influences in a multivariable framework. A survey of high-school students[28] found that most felt little or no pressure to drink. However, a study of younger (junior high school) Native American and Anglo-American students revealed that 53% and 38%, respectively, reported using alcohol because of peer pressure.[29] It may be that peer pressure is an age-dependent phenomenon, but such a generalization, not yet supported by existing data, awaits future analyses.

A second indicator of peer influence has been the perceived attitudes of one's contemporaries toward drinking. In general, a majority of those who reported that their friends disapproved of teenage drinking were abstainers, while at the opposite end of the spectrum, the greatest proportion of heavy drinkers was found among those who reported friends' approval of teenage drinking.[6] In a similar vein, problem drinkers reported significantly more approval of drinking by their friends than did nonproblem drinkers.[4]

The strongest relationships with adolescent drinking, however, have been with reported peer drinking levels. Study findings generally support the assertion that adolescent drinking behavior resembles that of their peers. The more one's peers use alcohol, the more likely one is to be a drinker, a heavy drinker, or a problem drinker.[4,6,10] Ninety-six percent of those whose friends were drinkers also drank, but only 35% of those whose friends did not drink were drinkers.[6] Well over half of those whose companions did not drink at all were abstainers, while one-third of those who reported all companions as drinkers were heavy drinkers.[6] In discriminant analysis, the proportion of friends who got drunk weekly was the strongest differentiator of abstainers and drinkers, and also was a significant positive predictor of mean daily alcohol consumption.[10] Multivariable analyses identified friends' use of alcohol as the strongest predictor of intensity of alcohol use,[2] and in another study, of any consumption of beer or liquor, as well as the frequency of intoxication.[21]

What is not clear, as Blane and Hewitt have pointed out, is the explanation for these findings: Do adolescents select friends on the basis of alcohol use behavior that is similar to their own, or to their intended eventual alcohol use behavior? Or is the peer group itself the stimulation for alcohol use? For the most part, data analyzed thus far have been cross-sectional, which has precluded determination of which alternative is the more likely. Longitudinal studies hold promise for resolving this issue, but thus far, we have been unable to identify a study that has monitored adolescents' intentions to use drugs along with examining peer group affiliations. Some longitudinal evidence is suggestive of an effect of the peer group itself. A 2-year follow-up study of nonusers of alcohol at the index interview revealed that commencing regular use of alcohol during the follow-up period was linked to a high degree of involvement in drug-using peer groups at the index interview.[27] It may still be that adolescents choose to become involved with drug-using peers because they intend to use drugs, even though the drug use itself may occur much later than affiliation with the group.

Evidence of the relative importance of peer, compared to parental, influences has favored peer influences as being the more important,[2,4,10,16] although one study suggested that positive parental influences may offset negative peer influences,[27] at least in relation to the initiation of weekly alcohol use. More research is needed to tease out the effect of peers, compared to that of parents, in relation to drinking levels, particularly problem drinking. In at least one study, problem drinkers ascribed more influence to their friends than to their parents,[4] bringing up the possibility of a group of adolescents that might be differentially vulnerable to peer suasion.

Finally, one study has partitioned types of peer influences in an effort to discern whether certain types of peer interactions may actually prevent alcohol use.[30] The authors found that adolescents with a high level of activity in ad hoc peer groups (defined as unsupervised, non-goal-directed activities) had significantly higher levels of alcohol and drug use than those not so involved. Furthermore, the analyses suggested that adolescents who were moderately to heavily involved in supervised, goal-directed activities had lower drug use than those with little involvement, although this effect did not appear to hold for those adolescents who were heavily involved in both types of group activities. Other factors that have been shown to be related to alcohol use, such as drug-using status of peers and parental and personality effects, were not included in these analyses, leaving open the question that perhaps the types of group affiliations are a surrogate for some of these other influences. However, the attempt to partition types of peer activities represents the type of investigation that is needed to identify the mechanisms underlying the effects of peers on adolescent drinking and other substance use.

5. Personality and Personal Values

Measures of Conventionality

Many studies have suggested that adolescents with a low degree of conventionality, as measured by infrequent church attendance, lower expectations for, attachment of little value to, and poor academic achievement, and low degree of conformity are more likely to be users of alcohol.[4–6,8–10,13,17,20,21,31,32] Blane and Hewitt[22] reported that the majority of studies found a negative relationship between school performance and level of drinking, with heavy drinkers having poor grades and abstainers having high grades. This is also true for recent studies.[2,6,8,10,21] Multivariable analyses have revealed that poor school performance persists as a significant influence on the likelihood of being a drinker and on frequency and quantity of alcohol consumed.[2,21] Compared to nonproblem drinkers, problem drinkers had significantly poorer school performance and placed less value on, and had lowered expectations for, academic achievement.[4] In addition, on 7-year follow-up,[20] poor school performance was found to predict both continuation of problem drinking behavior into adulthood and onset of problem drinking in young adulthood among former nonproblem drinkers.

Adolescents classified as having a low degree of religiosity, most typically measured by frequency of attendance of religious services, but also occasionally assessed by a religiousness scale, commitment to religion, and the importance of religion in one's life, were more likely to be drinkers than those who had a high degree of religiosity.[8,22] Some studies have also reported a strong relationship between degree of religiosity and intensity of alcohol use, with adolescents with low rather than high religiosity more likely to be frequent heavy or problem drinkers.[2,4] These findings, coupled with those on school achievement, attest to the fact that adolescents who subscribed to and valued conventional behaviors were less likely to drink alcohol or to be problem drinkers.

In addition to measures of conventional value systems, some surveys have included an appraisal of what might be broadly termed "happiness with self and with life," including such constructs as self-esteem and degree of alienation, along with indicators of stress, such as personal crisis and emotional distress.[1,5,12] Self-esteem is not a common consideration in most studies, but those that have assessed this construct have not found either a consistent or a positive relationship with any measure of alcohol use.[22] In general, results suggest that the prevalence of drinking increases with unhappiness.[22] However, relatively few studies have examined the relationships of these constructs with excessive alcohol use. White et al.,[2] reporting on a series of multivariable analyses, found that quantity and frequency of typical alcohol consumption increased with the number of stressful life events. As with all findings based on cross-sectional data, however, it is not possible to discern whether the stressful events led to an increase in alcohol use, or whether heavier drinkers either experienced or just reported more stressful life events than lighter drinkers.

6. Psychiatric Correlates

6.1. General Deviant Behavior

The counterpart to the earlier-discussed conventional behaviors are those behaviors regarded as deviant (such as stealing, truancy, fighting, property destruction, and school misconduct). As would be expected, these behaviors have a positive relationship with any alcohol use, initiating alcohol use, quantity of alcohol consumed, and problem drinking.[3,4,8,10,27] Donovan and Jessor[4] reported that problem drinkers engaged in significantly more deviant behaviors than did nonproblem drinkers, which was true for males and females, as well as for several definitions of problem drinking. In addition, their 7-year follow-up study[20] indicated that engaging in deviant behaviors might be a marker for persistent problem drinking or for development of problem drinking in young adulthood. Number of general deviant behaviors during adolescence among both those who maintained or who developed problem drinking during the follow-up period significantly exceeded that of either those whose problem drinking had remitted by, or those who remained nonproblem drinkers at, the follow-up interview. Another study found that number of school misconduct incidents during the past year not only distinguished drinkers from nondrinkers, but also predicted mean daily alcohol consumption; on both accounts those with more misconduct were drinkers and drank more.[10]

When substance abuse, based on DSM-III criteria[33] for drug or alcohol abuse or dependence, was the outcome variable of interest,[18] abusers were more likely to have had three or more conduct disorder behaviors (excluding those related to substance abuse) than nonabusers. In fact, 83% of abusers, compared to 17% and 47% of low users and nonabusing users, respectively, met lifetime criteria for a diagnosis of conduct disorder.

Robins,[34] using information on childhood behavior problems reported by adults in five communities in the United States who were also interviewed about lifetime psychiatric histories, explored the role of conduct problems in eventual development of substance abuse/dependence disorder (including alcohol and illicit drugs), defined by DSM-III criteria. She found that those with conduct problems were more likely than others to have used illicit drugs, which increased the proportion of those at risk for developing a substance abuse disorder by virtue of their greater exposure. In addition, the greater the number of conduct problems, the earlier the use of substances, which independently foreshadowed substance abuse.

6.2. Depressive Symptoms

Preliminary work has been suggestive of a relationship between depressive symptoms and adolescent alcohol use. Brook et al.[27] found that depressed mood at index interview was positively and significantly correlated with initiation of alcohol use at the follow-up interview. In a similar vein, Stiffman et al.[18] reported that substance abusers were more likely than either low users or nonabusing users to have three or more depressive symptoms (63% compared to 22% for the other two groups). Quantity of consumption of liquor, beer, and wine was significantly and positively correlated with the Beck Depression Inventory score.[35] Another study using 16- to 19-year-old students found that onset of depression tended to precede onset of alcohol abuse.[36] Kandel and Davies[37] found that a greater proportion of young adults who had been depressed as adolescents reported drinking four or more times per week, compared to their nondepressed peers, although the difference did not reach statistical significance. These findings suggest that alcohol use may be part of an effort to alter depressed mood.

7. Conclusion

As this review has shown, the correlates of adolescent alcohol use that have been identified in the current literature are generally consistent from study to study. Drinkers, and heavier drinkers, are more likely to be found among the ranks of males, older adolescents, whites, those of Catholic and Protestant persuasions, those with at least one regularly drinking parent, those who associate with peers who drink, those who are unconventional, perform poorly in school, and value academic achievement less, engage in deviant behavior, and manifest some depressive symptomatology. New ground has been broken by studies with detailed psychiatric information; these suggest strong links between a diagnosis of substance abuse and conduct and depressive symptomatology in particular.

Although this review has concentrated on adolescent alcohol use and problem use, one theme in the current literature is that problem drinking is part of a continuum of problem behaviors, including use of illicit substances, and therefore should not be considered in isolation.[3] In fact, a comparison of correlates of problem drinking and of marijuana use yielded very similar patterns.[31] Since there are such close ties between alcohol and illicit drug use, some have argued that adolescent substance use ought to be treated as a single phenomenon.[16] This trend is in marked opposition to the adult substance use literature, in which it is rare to find use of alcohol and of other substances studied concomitantly.[25]

Another movement in the adolescent substance use literature is directed away from assessment of specific correlates and toward an additive risk factor index to identify adolescents at high risk of involvement with substances.[32,38] Preliminary work has suggested the utility of this approach.[32]

Whether considered separately or in the aggregate, correlates of adolescent alcohol use will continue to receive attention, because of alcohol's pivotal role in illicit substance use. It seems reasonable to expect that a national antidrug policy will assign a high priority to curbing society's appetite for drugs, which begins in adolescence and in which alcohol plays an important part. In light of this, it is a propitious time to call for more intensive efforts to learn more about the theory and mechanisms underlying the correlates.

ACKNOWLEDGMENTS. This work was supported by Training Grant MH 17104 and the MacArthur Network on Risk and Protective Factors.

References

1. Yamaguchi K, Kandel DB: Patterns of drug use from adolescence to young adulthood. II: Sequences of progression. *Am J Public Health* 74:668–672, 1984.
2. White HR, Johnson J, Horwitz A: An application of three deviance theories to adolescent substance use. *Int J Addictions* 21:347–366, 1986.
3. Jessor R: Problem-behavior theory, psychosocial development, and adolescent problem drinking. *Br J Addiction* 82:331–342, 1987.
4. Donovan JE, Jessor R: Adolescent problem drinking: Psychosocial correlates in a national sample study. *J Stud Alcohol* 39:1506–1524, 1978.
5. Potvin RH, Lee C-F: Multi-strange path models of adolescent alcohol and drug use: age variations. *J Stud Alcohol* 41:531–542, 1980.
6. Rachal JV, Guess LL, Hubbard RL, et al. Vol. I: Adolescent drinking behavior: The extent and nature of adolescent alcohol and drug use: The 1974 and 1978 National Sample Studies. Final report to the National Institute on Alcohol Abuse and Alcoholism, ADM 281-76-0019. Research Triangle Park, NC, Research Triangle Institute, 1980.

7. Zucker RA, Harford TC: National study of the demography of adolescent drinking practices in 1980. *J Stud Alcohol* 44:974–985, 1983.

8. Bachman JG, Johnston LD, O'Malley PM: Smoking, drinking and drug use among American high school students: Correlates and trends, 1975–1979. *Am J Public Health* 71:59–69, 1981.

9. Kandel DB: Epidemiological and psychosocial perspectives on adolescent drug use. *J Am Acad Child Psychiatry* 21:328–347, 1982.

10. Barnes GM, Welte JW: Patterns and predictors of alcohol use among 7–12th grade students in New York State. *J Stud Alcohol* 47:53–62, 1986.

11. Boyle MH, Offord DR: Smoking, drinking, and use of illicit drugs among adolescents in Ontario: Prevalence patterns of use and sociodemographic correlates. *Can Med Assoc J* 135:1113–1121, 1986.

12. Napier TL, Carter TJ, Pratt MC: Correlates of alcohol and marijuana use among rural high school students. *Rural Sociol* 46:319–331, 1981.

13. Gibbons S, Wylie ML, Echterling L, et al: Patterns of alcohol use among rural and small-town adolescents. *Adolescence* 21:887–900, 1986.

14. Murray DM, Perry CL, O'Connell C, et al: Seventh-grade cigarette, alcohol, and marijuana use: distribution in a North Central U.S. metropolitan population. *Int J Addictions* 22:357–376, 1987.

15. Maddahian E, Newcomb MD, Bentler PM: Adolescents' substance use: impact of ethnicity, income, and availability. *Adv Alcohol Subst Abuse* 5:63–78, 1986.

16. Hansen WB, Graham JW, Sobel JL, et al: The consistency of peer and parent influences on tobacco, alcohol, and marijuana use among young adolescents. *J Behav Med* 10:559–579, 1987.

17. Schwartz RH, Hayden GF, Getson PR, et al: Drinking patterns and social consequences: a study of middle-class adolescents in two private pediatric practices. *Pediatrics* 77:139–143, 1986.

18. Stiffman AR, Earls F, Powell J, et al: Correlates of alcohol and illicit drug use in adolescent medical patients. *Contemp Drug Prob* Summer:295–314, 1987.

19. Hays RD, Stacy AW, DiMatteo MR: Problem behavior theory and adolescent alcohol use. *Addictive Behav* 12:189–193, 1987.

20. Donovan JE, Jessor R, Jessor L: Problem drinking in adolescence and young adulthood: A follow-up study. *J Stud Alcohol* 44:109–137, 1983.

21. Fors SW, Rojek DG: The social and demographic correlates of adolescent drug use patterns. *J Drug Educ* 13:205–222, 1983.

22. Blane HT, Hewitt LE: Alcohol and youth: an analysis of the literature 1960–1975. Rockville, MD, National Institute on Alcohol Abuse and Alcoholism. National Technical Information Service. Springfield, VA, PB-268968/AS, 1977, pp III-1–153.

23. Lowman, C: Facts for planning no. 1: Prevalence of alcohol use among U.S. senior high school students. *Alcohol Health Res World* 6:29–40, 1981.

24. Rachal JV, Guess LL, Hubbard RL, et al: Facts for planning no. 4: Alcohol misuse by adolescents. *Alcohol Health Res World* 6:61–68, 1982.

25. Bucholz KK, Robins LN: Sociological research on alcohol use, problems and policy. *Annu Rev Sociol* 15:163–186, 1989.

26. Welte JW, Barnes GM: Alcohol use among adolescent minority groups. *J Stud Alcohol* 48:329–336, 1987.

27. Brook JS, Whiteman M, Gordon AS, et al: Onset of adolescent drinking: A longitudinal study of intrapersonal and interpersonal antecedents. *Adv Alcohol Subst Abuse* 5:91–110, 1986.

28. Singer MI, Petchers MK: A biracial comparison of adolescent alcohol use. *Am J Drug Alcohol Abuse* 13:461–474, 1987.

29. Binion A, Miller CD, Beauvais F, et al: Rationales for the use of alcohol, marijuana, and other drugs by eighth-grade Native American and Anglo youth. *Int J Addictions* 23:47–64, 1988.

30. Selnow GW, Crane WD: Formal and informal group affiliations: Implications for alcohol and drug use among adolescents. *J Stud Alcohol* 47:48–52, 1986.

31. Jessor R, Chase JA, Donovan JE: Psychosocial correlates of marijuana use and problem drinking in a national sample of adolescents. *Am J Public Health* 70:604–613, 1980.

32. Newcomb MD, Maddahian E, Skager R, et al: Substance abuse and psychosocial risk factors among teenagers: Associations with sex, age, ethnicity, and type of school. *Am J Drug Alcohol Abuse* 13:413–433, 1987.
33. American Psychiatric Association Committee on Nomenclature and Statistics: *Diagnostic and Statistical Manual of Mental Disorder*, 3rd edition. Washington, DC, American Psychiatric Association, 1980.
34. Robins LN: Conduct problems as predictors of substance abuse, in Robins LN, Rutter M (eds): *Straight and Devious Pathways from Childhood to Adulthood*. Cambridge, Cambridge University Press, in press.
35. Kaplan SL, Landa B, Weinhold C, et al: Adverse health behaviors and depressive symptomatology in adolescents. *J Am Acad Child Psychiatry* 23:595–601, 1984.
36. Deykin EY, Levy JC, Wells V: Adolescent depression, alcohol and drug abuse. *Am J Public Health* 77:178–182, 1987.
37. Kandel DB, Davies M: Adult sequelae of adolescent depressive symptoms. *Arch Gen Psychiatry* 43:255–262, 1986.
38. Bry BH, McKean P, Pandina RJ: Extent of drug use as a function of number of risk factors. *J Abnormal Psychol* 91:273–279, 1982.

Drug Use and Its Social Covariates from the Period of Adolescence to Young Adulthood

Some Implications from Longitudinal Studies

Kazuo Yamaguchi

Abstract. This chapter presents a review and discussion of the dynamic relationship between drug use, especially the use of illicit drugs, and its social covariates from the period of adolescence to young adulthood. The discussion is based primarily on longitudinal studies. In particular, I include a review and discussion of my collaborative studies with Kandel, in which we employ life-course perspectives for the analysis of natural drug and life histories of individuals based on event-history models. Specifically, I discuss five covariates: (1) age, (2) onset age of drug use, (3) historical period, (4) family and work roles, and (5) influence of significant others, with the dynamic interdependence between drug use and family and work roles as the major topic of discussion. The discussion also includes some insights into the issue of causation vs. selection effects regarding the influence of drug use on life-course pattern, and presents a novel aspect of indirect effects in the analysis of the determinants of drug use progression.

1. Introduction

This chapter presents a review and discussion regarding social covariates of drug use from the period of adolescence to young adulthood. By social covariates, I imply sociodemographic and social contextual variables that covary with drug use in natural life histories of individuals. I specifically discuss (1) age, (2) onset age of drug use, (3) historical period, (4) family and work roles, and (5) influence of significant others. The discussion of the fourth factor, family and work roles, is more extensive than that of other factors because of its centrality in my collaborative research with Kandel.

Kazuo Yamaguchi • Department of Sociology, University of California–Los Angeles, Los Angeles, California 90024.

Sociodemographic factors that do not vary with time, such as race, ethnicity, and cohort, are not included in the discussion because the chapter is concerned with possible causal relationships between drug use and its social covariates. The effects of time-constant sociodemographic variables cannot be distinguished from the effects of latent population heterogeneity. Therefore, it is difficult to examine their causal effects. However, I include gender in my discussion because it is a major interacting variable in the dynamic relationship between drug use and its social covariates.

The chapter includes a review of my collaborative studies with Kandel, studies by others that are directly related to our studies in terms of their content, and additional studies that pertain to the five covariates of drug use mentioned. This chapter also includes discussions of the implications of these studies. The studies reviewed and discussed here are also primarily longitudinal, because the dynamic relationship between drug use and its social covariates can be analyzed only by longitudinal data. Longitudinal studies have advantages over cross-sectional studies in many substantive respects. First, the determinants/predictors of initiation, cessation, and resumption of drug use can be analyzed separately in longitudinal studies. Such studies can also identify the determinants/predictors of the timing of those events. The timing of initiation is particularly important in predicting a further progression in drug use. Second, since social covariates of drug use also change over time in individual life histories, it is important to take into account the relative timing between the drug and life events to analyze their dynamic relationship.

Although causal inference is difficult to make for the analysis of natural histories of individuals because of the selection bias and the effects of unobserved population heterogeneity which are necessarily involved in the analysis of nonexperimental data, longitudinal studies have some notable advantages over cross-sectional studies regarding the causal inference. First, longitudinal studies can focus on changes in drug use rather than levels of use. Changes in use are analytically independent from any unobserved time-constant individual differences, while levels of use are not. Second, some methods for the analysis of longitudinal data can be employed to take into account the effects of unobserved population heterogeneity.[1]

2. Social Covariates of Drug Use

2.1. Age

Age reflects not only maturational and other individual aspects of changes, but also social aspects of changes associated with the transition from adolescence to young adulthood. During the transition, individuals experience major changes in the participation of social roles as is represented by the transition from school to work and then to adult family roles.[2] Age also reflects changes in perceived normative expectations associated with the assumption of adult roles.

Age has been known to be one of the most significant predictors of the use of illicit drugs. Adolescents enter the risk of initiating each illicit drug during certain ages, subsequently experience age periods of high risks, then experience a gradual decline of risks, and they eventually "mature out." Kandel[3] once wrote that "the period of risk of initiation into illicit drug use is over by the mid-20s." Kandel and Logan[4] subsequently reported for both men and women that the hazard rate of initiating the use of licit drugs (i.e., cigarettes and alcohol), and many illicit drugs (e.g., marijuana and psychedelics) peaks at age 18 and declines thereafter.

The prevalence rate of drug use as a function of age depends on three age-specific rates: the rates of initiation, cessation, and resumption of drug use. Yamaguchi and Kandel[5] observe that during ages 16–25, the hazard rate of stopping marijuana use increases at 22 and over, especially 24 and over. The increase in the rate of stopping at age 24 and over apparently explains a decline in the prevalence rate of marijuana use at age 24 and over for both men and women.[4] One the other hand, the rate of resuming marijuana use did not depend significantly on age[5] and the age patterns of the rates of stopping and resuming marijuana use remain largely unchanged, controlling for unobserved population heterogeneity.[1]

Two factors, however, limit definitive interpretations of observed age effects: (1) the effect of unobserved population heterogeneity for findings about the rate of initiation, and (2) possible confounding with period effects. Adolescents are heterogeneous regarding individual risks of initiating the use of a drug, and since those who have higher risks tend to initiate earlier, the average extent of risks among those who remain nonusers of the drug declines with age. The decline of the hazard rate of initiation after age 18 reflects, to a certain significant extent, a result from a changing composition of people who never used the drug.

The study of Kandel and her colleagues is based on the analysis of a single cohort for which age effects cannot be separated from period effects. O'Malley et al.[6] analyze longitudinal data of multiple cohorts and report that the decline in marijuana use at age 24 and over observed by Kandel and Logan[4] coincides with the period of historical decline in marijuana use that started in 1979 and is better interpreted as a consequence of the period effect. Generally, the age at which a gradual decline in the use of each drug begins needs further research based on longitudinal data of multiple cohorts.

2.2. Age of Onset

The onset age of use of a given drug predicts three direct consequences. First, an earlier onset of a drug will, on average, lead to a longer period of lifetime use of this drug. Second, onset at an earlier age will lead to a longer period of high risk for making a further progression of drug use. Third, among those who initiated a drug, its onset at an earlier age may lead to a still higher hazard rate of making a further drug-use progression.

Yamaguchi and Kandel[7] studied the last two aspects of drug use progression by analyzing hazard rates of initiating the use of marijuana and other illicit drugs and the medically prescribed use of psychotropic drugs. It was found that during the period of transition from adolescence to young adulthood, current and former uses of alcohol as time-varying states predict higher hazard rates of initiating marijuana use at each month, and that the onset age of alcohol drinking does not have any effect on the hazard rate, when the current and former uses of alcohol are taken into account. Thus, an earlier onset of alcohol drinking puts a person in a high hazard period regarding the initiation of marijuana use at an earlier age and thereby increases the proportion of persons who initiate marijuana use by age 25. In the case of initiating the use of illicit drugs other than marijuana, current and former uses of marijuana as time-varying states predict higher hazard rates of initiation. In addition, among current and former users of marijuana, an earlier onset age of marijuana use predicts a still higher hazard rate of initiating the use of other illicit drugs. Hence, an early onset age of marijuana use not only lengthens the high-risk period of initiating the use of other illicit drugs, but the level of the high risk at each month is augmented for the earlier onset age of marijuana use.

These findings have the following implications. If this pattern of hazard rates remains the same, postponing the onset age of alcohol drinking will lead to a smaller proportion of persons who initiate marijuana use by a given age because it shortens the period of high risk (i.e., the period of ever used alcohol) for initiating marijuana use. Second, under the same assumption, postponing the onset age of marijuana use will lead to a smaller proportion of persons who initiate the use of other illicit drugs by a given age because of two consequences: (I1) a shortened period of high risk (i.e., period of ever used marijuana) for the initiation and (I2) a lowered level of hazard rate for the period of high risk by selectively reducing the portion of higher risks in the high-risk period.

A possible limitation for these inferences, however, is that the patterns of hazard rates may not remain the same under a change in the onset ages of alcohol and marijuana use. Specifically, one may argue that (C1) if the onset age of marijuana use becomes larger, there will be more initiators of other illicit drugs without a prior use of marijuana. The same thing will be true for the relationship between alcohol drinking and marijuana use. It also could be argued that (C2) even if the onset age of marijuana use becomes larger, the average level of high risk among those who initiated marijuana use will not be affected because the effect of the age of marijuana onset likely reflects population heterogeneity, such that those who start marijuana use early are more deviant initially than those who start late.

In order to make these counterarguments clearer, let me denote by H1 the hazard rate of initiating use for a drug without initiating the use of its lower-stage drug (alcohol for marijuana, and marijuana for other illicit drugs), and by H2 the hazard rate of initiating use for a drug after the initiation of its lower-stage drug. By definition, H1 < H2 holds true. My two initial inferences are (I1) a delay in initiating the use of the lower-stage drug lengthens the period of H1 and shortens the period of H2 and consequently leads to a lower prevalence rate of the higher-stage drug by a given age, and (I2) since it selectively eliminates higher values of H2, the average level of H2 becomes lower. On the other hand, counterargument C1 suggests that my inference I1 may not hold true because a delay in the onset of lower-stage drug use may make H1 higher. Counterargument C2 suggests that my inference I2 may not hold true because delaying the onset of lower-stage drug use may shift higher levels of H2 to later ages rather than eliminate them, thereby keeping the same average level of H2. The two counterarguments have different theoretical implications. Counterargument C1 assumes that sequencing in drug use progression is spurious and is the result of some common causes and drug-specific age effects on initiation, and therefore, the relationship between the use of two drugs will not be sustained under the modification for the onset age of the drug that normally starts earlier. Counterargument C2 accepts sequencing in drug use progression but considers the effect of the age of marijuana onset on the hazard rate of initiating the use of other illicit drugs as spurious and due to uncontrolled population heterogeneity.

We cannot test these counterarguments without social experimentations. However, an evaluation of counterargument C1 is possible from what we can observe among various groups which represent different onset ages of using the lower-stage drug. If counterargument C1 holds true, we should expect that sequencing between the lower- and higher-stage drugs will become weaker for groups with relatively later onset ages of using the lower-stage drug compared with those with relatively early onset ages. This tendency somewhat exists in the sequencing of alcohol and marijuana but is almost absent in the sequencing of marijuana and other illicit drugs.[7–9] Hence, sequencing of alcohol and marijuana may in part be spurious, but sequencing of marijuana and other illicit drugs is unlikely to be spurious.

Counterargument C2 is more difficult to test and remains to be examined. However, the acceptance of this argument does not affect the major implication of our findings that a delay in the onset of lower-stage drug use leads to a shortened high-risk period for initiating the use of the higher-stage drug and will lead consequently to a lower prevalence rate of the higher-stage drug.

2.3. Historical Period

In comparison with age effects, period effects reflect more social factors because it is impossible for the average individual vulnerability to drug use or other averages of individual risk factors in the population to change rapidly over time. Yet, the period effect is only an indicator of some unobserved changes in the social causes of drug use. O'Malley et al.[6] made an analysis of period, age, and cohort effects and reported the significance of period effects for most of the drugs.

It is rather surprising that in spite of its importance, underlying determinants of the period effects are not well known. The majority of research in drug use focus on who becomes a drug user and why, rather than why the population as a whole, or particular social groups, experience an average increase/decrease in the use of drugs over time.

Interestingly, two longitudinal studies on the historical trends of drug use focused on the decline in drug use rather than the rise of drug use. Although these two studies were based on different samples and analyzed the use of different drugs, they reached somewhat similar conclusions. Backman, Johnston, and O'Malley[10,11] studied a decline of marijuana use from 1979 to 1986 with their Monitoring the Future samples. They found that while life-style factors (such as religious commitment and truancy) explained individual differences in marijuana use, they could not account for the historical decline in marijuana use during the period. Johnston[10] also reported for the same sample that the possible change in the availability of drugs over time did not explain the historical decline, either. Instead, Backman et al.[11] found that an increase in the perceived risks and personal disapproval associated with regular marijuana use explained the historical decline.

Boyle and Brunswick[12] studied a decline of heroin use during 1970–1976 with a longitudinal sample of Harlem black youth. They identified three factors that contributed to the decline: (1) an effect of cohort shift—cohorts with high prevalence rates being replaced by cohorts with low prevalence rates, (2) an increase in the rate of stopping heroin use, and (3) a decrease in the rate of initiating heroin use. They then analyzed reasons for stopping and not progressing heroin use and concluded that the increased perception of negative consequences of heroin use was the likely cause of the historical decline in use.

In discussing the implications from these studies, references to other studies that attempted to explain differences in drug use among social groups, which are characterized by relatively frequent within-group social interactions, are useful. Unless we assume that group differences are reducible to differences of individuals, these studies have relevance for the analysis of trends observed in the population because they suggest the determinants of drug use at the group level, rather than at the individual level.

The well-known influence of significant others in drug use, the influence of peers and parents in particular, is relevant here because the influence of significant others in part explains group differences in drug use among families and schools. Kandel[3,13] identifies two distinct patterns of influence: modeling and reinforcement. In modeling, individuals simply imitate significant others' behavior. In reinforcement, individuals respond to specific attitudes of significant others regarding drug use.

Another relevant factor is the availability of drugs from peers. A recent study by Maddahian et al.[14] shows that differences in drug use among ethnic groups of adolescents in Los Angeles County are largely explained by differences among the groups in the availability of drugs from peers.

The importance of both availability of drugs from peers and modeling of a peer's drug behavior in explaining group differences in drug use indicates that the opportunity to have personal contacts with drug-using peers is a major determinant of the group differences. It seems that this factor is also a major *endogenous* covariate of the historical increase in the use of illicit drugs because an increase in the number of drug users leads to an increase in the opportunity for nonusers to have personal contacts with drug-using peers, which will subsequently lead to a further increase in the number of drug users. This factor, more than any exogenous social covariates that vary with time, may explain the historical rise of drug use, though this speculation remains to be tested empirically.

On the other hand, the Backman et al. study and the Boyle–Brunswick study documented that perceived harms/risks of drug use and personal disapproval of drug use seem to contribute to historical declines in the use of illicit drugs. Changes in personal disapproval and the perception of harms/risks can arise from the informal influence of changes in significant others' disapproval/perception, as well as from changes in one's perception due to acquiring new information from formal means such as education and mass media. Johnston[10] suggests that personal disapproval is more a cause than a consequence of perceived peers' disapproval, but the determinants of changes in personal disapproval and the perception of risks need further research.

Finally, Jessor,[15] in his comments on Johnston's paper, notes that changes in personal disapproval and the perception of harms/risks can be consequences rather than causes of the decline in drug use. Hence, possible reciprocal effects and potential spuriousness in the effects of changes in the perception need to be examined with individual-level longitudinal data.

2.4. Family and Work Roles

Kandel and I[5,16,17,18] conducted a series of studies that analyzed dynamic relationships between the use of illicit drugs and participation in family and work roles using event-history analysis and Kandel's longitudinal sample of a cohort of former New York State public high-school students for the period 1972–1980. The period covers ages 16–25 for the cohort. Several general life course characteristics of the users of illicit drugs became clear: (1) tendency to avoid potential incompatibilities between the use of illicit drugs and conventional family roles by two methods, role selection and role socialization; (2) instability of attained statuses; and (3) deviant sequencing of family role events prior to marriage.

The resolution of potential incompatibilities between conventional family roles, i.e., marriage and parenthood in marriage, and marijuana use was examined by specifying distinct pathways of resolution by either role selection or role socialization.[5] Role selection refers to a purposeful commitment to roles that agree with one's drug use pattern, and role socialization refers to changing one's drug involvement so as to make the behavior compatible with the expectations from one's social roles. We also took into account the possibility of anticipatory socialization such that the expected change in drug behavior might occur prior to entry into the role. We assumed that anticipatory socialization might occur during 1 year prior to the entry into the role.

Three hypotheses were tested for role selection. Controlling for other determinants of entry into and exit from marriage and entry into parenthood in marriage:

> H1: Current marijuana use postpones the timing of marriage and/or reduces the rate of getting married.
>
> H2: Current marijuana use during marriage further postpones the timing of parenthood and/or reduces the rate of becoming a parent.
>
> H3: Marijuana use during marriage increases the rate of separation or divorce.

On role socialization, six hypotheses were tested. Controlling for other determinants of marijuana use:

> H4: Marriage increases the rate of stopping marijuana use.
>
> H5: Becoming a parent after marriage further increases the rate of stopping marijuana use.
>
> H6: Marriage decreases the rate of initiating/resuming marijuana use.
>
> H7: Becoming a parent after marriage further decreases the rate of initiating/resuming marijuana use.
>
> H8: Separation or divorce decreases the rate of stopping marijuana use.
>
> H9: Separation or divorce increases the rate of initiating/resuming marijuana use.

Of the nine hypotheses, H1–H7 were supported for at least one gender. The three hypotheses on role selection, H1–H3, were supported for both men and women. The two hypotheses on the effects of entry into family roles on the stopping of marijuana use, i.e., H4 and H5, were supported for both men and women either as anticipatory socialization or as socialization after entry. As for the effect of role entry on initiation/resumption of marijuana use, H6 and H7, the effect of marriage which reduces the rate of initiation was found for women. The latter two findings indicate that except for the tendency that women are less likely to initiate marijuana use after marriage, role socialization effects of marriage and parenthood operate by increasing the rate of stopping rather than decreasing the rate of initiation/resumption.

The tests of H8 and H9 were insignificant and indicate that leaving marriage may not reverse the prior socialization in marriage.

The test was also made for the use of illicit drugs other than marijuana regarding whether their use further increased the tendency to resolve incompatibilities with family roles. The use of other illicit drugs predicted a further postponement of marriage for women. Other effects of other illicit drugs were insignificant when marijuana use was taken into account.

The tendency to resolve potential incompatibilities between the use of illicit drugs and conventional family roles were further tested by Kandel and I in analyses of dynamic relationships between the use of illicit drugs and premarital cohabitation and pregnancy.[16,17] Assuming that cohabitation is compatible with the use of illicit drugs and will become a temporary substitute for marriage, we hypothesized that (1) users of illicit drugs are more likely than nonusers to cohabit premaritally, and (2) among those who cohabit, users of illicit drugs are less likely than nonusers to marry with the partner. The first hypothesis was supported for both male and female marijuana users and this tendency became stronger for female users of other illicit drugs. On the other hand, the second hypothesis was insignificant.[16]

Given the assumption that being single without a partner and living with an unmarried partner are both compatible with the use of illicit drugs, it is difficult to specify the effect of premarital cohabitation on their use. Our analysis showed that the effects of cohabitation on both stopping and resuming marijuana use were absent for men. However, for women, cohabitation reduced the rate of resuming marijuana use, though it did not affect the rate of stopping marijuana use. Hence, for women, living with spouse and living with unmarried partner both tend to reduce marijuana use.

Using the sample of women who ever had a premarital pregnancy, another set of hypotheses was tested for role selection to resolve the incompatibility of illicit drug use with marriage and parenthood.[17] First, three outcomes for premarital pregnancy were distinguished: (1) abortion, (2) premarital birth, and (3) postmarital birth for which marriage occurs before the birth of a child. We then hypothesized that compared with nonusers, users of illicit drugs who become pregnant premaritally are (1) more likely to have an abortion and (2) less likely to have a postmarital birth. These hypotheses are based on the reasoning that drug users will most prefer to avoid both parenthood and marriage (abortion), will least prefer to assume both parenthood and marriage (postmarital birth), and will take the middle position for the assumption of parenthood only (premarital birth). Both hypotheses were empirically supported for the use of illicit drugs other than marijuana compared with nonuse, but not for the use of marijuana. Thus, the tendency to resolve potential incompatibilities between conventional family roles and illicit drug use is found in various aspects of family role transitions. The second characteristic among the users of illicit drugs is a high incidence of having two deviant sequencing of family role events prior to marriage, namely, premarital cohabitation and premarital pregnancy, controlling for major determinants of the timing of marriage. I have already reported the higher hazard rate of getting premaritally cohabited among male and female marijuana users. As for premarital pregnancy, a higher hazard rate of having this event was found among women who use illicit drugs other than marijuana but not for users of marijuana only.

The third general life course characteristic of illicit drug users compared with nonusers is instability of attained statuses. In separate papers, instability was examined for three statuses: marriage, cohabitation, and work.[5,16,18] In addition to the increased rate of divorce among marijuana-using men and women that was mentioned earlier, instability was found for the other two statuses as well. Once cohabited, male and female users of illicit drugs other than marijuana had a higher hazard rate of separation from the partner than nonusers.[16] The use of illicit drugs other than marijuana also predicted a higher hazard rate of having interfirm job separations for both men and women.[18] More specifically, the use of other illicit drugs predicted higher hazard rates of both interfirm job changes and job losses.

Kandel and I (unpublished reference table for Ref. 18) also examined a possible reciprocal effect of work roles on the use of illicit drugs. Some cross-sectional studies had documented the association between illicit drug use and unemployment.[19,20] Our results indicate that employment and schooling statuses, which includes loafing (not married, not working, and not in school), have no effects on the rates of initiating/resuming and stopping marijuana use for both men and women. Having a job separation during the preceding year did not affect these rates either. Hence, while the dynamic relationship between illicit drug use and family roles is reciprocal, the dynamic relationship between illicit drug use and work roles seems rather unidirectional, with drug use leading to job instability and unemployment.

Other researchers also investigated the relationships between family and work roles and drug use. Backman et al.[21,22] studied the effects of living arrangements and employment/education experiences on the use of licit and illicit drugs using their Monitoring the Future sample. They hypothesized that compared with drug use at the end of high school, drug use in the following few years would be (1) decreased among those living with spouse, (2) relatively unchanged among those still living with parent(s), and (3) increased among those living in dormitories or other arrangements involving few adults. The results supported the three hypotheses, except for a slight modification of the third. Those with unmarried partner showed a consistently high level of use but no change, while others in the third category showed, as hypothesized, an increase in drug use. Backman et al.[21,22] also investigated the effects of employment/student/homemaker status on drug use. Those who remained students after graduation from high school increased the use of alcohol and illicit drugs compared with their use at the end of high school, but these increases can be described as "catching up" because their initial levels of using these drugs were lower than those who did not continue schooling after high school. Those in full-time civilian jobs showed little or no increase in use, though their initial level of use was relatively high. Full-time homemakers decreased their drug use significantly. Finally, it was found that those who were unemployed slightly decreased their drug use.

In a pair of papers, Newcomb and Bentler[23,24] analyzed dynamic relationships between drug use and living arrangements and drug use and career direction/career pursuit. In one paper they focused on the effect of high-school drug use on the living arrangements and career direction in young adulthood, i.e., the aspect of role selection.[23] They found nonfrequent use or nonuse of licit and illicit drugs in high school was associated with living with parent(s) or in dormitory 4 years later, and frequent drug use in high school was associated with living with spouse and, more strongly, with living with unmarried partner 4 years later. Newcomb and Bentler also found that non-frequent use or no use of drugs in adolescence was associated with military and university life pursuit, while frequent drug use in adolescence was associated with full-time work and "no life pursuit."

Newcomb and Bentler's finding that drug users in adolescence are more likely to have an early marriage may appear to contradict Yamaguchi and Kandel's finding that marijuana users tend to postpone marriage. In fact, the contradiction does not exist. Newcomb and Bentler's analysis of the effects of drug use in high school on later living arrangements did not control for other determinants of the living arrangements. On the other hand, Yamaguchi and Kandel's analysis of the effect of marijuana use on entry into marriage is based on multivariate hazard rate models which control for time-varying education and employment statuses simultaneously. Drugs users include, on average, more high-school dropouts and fewer college students/graduates. On the other hand, being in school full time strongly reduces the rate of getting married, controlling for age.[5] Users of illicit drugs appear to have a tendency to marry early because they have, on average, a shorter period of full-time schooling. Yet, compared with nonusers with similar timings of leaving full-time schooling, they tend to postpone marriage.

A companion paper of Newcomb and Bentler[24] focused on role socialization. They analyzed levels and changes in drug use as a function of living arrangements and "life pursuit" for the period of transition from adolescence to young adulthood. They found that living with spouse inhibited the use of cannabis and hard drugs and increased alcohol use. They also found that living with unmarried partner generated the same pattern of changes in drug use, though the level of use was consistently higher than that of those living with spouse for all drugs. Hence, their findings about the effects of marriage and cohabitation on the use of illicit drugs are consistent with those of the Yamaguchi and Kandel study.[5,16] In an analysis of the effects of different current life pursuits on drug use, they found that the pursuit of "none," which was found only for women and which they interpret as the pursuit of a full-time housewife, significantly reduced the use of all drugs, except for medically prescribed drugs. This finding is consistent with that of Backman et al.[22] The effects of having other life pursuits (i.e., various types of schooling and employment pursuits) are either modest or none.

Thus, the findings from three studies, Yamaguchi–Kandel, Newcomb–Bentler, and Backman et al., are thus largely consistent. In particular, these researchers commonly observed a fairly strong socialization effect of marriage on reducing or stopping the use of illicit drugs.

2.5. Causation and Selection Effects of Illicit Drug Use on Drug Users' Patterns of Role Transitions

The findings made by Kandel and myself regarding the effects of illicit drug use on entry into and exit from family and work roles are based on event history analysis where the use of marijuana and other illicit drugs is a time-varying predictor of life events. Generally, drug use predicts higher or lower hazard rates of entry into or exit from a particular role due to one or both of two reasons, causation and selection. The selection effect of drug use discussed in this section is different from the effect of drug use on role selection discussed earlier, and their conceptual difference should be clearly recognized: The first concept is concerned with the spurious effect as opposed to causal effect of drug use; the second concept refers to the tendency for drug users to take certain patterns of role transition to make their roles compatible with drug use. The causation effect implies that drug use influences the hazard rate of entry into or exit from the role, and the selection effect implies that those who become drug users are different initially and the observed effects of drug use are, in fact, the result of a selection of certain people into drug use.

In the analysis of empirical data, the distinction between the causation and selection effects of drug use is difficult to establish. Kandel and I employed the following procedure to operationalize this.[16] First, we distinguished three time-varying states for the use of each given class of drugs: (1) never used before, (2) currently using, and (3) formerly used. Then we made two assumptions: (1) heterogeneity between those who become users of each class of drugs and those who do not become users and (2) homogeneity among current and former users of each class of drugs, controlling for various individual differences observed when they were high-school students. We specified marijuana and other illicit drugs as two classes of drugs. Suppose that the effects of current use and former use are measured by comparing these states with the state of never used before, then the assumptions lead to an expectation that (1) the causation effect will be revealed as the difference in the effect of current use compared with the effect of former use, and (2) the selection effect will be revealed as the commonality between the effects of current and former use.

However, this operationalization has three limitations. First, uncontrolled differences between those who stop using drugs and those who continue to use will exist. Hence, the difference between the effects of current use and former use may also reflect the selection effect. Thus, by assuming the difference between the effects of current and former use as the causation effect, we may overestimate the causation effect and underestimate the selection effect. Second, the effects of drug use may be chronic rather than acute. Then the effect of former use may involve the causation effect of drug use. In this respect, we may underestimate the causation effect and overestimate the selection effect. Finally, since the data on drug use and nonuse periods are obtained from retrospective recall, which is subject to measurement errors that introduce certain randomness regarding the distinction of the three drug use states, the difference between the effects of current and former use (i.e., causation effect) will be, on the average, underestimated. The difference between current use and never used before (i.e., the sum of causation and selection effects) will also be underestimated. With these limitations for the distinction between the causation and selection effects in mind, I propose to assess these two effects as follows.

First, I propose that the causation effect exists when the effect of current use is significantly stronger than the effect of former use. Second, I propose that the selection effect exists if the effect of former use compared with the state of never used before is significant. Given this definition, both causation and selection effects can be simultaneously included in an effect of a drug. Empirically, however, we did not find any such case. Finally, I propose that the effect of drug is ambiguous when the effect of current use is significant and that of former use is insignificant and, in addition, the effect of current use is not significantly larger than the effect of former use. It is ambiguous because neither the causation effect (the effect of current use minus the effect of former use) nor the selection effect (the effect of former use) is significant by itself, but the sum of the two effects (the effect of current use) is significant. The ambiguous effect may represent one of these two effects, or both, without identifying which is the case.

Table I summarizes the effects of the use of marijuana and other illicit drugs separately for men and women using the distinction between causation, selection, and ambiguous effects as defined earlier. These results are based on the analyses from hazard rate models that Kandel and I employed previously in four separate papers[5,16–18] plus the new definition of the distinction between the three effects I have described here.

Table I indicates that the patterns of the effects are largely, if not completely, consistent between men and women. The results summarized in Table I substantively show:

1. For role selection to avoid incompatibilities between family roles (marriage and parenthood) and the use of illicit drugs, i.e., for rows 1, 2, and 3 in Table I, the causation effects of marijuana use exist. The finding confirmed the generally hypothesized incompatibility between marijuana use and conventional adult family roles. The use of other illicit drugs has no additional causation effects.

2. With regard to role selection as a consequence of premarital pregnancy, i.e., rows 7 and 8, it is ambiguous whether the observed effect of other illicit drugs is the result of causation or selection effects.

3. With regard to the effects of drug use on instability of attained family and work roles, i.e., rows 3, 5, 9, and 10, the effects are causation effects for instability of family roles and selection effects for instability of work roles. The relevant drugs, whether marijuana or other illicit drugs, also vary with the role: marijuana for marriage and other illicit drugs for cohabitation and work.

Table I.   Patterns of Drug Effects[a]

	Causal effect		Selection effect		Ambiguous effect	
	Men	Women	Men	Women	Men	Women
1. On postponement of marriage	MJ	MJ		OID		
2. On postponement of parenthood	ID[b]	ID[b]				
3. On divorce	MJ	MJ				
4. On entry into cohabitation			MJ	MJ OID		
5. On separation from the partner	OID	OID				
6. On premarital pregnancy	n/a		n/a	OID	n/a	
7. On increased abortion, given premarital pregnancy	n/a		n/a		n/a	OID
8. On decreased postmarital birth, given premarital pregnancy	n/a		n/a		n/a	OID
9. On job loss				OID	OID	
10. On job change			OID	OID		MJ

[a]Causal effect: the effect of current use is significantly larger than the effect of former use. Selection effect: the effect of former use is significant. Ambiguous effect: the effect of current use is significant and the effect of former use is insignificant and the difference between the two is insignificant. MJ: marijuana; OID: other illicit drugs; ID: illicit drugs; n/a: not applicable.
[b]The effects of marijuana and other illicit drugs are not separated because of inefficiency in the estimation of the separate effects.

4. For deviant sequencing of family role events prior to marriage, i.e., rows 4 and 6, the effects of drugs are selection effects. Latent antecedents of marijuana use seem to predict premarital cohabitation and latent antecedents of other illicit drugs seem to predict premarital pregnancy.

2.6. Influence of Significant Others

The influence of significant others on drug use has been well documented for various drugs, including alcohol, cigarettes, marijuana, and other illicit drugs.[13,25–32] This is an important topic that has many aspects, a full discussion of which is beyond the space constraint of this chapter. Hence, I will comment on only a few selective points.

First, the influence of significant others has been studied primarily for parents and peers, and occasionally for siblings,[31] but the influence of spouse and partner's drug attitude/behavior is little studied. Because of its relevance as a potential modifier of socialization in family roles, study of this topic is important.

Second, by identifying influence and homophily (i.e., the tendency to choose others with similar drug behavior as friends) as two causes of the association between subjects' and friends' drug use, Kandel[13,29] concluded that these two factors have almost equal importance in explaining the association in marijuana use. However, adolescents will choose others like themselves not only with respect to the use of a particular drug in question, but also with respect to similarities in individual risk factors of drug use (such as, use of other drugs, nonconformity, and low achievement orientation). Hence, homophily tends to be underestimated and influence tends to be overestimated in explaining the association of subjects' and friends' drug use.

Third, homophily tends to be regarded simply as a confounding factor of peers' influence for the analysis of subjects' drug use. Yet, homophily will (1) reinforce the existing pattern of drug attitude/behavior and (2) reduce opportunities to be exposed to the influence of dissimilar others in close cohorts. Hence, homophily can be a major modifier of "social contagion" and contextual effects of drug use at the group level.

Fourth, Kandel identifies reinforcement and modeling as two patterns of significant others' influence. We may regard as a third pattern the influence of parents' dysfunctional parental–marital behaviors, such as family conflicts and parent coldness. This factor predicts children's later drug involvement, the use of illicit drugs other than marijuana in particular.[33] Although parents' dysfunctional marital–parental behaviors are expected to increase children's behavioral/attitudinal risk factors of drug use initiation, they also lead to the children's lack of positive role models of married partnership and parenthood. Hence, they also lead to a reduced socialization effect on stopping illicit drug use when some of those children who become drug users enter their own adult family roles later.

Fifth, an early study by Kandel[30] reports that high peer activity predicts marijuana use, while the relative isolation from peers characterizes the use of other illicit drugs among high-school students. This suggests that peer influence would be more important for marijuana use than for the use of other illicit drugs. However, recent studies by Newcomb and Bentler[32,34] show that peer influences through modeling, availability, and reinforcement are all important for cocaine use. Although this may reflect, in part, the compositional change among users of hard drugs over time, peer influence now seems to be an important causal factor for the use of hard drugs as well as of marijuana.

2.7. Indirect Effects in the Dynamic Relationship between Drug Use and Life Events

Some conceptually new aspects of indirect effects of drug use on life events became apparent from our event history analysis of drug use. In the traditional conceptualization, an indirect effect of variable A on variable C exists if variable A influences variable B and variable B influences variable C.

A distinct kind of indirect effect exists for the effects of drug use on life events when drug use influences the risk period of having a life event and thereby having an indirect effect on the lifetime probability of the occurrence of the life event. For example, Kandel and I find that using marijuana tends to lead to a postponement of marriage, controlling for education and other determinants of the timing of marriage. Hence, marijuana use has an indirect positive effect on the occurrence of premarital cohabitation by postponing the termination of the risk period of having the event.[16]

Another example is the effect of other illicit drugs on the occurrence of premarital pregnancy. Although we concluded that this effect was a selection effect rather than a causation effect, this selection effect of the use of other illicit drugs also predicts a higher hazard rate of having the first premarital sexual intercourse. (unpublished reference table for Ref. 17). Hence, in this case, an indirect effect on the occurrence of premarital pregnancy exists through acceleration of the entry into the risk period of having the event.

Generally, a variable can indirectly influence the occurrence of an event by either accelerating or postponing the timing of entry into, or exit from, the risk period of having the event. This notion has an important generalization when we modify its definition by replacing "the risk period" by "the period of high risk." This generalized notion has an importance use in the analysis of drug use progression.

The period of high risk for the initiation of a drug can be described not only in terms of age, but in terms of risk factors that can be changed. For example, subjects are at higher risk, than otherwise, when they are using the lower-stage drug, are single, and have drug-using friends. Although the use of alcohol has no direct effect on the hazard rate of initiating illicit drugs other than marijuana when the use of marijuana is taken into account,[7] it has an indirect effect on the initiation of use of other illicit drugs. By accelerating the initiation of marijuana use, the use of alcohol in early adolescence tends to lengthen the high-risk period of initiating the use of other illicit drugs.

Post-high-school education also plays a role here. Post-high-school education strongly affects the postponement of marriage. By lengthening the period of being single prior to marriage and keeping people under a social context that is particularly susceptible to peer influence, post-high-school education lengthens the high-risk period of drug use. The "catching up effect" that Backman et al.[21,22] found among those who continue education after high school reflects this indirect effect.

Thus, the consideration of indirect effects provides some further implications regarding causal factors of drug use progression.

3. Concluding Remarks

The findings of the longitudinal studies discussed in this chapter have several important implications for the prevention of drug use progression.

First, they indicate that the timing of initiation is important, especially for marijuana use, in making further progression into the use of other illicit drugs. If we could delay the timing of marijuana use initiation, even when we could not stop the initiation of marijuana use, we would reduce the high-risk period for initiating the use of other illicit drugs, which would lead eventually to a lower prevalence rate of the use of other illicit drugs.

Second, the progression from marijuana use to the use of other illicit drugs may depend on risks that existed even prior to marijuana initiation, such as parents' dysfunctional marital–parental behaviors. Resources may be allocated more efficiently by giving more prevention efforts to adolescents with such additional risk factors among those who initiated marijuana and/or alcohol use.

Third, we observed that young adults tend to resolve incompatibility between illicit drug use and conventional family roles either by role selection or by role socialization. Whereas role selection leads to a continuation of drug use, role socialization is realized primarily by stopping drug use. Little, however, is known about who resolves by role socialization as opposed to role selection. Efforts should therefore be made to identify the determinants of these alternative modes of the resolution of incompatibilities and, furthermore, the way in which we can increase the tendency for young adults to resolve the incompatibility by role socialization. Researchers found that those who make progression into the use of illicit drugs other than marijuana tend to have dysfunctional marital/parental role models in childhood. Hence, efforts should be made for these adolescents to somehow overcome their lack of positive family role models because the role socialization will not be successful without them.

Fourth, the drug use progression also depends indirectly on factors that shorten/lengthen the period of high risk at making a further progression in drug use. Determinants of the onset age of alcohol drinking, the timing of marriage, and the length of period during which people are under the strong influence of drug-using and/or drug-approving peers are examples of factors that are relevant in this respect. Further studies of indirect effects should be made to identify the possible pathways to reduce the high-risk periods of drug use progression.

Fifth, efforts should be made to identify the determinants of changes in the perception of harms/risks of drug use and personal disapproval of drug use in the population over time, because studies of the historical decline in the use of some illicit drugs suggest them as major covariates of the decline.

ACKNOWLEDGMENT. Preparation of this chapter was supported in part by the Academic Senate Grant of the University of California–Los Angeles. My collaborative research with Kandel, whose findings are reviewed in this chapter, was supported by NIDA grants DA01097, DA02867, and DA03196 to Denise B. Kandel at Columbia University. Research assistance of Mang-King Cheung and Anna Y. Leon-Guerrero is greatly appreciated.

References

1. Yamaguchi K: Alternative approaches to the problem of unobserved heterogeneity in the analysis of repeatable events, in Tuma NB (ed): *Sociological Methodology 1986*. Washington DC, American Sociological Association, 1986, pp. 213–249.
2. Hogan DP: Variable order of events in the life course. *Am Sociol Rev* 43:573–586, 1978.
3. Kandel DB: Convergences in prospective longitudinal surveys of drug use in normal populations, in Kandel DB (ed): *Longitudinal Research on Drug Abuse*. New York, Wiley, 1978, pp. 3–37.
4. Kandel DB, Logan JA: Patterns of drug use from adolescence to young adulthood: I. Periods of risk for initiation, continued use and discontinuation. *Am J Public Health* 74:660–667, 1984.
5. Yamaguchi K, Kandel DB: On the resolution of role incompatibility: A life event history analysis of family roles and marijuana use. *Am J Sociol* 90:1284–1325, 1985.
6. O'Malley PM, Backman JG, Johnston LD: Period, age and cohort effects among American Youth 1976–82. *Am J Public Health* 74:682–688, 1984.
7. Yamaguchi K, Kandel DB: Patterns of drug use from adolescence to young adulthood: III. Predictors of progression. *Am J Public Health* 74:673–681, 1984.
8. Yamaguchi K, Kandel DB: Patterns of drug use progression from adolescence to young adulthood: II. Sequences of progression. *Am J Public Health* 74:668–672, 1984.
9. Kandel, DB, Yamaguchi K: Developmental patterns of the use of legal, illegal and medically prescribed psychotropic drugs from adolescence to young adulthood, in Jones CR, Battjes RJ (eds): *Etiology of Drug Abuse: Implications for Prevention*. Rockville, MD, National Institute on Drug Abuse, 1985, pp. 193–235.
10. Johnston LD: The etiology of prevention of substance use: What can we learn from recent historical changes? in Jones CR, Battjes RJ (eds): *Etiology of Drug Abuse: Implications for Prevention*. Rockville, MD, National Institute on Drug Abuse, 1985, pp. 155–177.
11. Backman JG, Johnston LD, O'Malley PM: Explaining the recent decline in marijuana use: Differentiating the effects of perceived risks, disapproval and general life style factors. *J Health Soc Behav* 29:92–112, 1988.
12. Boyle JM, Brunswick AF: What happened in Harlem? Analysis of a decline in heroin use among a generation unit of urban black youth. *J Drug Issues* 10:109–131, 1980.
13. Kandel DB: On processes of peer influence in adolescent drug use: A developmental perspective. *Adv Alcohol Substance Abuse* 5:139–163, 1985.
14. Maddahian E, Newcomb MD, Bentler PM: Adolescents' substance use: Impact of ethnicity, income, and availability. *Adv Alcohol Substance Abuse* 6:63–79, 1986.
15. Jessor R: Bridging of etiology and prevention in drug abuse research, in Jones CR, Battjes DSW (eds): *Etiology of Drug Abuse: Implications for Prevention*. Rockville, MD, National Institute on Drug Abuse, 1985, pp. 257–268.
16. Yamaguchi K, Kandel DB: Dynamic relationships between premarital cohabitation and illicit drug use: An event history analysis of role selection and role socialization. *Am Soc Rev* 50:530–546, 1985.
17. Yamaguchi K, Kandel DB: Drug use and other determinants of premarital pregnancy and its outcome: A dynamic analysis of competing life events. *J Marriage Family* 49:257–270, 1987.
18. Kandel DB, Yamaguchi K: Job mobility and illicit drug use: An event-history analysis. *Am J Sociol* 92:836–878, 1987.
19. Backman, JG, O'Malley PM, Johnston, LD: *Youth in Transition, Vol. IV: Adolescence to Adulthood—A Study of Change and Stability in the Lives of Young Men*. Ann Arbor, MI, Institute for Social Research, 1978.
20. Kandel DB: Drug and drinking behavior among youths. *Annu Rev Sociol* 6:235–285, 1980.

21. Backman JG, O'Malley PM, Johnston LD: *Changes in Drug Use after High School as a Function of Role Status and Social Environment* (Monitoring the Future Occasional Paper 11). Ann Arbor, MI, Institute for Social Research, 1981.
22. Backman JD, O'Malley PM, Johnston LD: Drug use among young adults: The impacts of role status and social environment. *J Personal Soc Psychol* 47:629–645, 1984.
23. Newcomb MD, Bentler PM: The impact of high school substance use on choice of young adult living environment and career direction. *J Drug Education* 15:253–261, 1985.
24. Newcomb MD, Bentler PM: Changes in drug use from high school to young adulthood: Effects of living arrangement and current life pursuit. *J Appl Dev Psychol* 8:221–246, 1987.
25. Downs, WR: A panel study of normative structure, adolescent alcohol use and peer alcohol use. *J Stud Alcohol* 48:167–175, 1987.
26. Huba GJ, Bentler PM: The role of peer and adult models for drug taking at different stages in adolescence. *J Youth Adolescence* 9:449–465, 1980.
27. Huba GJ, Wingard JA, Bentler PM: Longitudinal analysis of role of peer support adult models, and peer subcultures in beginning adolescence substance use: An application of setwise canonical correlation methods. *Multiple Behav Res* 15:259–279, 1980.
28. Jessor R, Jessor S: Theory testing in longitudinal research on marijuana use, in Kandel DB (ed): *Longitudinal Research on Drug Use: Empirical Findings and Methodological Issues.* Washington DC, Hemisphere, 1978, pp. 41–71.
29. Kandel DB: Homophily, selection, and socialization in adolescent friendships. *Am J Sociol* 84:427–436, 1978.
30. Kandel DB, Kessler, RC, Margulies RZ: Antecedents of adolescent initiation into stages of drug use: A developmental analysis, in Kandel DB (ed): *Longitudinal Research on Drug Use: Empirical Findings and Methodological Issues.* Washington DC, Hemisphere, 1978.
31. Needle R, McCubbin H, Wilson M, Reineck R, Lazar A, Mederer H: Interpersonal influences in adolescent drug use—The role of older siblings, parents and peers. *Int J Addict* 21:739–766, 1986.
32. Newcomb MD, Bentler PM: Cocaine use among adolescents: Longitudinal associations with social context, psychopathology, and use of other substances. *Addict Behav* 11:263–273, 1986.
33. Simcha-Fagan O, Gersten JC, Langner TS: Early precursors and concurrent correlates of patterns of illicit drug use in adolescence. *J Drug Issues* 16:7–28, 1986.
34. Newcomb MD, Bentler PM: Cocaine use among young adults. *Adv Alcohol Substance Abuse* 7:73–97, 1987.

7

Longitudinal Patterns of Alcohol Use by Narcotics Addicts

Yih-Ing Hser, M. Douglas Anglin, and Keiko Powers

Abstract. Longitudinal patterns of alcohol use by narcotics addicts sampled from a drug-free treatment program and from several methadone maintenance treatment programs were examined. Overall, a high prevalence of alcohol use was found in both samples across several stages of the addicts' careers. Many addicts were also using nonnarcotic drugs and marijuana concurrently. Generally, levels of alcohol, as well as of other substances use, decreased as the narcotics addiction career began. Unlike other drug use, however, only alcohol consumption increased whenever a decrease occurred in narcotics use. Effects of ethnicity, gender, parental alcohol problems, and opiate and alcohol use onset sequence on the alcohol- and narcotics-related behavior are examined in detail. A pattern of early onset of heavy alcohol consumption before initial narcotics addiction was more common among Chicanos and was associated with a positive parental alcohol history. Women addicts typically had a much lower alcohol consumption level than their male counterparts. Among the 160 deaths of the original 581 addicts followed during the 20 years of the study, alcohol-related deaths accounted for 17.5% of the total. Treatment implications for addicts with an alcohol problem are discussed.

1. Introduction

The high prevalence of alcohol use among opiate users and the related health and social problems have been matters of concern to researchers and to clinical practitioners for decades. Furthermore, an increasingly common pattern of multiple substance use, particularly where opiates and alcohol are concerned, has been associated with many severe consequences, including high rates of morbidity and mortality.[1] Reports of high rates of multiple substance use, however, tend to be based on anecdotal or cross-section data; longitudinal studies of opiate users that delineate patterns of opiate and alcohol use and the antecedents and correlates of such use are rare.

Yih-Ing Hser, M. Douglas Anglin, and Keiko Powers • UCLA Drug Abuse Research Group, Neuropsychiatric Institute, University of California–Los Angeles, Los Angeles, California 90024.

The individual and social consequences of narcotics and alcohol use can be severe. A careful analysis of existing research findings is crucial for understanding the phenomenon sufficiently to design effective prevention and intervention strategies, as is also the delineation and execution of further research to clarify unresolved issues.

This chapter discusses some of the factors identified in the literature as important for understanding alcohol use among opiate addicts. Such factors include demographic characteristics (e.g., race, sex, and onset age), family alcohol history, and temporal relationship between narcotics and alcohol use. Longitudinal data collected in two long-term follow-up studies of narcotics addicts are also presented to further enrich our knowledge of the patterns of alcohol consumption and related behavior by opiate addicts.

2. Literature Review

2.1. Considerations of Background Characteristics

The compulsive use of drugs or alcohol is considered to be a behavioral disorder, the origins of which are complex, involving biological, societal, family, and psychological factors. Across hundreds of studies, no single genetic, social, developmental, or personality factor has been found to be consistently associated with drug dependence, although evidence implicating variables in all of these areas has been reported.[2]

2.1.1. Ethnicity and Gender Factors. From the findings of many studies, ethnicity and gender have emerged as two of the major variables, along with age, that define patterns of alcohol use and incidence of alcohol-related problems.[3] Because the research to be reported is limited to Anglos and Mexican–Americans, only these two ethnic groups will be considered here.

Cultural variation in norms related to alcohol consumption and patterns of alcohol use are well documented.[4,5] Comparisons between Anglo and Mexican–American samples usually show that Anglo men have a slightly lower alcohol use prevalence and lower overall consumption levels than Mexican–American men; for women, the opposite is true.[6–8] The relationship between age and alcohol abuse or alcohol problems among Mexican–American men is very different from that for men in the general population, where heavy drinking behavior, alcohol-related social problems, and alcohol dependency symptoms are at their highest in the years between 18 and 29, dropping progressively in older age groups.[9,10] This progressive dwindling of heavy alcohol use and problem sequelae does not take place to the same degree among Mexican–American men. Some studies have shown[11,12] that a sizable percentage of Mexican–American men in their 30s or 40s drink heavily.

Research findings on gender differences usually show a lower prevalence of illicit drug use and alcohol consumption among women. However, antecedents and correlates of use often vary between the genders during both childhood and adulthood. Several studies have found that more female alcoholics report parental drinking problems, especially for the father.[13–15] As children, male alcoholics tend to be more antisocial and encounter more school problems than female alcoholics.[16,17] As adults, the prevalence of conduct-related psychopathology continues to be higher, in general, among men than among women alcoholics, whereas affective disorders are more common among women than men.[3] The natural history of opiate addiction and alcoholism also seems to differ between men and women.[3,18] Women usually begin use of both drugs at a later age than men. The progression from first use to the development of problem use and the subsequent progression to entering treatment are typically more rapid for women than for men.

2.1.2. Family of Origin. A developmental factor found to be of some significance in substance abuse is parental loss, whether through death, desertion, marital breakup,[19–21] or inability of parents to relate emotionally to their children.[22,23] Substance abuse by parents may also provide a model for similar behavior in children,[24,25] and the degree to which nonconformity is tolerated in the home may be a contributing factor. Francis et al.[26] and Schuckit[27] have shown that familial alcoholics (i.e., alcoholics with a family history of alcoholism) had more antisocial behavior, poorer academic performance, and more severe alcoholism symptoms than other categories of alcoholics. Penick et al.[28] found that alcoholics with alcohol-abusing parents or grandparents began drinking at an early age and had severe social and personal problems. Apparently, as is true in the general population, a family history of alcoholism among narcotics addicts is a risk factor for the development of alcoholism.[29]

2.2. Patterns of Alcohol Use among Opiate Users

Temporal patterns of alcohol and narcotics abuse, including sequential, concurrent, and alternating patterns, have been described among opiate addicts.[30] Despite the lack of rigorous research findings, it is clear that this form of multiple substance abuse has been an ongoing phenomenon for many decades. Particularly during the past 20 years, the proliferation and availability of greater numbers of drugs have increased medical and social interest in multiple substance abuse and related problems generally. Because of the long-standing relationship between alcohol and narcotics use and the frequent problems resulting from joint use, alcohol use has become a significant research and clinical focus. Specifically, alcohol is almost invariably the first psychoactive agent abused by adolescents,[31] including those who later become opiate addicts.[32] Moreover, evidence indicates that initial alcohol use tends to occur at earlier ages in those who later abuse alcohol and/or other drugs.[20]

2.2.1. Sequence of Opiate and Alcohol Use Onset. Alcohol abuse prior to the development of illicit drug addiction is a common occurrence. Weppner and Agar[33] reported evidence of alcohol abuse prior to narcotics addiction in approximately 22% of 738 addicts. Of the 446 addicts (60.4%) who had been physically dependent on another drug prior to their heroin addiction, nearly 18% reported that alcohol abuse was an "immediate precursor" to heroin dependence.

In a study examining the precursor role of alcohol in narcotics addiction, Rosen et al.[34] reported that 68% of a sample of predominantly white narcotics addicts in treatment had abused alcohol prior to becoming dependent on any other drug. These researchers defined abuse as loss of control over drinking and the occurrence of alcohol-related medical or psychosocial problems. Demographic analyses by other researchers indicated that their addict subgroup, which reported prenarcotic histories of alcohol dependence, tended to include more blacks, women, and older individuals.[33]

2.2.2. Concurrent and Alternating Patterns of Opiate and Alcohol Use. Several studies of addicts who had been withdrawn from heroin[34] reported that alcohol abuse frequently occurs during periods of abstinence from opiates (an alternating abuse pattern), although a small proportion of the addicts continued to drink excessively while addicted (a concurrent abuse pattern). It is common for addicts to abuse a number of drugs for a variety of reasons, using them simultaneously to enhance effects, subsequently to counteract undesirable effects, or alternately as substitutes for preferred drugs temporarily not available. Alcohol appears to be used for all of these reasons. O'Donnell's[35] follow-up study of narcotics addicts showed that at some point during follow-up, 17% of 122 addicts had become addicted to barbiturates or alcohol (no distinction made). Vaillant[36] studied 30 opiate addicts who had maintained "stable abstinence" from heroin for at least 3 years. Most of these individuals were found to have substituted a variety of substance use behaviors for previous heroin-related activities. In 47% of the cases, the major substitute was alcohol. Some of the addicts drank to excess only during the first year of abstinence, but four addicts sustained "heavy drinking" practices over the years, and six others used alcohol to such an extent as to impair health or social functioning. Anglin et al.[37] confirmed the inverse relationship between consumption levels of alcohol and heroin suggested by literature findings. An inverse relationship, consistent across ethnic and gender subgroups, persisted throughout the addiction career in several samples of chronic heroin addicts.

2.3. Abuse of Alcohol by Opiate Addicts Maintained on Methadone

Alcohol abuse among clients maintained on methadone has often been reported; such abuse has been associated with the rapid development of medical problems and with higher-than-average rates of treatment failure.[38] Although methadone maintenance (MM) treatment has been suggested as contributing to alcohol abuse, assessment of the prevalence rates reported in most studies suggests that there is little difference between the alcohol abuse rates occurring during long-term MM periods and those occurring during pretreatment periods.[39,40]

The prevalence of alcohol abuse among heroin addicts applying for methadone treatment is estimated by some[30] to be between 10 and 30%; generally, these prevalence rates do not necessarily increase during treatment. For example, Maddux and Elliott[40] observed high rates of problem drinking among Mexican–American addicts in MM treatment, but for their group, alcohol abuse was common before they entered methadone treatment. One study, however, has suggested that alcoholism rates may increase during methadone maintenance treatment.[41] This study of a random sample of 120 predominantly Mexican–American patients in an MM program reported that 25% had drinking problems. In contrast, only 5% of a sample of 60 consecutive new admissions to the program fulfilled the same criteria. The comparison suggests that a significant increase in alcoholism occurred during the average 15 months of methadone treatment for the former group.

On the other hand, Anglin et al.[37] compared the patterns of alcohol and heroin use by narcotics addicts from the nonmethadone (drug-free) California Civil Addict Program (CAP) with those from Southern California MM programs. These authors demonstrated that alcohol and heroin consumption were inversely related throughout the addicts' careers, regardless of treatment modality, ethnicity, or stage of addiction career. They concluded that MM participation itself should not be considered a cause of increased alcohol consumption. Rather, alcohol consumption consistently increased under any condition where heroin consumption declined.

Heavy alcohol consumption by methadone maintenance patients has been attributed by researchers to at least two motivations, one based on underlying psychiatric and psychosocial adjustment problems and the other on a desire for a psychoactive effect, or "high." For example, patients may drink alcohol in order to quell the anxiety associated with difficulties in adjusting to the "straight" world, or, alternatively, simply to obtain a psychoactive effect to replace that denied them by MM. Both hypotheses are valid as partial explanations of the same phenomenon.

2.4. Consequences of Alcohol and Opiate Use

The risk of medical consequences and the potentially lethal effects associated with the concurrent abuse of more than one psychoactive agent have been well documented,[42–45] particularly with respect to alcohol use among heroin addicts. The death rate of MM patients who drink heavily is as much as 10 times that of patients who abstain. The potentially life-threatening nature of alcohol abuse by opiate addicts has been attributed to two factors. One is the synergistic depressant effect of alcohol and heroin on the central nervous system. The depressant effects of alcohol and opiates are additive, if not superadditive, and the cumulative effect can be deadly. The other main contribution is related to the more careless preparation and use of heroin by individuals already under the influence of alcohol. It is obvious that these two factors can, and probably do at times, operate simultaneously.

Both alcohol and adulterated street heroin can damage the liver. Heroin use may introduce hepatitis B infection through contaminated injections. Alcohol excess induces alcoholic hepatitis and cirrhosis, a combination that can lead to fulminating liver disease.[40] For example, over 20% of a sample of New York City heroin addicts showed evidence of chronic alcoholism at autopsy.[46]

Furthermore, for persons addicted to both narcotics and alcohol, withdrawal effects become much more complicated and the prognosis for recovery is more negative.[47] In addition, dual addicts are typically a more disturbed and antisocial group, and their behavior is more aberrant, thus requiring greater treatment effort. Concurrent drug/alcohol abuse is also associated with traffic violations and accidents. Thus, alcohol abuse by drug-dependent individuals is associated not only with increased social dysfunction and failure in treatment programs, but also with illness and accidents.

Although many studies have examined the antecedents and consequences of alcohol use by opiate addicts, few have examined the simultaneous patterns of use of both substances across time and the associated long-term consequences. Data from two studies performed at UCLA allow an examination of such patterns in addicts sampled from both drug-free and methadone maintenance treatment programs. Research findings pertinent to the topic are presented in the next section.

3. Longitudinal Patterns of Alcohol Use and Related Behaviors among Narcotics Addicts

One of the UCLA studies used data collected from 581 male addicts admitted to the California Civil Addict Program (CAP) in 1962–1964.[48,49] The other study collected information from 720 narcotics addicts who entered MM programs in Southern California in the years 1971–1978. The CAP was a drug-free treatment program established in 1961 by California legislation and administered under the Department of Corrections. This program provided the only major treatment available to addicts in California during the 1960s. After 1970, community MM treatment clinics became popular in California and nationwide. Even though there are differences in sample selection and sample characteristics that preclude direct comparisons between these two samples in absolute terms, patterns of substance use that can be replicated may suggest common behaviors generalizable to clients of both drug-free and methadone maintenance programs.

Both studies obtained background characteristics and retrospective longitudinal information starting the year before the first use of narcotics and continuing through the treatment and posttreatment periods. These self-reported data include measures of narcotics, heavy alcohol,* and other drug use, as well as measures of employment, marital status, property crime involvement, drug dealing involvement, and so on.† Because polydrug use is a common and an important pattern among these addicts,[50] daily use of marijuana and other nonnarcotic drugs‡ was included in the following analyses whenever applicable. Decreased social productivity or employment and increased property crime involvement are social consequences also likely to be associated with narcotics and alcohol use; these social consequences are included for examination.

Although most of the information collected from the CAP and MM samples is similar, because the studies were conducted at different times they do not necessarily contain exactly the same set of variables. In general, richer information on alcohol use is available for the CAP sample because respondents were interviewed twice, 10 years apart. In order to make observational comparisons between the two samples, however, the analysis conducted for each sample will include, as much as possible, parallel dependent variables. Statistical analyses performed for each dependent variable include multiway frequency loglinear tests if the dependent variable was categorical and three-way ANOVAs if the dependent variable was continuous. Because of the unbalanced design, ANOVAs were tested using the General Linear Models (GLM) procedure available in statistical package (SAS).

3.1. Sample Characteristics

3.1.1. Civil Addict Program. The CAP sample consisted of 581 male narcotics addicts selected from admissions to the program in 1962–1964. Subjects were located and interviewed twice in follow-up studies conducted in 1974–1975 and 1985–1986. The experimental design and procedures are described in detail in Anglin et al.[49] Interview completion statistics are presented in Table I. Background characteristics and substance use behavior of the 405 Anglo and Chicano** male addicts who were interviewed in 1974–1975 are presented in Table II. Additional information obtained in 1985–1986 is presented in Table III and provides another assessment 10 years after the first.

---

*Heavy alcohol use is operationally defined as getting high on alcohol at least twice a week, where getting high means drinking at least a six-pack of beer, or a bottle of wine, or seven drinks of liquor over a 6-hr period.

†Detailed descriptions of interview procedures have been given in previous papers.[48,51]

‡Nonnarcotic drugs examined include inhalants, amphetamines, barbiturates, cocaine, tranquilizers, and PCP.

**Because black clients constitute a small percentage of California treatment patients, they are excluded from the present study to avoid the possible misinterpretation that the data could be representative of blacks.

Table I. Locating and Interviewing Results for 1974/1975 and 1985/1986 Studies

	1974/1975		1985/1986		Both studies	
	N	%[a]	N	%	N	%[a]
Number selected	581	100	581	100	581	100
Number interviewed	439	76	354	61	328	56
Anglo	150	(34)	122	(34)	116	(35)
Chicano	255	(58)	204	(58)	187	(57)
Black	34	(8)	28	(8)	25	(8)
Number not interviewed	142	24	227	39		
Deceased	70	12	160	28		
Incapacitated	0	0	5	1		
Refused	30	5	26	4		
Not located	42	7	30	6		

[a]Parentheses indicate percentages are calculated based on number interviewed.

Three variables expected to be related to alcohol use patterns were chosen to be examined: race (Anglo vs. Chicano), parental alcohol history (either father or mother reported as having an alcohol problem vs. neither), and sequence of heroin and alcohol* onset (self-reported heavy alcohol use before narcotics addiction, addiction before heavy alcohol use, or no heavy alcohol use). These three variables are included as between-subject, or grouping, variables wherever applicable in the analyses.

   3.1.1a. Assessment at First Interview.   About one-third of each of the two ethnic groups reported a positive parental alcohol problem history (Table II). Onset sequence was found to be significantly associated with race as well as with parental history. Forty-five percent of the Chicanos started heavy alcohol use before their narcotics addiction, while only 33% of the Anglos did so; in contrast, 48% of the Anglos started narcotics addiction first, as compared to 34% of the Chicanos. Addicts reporting parents with a history of alcohol problems were not any more likely than those without such family influence to start heavy alcohol use first, but were more likely to self-report heavy alcohol use. Only 13% of addicts with a history of parental alcohol problems reported no heavy personal use of alcohol; 24% of addicts with no history of parental problems with alcohol reported no heavy personal use.

   Ages at first narcotics use, first period narcotics addiction (defined as daily use for 30 consecutive days), first drunk, first heavy alcohol use, first marijuana use, first regular marijuana use, and first arrest for the 405 CAP narcotics addicts are presented in Table II by ethnicity, parental history, and sequence, as well as for the total sample. Overall, the total sample reported first drunk as early as 13.6 years old and first marijuana use at 14.7. Mean age of first arrest was 15, regular use of marijuana generally began at 15.5, first narcotics use at 18.4, and narcotics addiction at 20.2. Many of the addicts also

---

*Age at the start of period of heaviest drinking.

Table II. Heroin Use, Alcohol Use, and Other Critical Events (Information Collected at the First Interview: CAP Sample)

Race (R)	Anglo (N = 150) (37%)						Chicano (N = 255) (63%)							
Parental alcohol problem (P)	Positive (N = 58) (39%)			Negative (N = 92) (61%)			Positive (N = 97) (38%)			Negative (N = 158) (62%)			Total	Statistical results[e]
Relative onset sequence (S)	Alcohol first	Narcotics first	No alcohol	Alcohol first	Narcotics first	No alcohol	Alcohol first	Narcotics first	No alcohol	Alcohol first	Narcotics first	No alcohol		
N	17	34	7	32	38	22	45	39	13	71	48	39	405	R*S, P*S
% of parental use	29	59	12	35	41	24	46	40	14	45	30	25	25.0	R
Age at CAP entry	24.7	24.8	22.6	24.1	24.6	23.9	24.7	26.4	25.8	24.9	26.7	24.1	25.0	R
Age at first interview	36.0	36.2	34.7	35.4	36.0	35.4	36.2	37.7	37.8	36.2	38.1	35.6	36.4	
Narcotics use														
Age at FN[a]	19.4	18.0	18.4	18.6	17.9	18.2	18.8	17.6	18.9	18.8	17.6	18.3	18.4	S
Age at FDU[b]	21.7	20.1	20.0	20.5	19.5	19.1	21.1	19.3	19.4	21.0	19.4	20.3	20.2	S
Age at LDU[c]	31.5	30.1	26.6	30.3	29.9	28.6	32.2	31.8	31.5	33.4	32.9	30.7	31.4	R, S
Addiction career length (years)[d]	9.7	10.0	6.6	9.8	10.4	9.4	11.2	12.5	12.1	12.4	13.5	10.4	11.2	R
Alcohol use														
Age first drunk	12.9	12.6	13.8	13.5	13.7	15.7	12.8	13.2	16.3	13.4	13.7	13.8	13.6	P, S, R*P*S
Age first heavy drink	16.9	29.6	—	18.5	28.6	—	16.2	30.1	—	17.4	29.1	—	23.2	S
Duration (months)	23.5	22.2	—	20.6	20.1	—	25.1	16.2	—	19.8	21.9	—	21	
Oz used/week	103.3	179.2	—	80.8	138.9	—	103.8	112.9	—	103.5	109.8	—	115.5	S, R*S
Ever hospitalized for a drinking problem (%)	0.0	20.6	14.3	3.1	13.2	0.0	4.4	20.5	7.7	11.3	10.4	0.0	9.4	S
Ever arrested due to drinking (%)	64.7	85.3	85.7	68.8	63.2	22.7	86.7	66.7	38.5	80.3	68.8	48.7	68.1	
Drinking in the week before first interview														
Oz consumed	15.9	19.5	4.1	13.1	38.5	2.3	21.3	26.0	10.8	11.6	11.0	4.2	16.1	S, R*P
# of times high	0.4	0.7	0.0	0.2	0.9	0.0	0.5	0.8	0.5	0.4	0.3	0.0	0.4	S

(continued)

Table II. (Continued)

Race (R)	Anglo (N = 150) (37%)						Chicano (N = 255) (63%)							
	Positive (N = 58) (39%)			Negative (N = 92) (61%)			Positive (N = 97) (38%)			Negative (N = 158) (62%)				
Parental alcohol problem (P)														
Relative onset sequence (S)	Alcohol first	Narcotics first	No alcohol	Alcohol first	Narcotics first	No alcohol	Alcohol first	Narcotics first	No alcohol	Alcohol first	Narcotics first	No alcohol	Total	Statistical results[e]
Marijuana use														
Ever used (%)	100	100	100	100	100	91	98	100	92	98	100	95	98	
Mean age first use	14.5	15.3	15.4	15.5	14.7	16.4	14.1	13.9	14.5	14.5	14.6	14.4	14.7	R
Ever daily use (%)	82	82	86	87	74	72	87	69	54	70	81	59	75	
Mean age first daily use	14.6	16.7	16.0	16.1	15.7	17.4	14.7	15.1	14.1	15.4	15.5	14.9	15.5	R
School/family-related events														
Education (year)	9.9	10.7	10.0	10.7	11.2	12.0	9.6	10.0	8.5	10.2	10.0	10.3	10.3	R, P, P*S
Socioeconomic status of family (%)														
Poor	13	8	14	16	4	0	14	23	18	17	11	12	13.9	R
Working class	60	32	28	16	11	29	46	46	45	37	31	50	38.2	
Middle class	13	52	28	48	44	59	23	23	36	39	49	31	40.0	
Upper-middle class	13	8	28	20	41	12	17	7	0	7	9	8	7.8	
Age left home	16.8	17.3	18.3	18.1	17.6	18.0	17.4	16.9	19.1	17.5	17.6	17.4	17.6	R
Main occupation														
Skilled	53.5	60.0	14.3	56.6	55.6	52.9	34.3	53.8	27.3	18.5	22.9	23.1	38.0	
Semiskilled	47.7	36.0	85.7	44.0	37.0	35.3	42.9	26.9	54.5	57.4	45.7	38.5	44.2	
Unskilled/unemployed	0.0	4.0	0.0	0.9	7.4	11.8	22.9	19.2	18.2	24.1	31.4	38.5	17.8	
Legal system involvement														
Age at first arrest	14.2	14.8	17.7	15.2	15.7	15.2	14.4	14.2	16.8	15.2	15.2	13.9	15.0	P*S
Age at first legal supervision	22.0	22.2	22.2	21.8	21.9	20.8	22.3	22.5	23.2	22.9	24.0	22.4	22.5	

[a] FN represents date of first narcotics use.
[b] FDU represents first daily use for 30 days or more.
[c] LDU represents last daily use.
[d] Addiction career length represents years from first daily use to last daily use, or to the time of interview if still using.
[e] Variables significant at $p < 0.05$. * represents interaction between factors.

tried other nonnarcotic drugs, such as amphetamines and barbiturates, at a mean age of 17 or 18, and cocaine at a later age of 25.6.

Onset sequence of narcotics addiction and heavy alcohol use was clearly related to many of the variables reported in Table II. For those whose heavy alcohol use occurred before narcotics addiction (Alcohol-First Group), heavy alcohol consumption started at an average of 17.2 years old; those whose narcotics addiction occurred first (Narcotics-First Group) started drinking heavily at the age of 29.3. On the other hand, members of the Alcohol-First Group started their narcotics addiction career a year or two later than either the Narcotics-First or No-Alcohol Group. Members of the No-Alcohol Group were the least likely among the three sequence groups to have been hospitalized for a drinking problem. However, many of these addicts reported at least one arrest due to drinking; even so, their percentages were much lower than among the other groups.

Parental alcohol history affected only a few variables. Positive parental alcohol use history seemed to be associated with earlier age of first drunk, earlier age of first arrest, and lower education achievement.[29] Racial differences, in general, showed that Chicanos had their first drunk at a younger age, consumed alcohol typically at a higher level, had a lower education achievement level and longer addiction careers, and were slightly older, both at treatment entry and at time of interview.

3.1.1b. Assessment at Second Interview. The second follow-up interview, which was conducted in 1985–1986 among those of the original 581 who were still alive, provided an opportunity to assess current narcotics and alcohol use status for a sample group that had reached middle age and had been followed for more than 20 years. These data are reported in Table III. At this interview point, only one-third of the sample had not been using narcotics in the year before the interview; the remaining addicts were either incarcerated, in MM treatment, or had not ceased the use of narcotics. Chicanos reported overall higher levels of narcotics consumption. Self-reported current drinking level did not show differences among the groups; however, the overall amounts consumed and the number of alcohol highs experienced during the week before the interview seemed to be higher for several groups than the comparable measures taken at the first interview 10 years earlier (Table II).

Except for the few ethnic differences mentioned earlier, parental alcohol problem history and onset sequence did not seem to influence the outcome variables measured at this interview point. One item worthy of notice is the self-reported use of different coping strategies for stress.* Addicts who developed heavy alcohol use later than their narcotics addiction tended to drink more alcohol when under stress. Addicts also reported increased use of narcotics in coping with stress, and this tendency varied depending on parental alcohol history as well as onset sequence. In general, those who did not report heavy alcohol use either by themselves or by their parents were more likely to increase narcotics use under stress.

*Measured by 0–4 self-rating (corresponding to never, rarely, sometimes, often, and always) on how frequently the addict used various methods of coping with stressful situations.

Table III. Current Drinking Patterns and Related Status (Information Collected at the Second Interview: CAP sample)

Race (R)	Anglo (N = 116)						Chicano (N = 187)							
Parental alcohol problem (P)	Positive (N = 47)			Negative (N = 69)			Positve (N = 72)			Negative (N = 115)				
Relative onset sequence (S)	Alcohol first	Narcotics first	No alcohol	Alcohol first	Narcotics first	No alcohol	Alcohol first	Narcotics first	No alcohol	Alcohol first	Narcotics first	No alcohol	Total	Statistical result[c]
N	15	25	7	25	27	17	35	26	11	54	35	26	303	
Age at second interview	46.3	46.9	45.6	47.2	45.8	46.2	47.6	48.5	49.6	46.5	49.6	45.4	47.2	R
Status at interview (%)														
Incarcerated	20.0	40.0	14.3	12.0	7.4	11.8	22.9	15.4	18.2	14.8	20.0	26.9	18.8	R
On MM	13.3	4.0	28.6	16.0	18.5	17.7	11.4	15.4	18.2	13.0	8.6	15.4	13.5	
Not on MM														
Using daily	6.7	0.0	0.0	8.0	7.4	11.8	5.7	23.1	27.3	20.4	17.1	3.9	11.9	
Irregular use	13.3	12.0	14.3	4.0	7.4	17.7	20.0	7.7	0.0	16.7	20.0	19.2	13.9	
No use, no MM, no incarceration in last 12 mo.	46.7	40.0	42.9	56.0	40.7	41.2	25.7	38.5	9.1	24.1	28.6	30.8	34.0	
Others	0.0	4.0	0.0	4.0	18.5	0.0	14.3	0.0	27.3	11.1	5.7	3.9	7.9	
Alcohol use														
Current drinking level (%)														
None	53.3	52.0	14.3	40.0	29.6	47.0	34.3	23.1	63.6	35.2	40.0	46.2	38.9	
Below average amount	13.3	12.0	57.1	12.0	22.2	11.8	17.1	19.2	9.1	20.4	14.3	15.4	17.2	
Average amount	13.3	16.0	14.2	36.0	37.0	29.4	28.6	38.5	18.2	33.3	20.0	30.8	28.4	

Above average/out of control	20.0	20.0	14.3	12.0	11.1	11.8	20.0	19.2	9.1	11.1	25.7	7.7	15.5
Drinking in last 7 days													
Oz of alcohol	27.9	11.5	17.4	23.7	11.0	8.5	9.1	17.8	1.5	7.9	15.8	8.9	12.8
No. times high	0.7	0.5	0.7	0.3	0.7	0.1	0.7	1.2	0.0	0.4	0.9	1.0	0.6
Ever hospitalized for alcohol problem (%)	13.3	33.3	28.5	16.0	18.5	5.9	22.9	16.7	9.1	11.1	8.8	0.0	14.5
Current physical health													
Poor	20.2	8.0	0.0	12.0	3.7	5.9	5.7	7.7	18.2	3.7	20.0	0.0	8.2
Fair	13.3	20.0	28.6	32.0	22.2	11.8	40.0	19.2	18.2	27.8	14.3	15.4	23.1
Good	33.3	68.0	28.6	40.0	51.9	52.9	42.9	65.4	54.6	55.6	57.1	61.5	53.1
Excellent	33.3	4.0	42.9	16.0	22.2	29.4	11.4	7.7	9.1	13.0	8.6	23.1	15.5
Disabilities (%)	13.3	32.0	28.6	20.0	25.9	11.8	28.6	11.5	36.4	11.1	28.6	15.4	20.8
Coping with stress													
Drink more	1.57	1.59	1.00	1.00	1.52	0.88	1.43	1.38	0.45	1.11	1.63	0.77	1.25
Narcotics use	2.07	1.82	1.00	1.08	1.74	1.94	1.97	1.81	2.00	1.54	1.91	2.46	1.79

S
P*S

3.1.2. Methadone Maintenance (MM) Sample.   Because MM has become one of the major treatment modalities for narcotics addiction in the United States, and because MM participation has been related to alcohol abuse in the literature, an addict sample selected from admissions to Southern California MM clinics was examined to further address the issues developed in the literature review. This sample of 720 narcotics addicts consisted of 251 Anglo men, 283 Anglo women, 141 Chicanos, and 45 Chicanas.[51,52] The research results reported in the preceding section were for men only. This sample allowed investigators to compare longitudinal narcotics and alcohol consumption patterns between women and men addicts.

Background characteristics and ages at critical events such as first narcotics use, first daily use, first arrest, and several other significant variables are presented in Table IV. In general, this group of addicts reported age first drunk at 14.0 years old and first marijuana use at 15.7, began regular use of marijuana at 16.7, were first arrested at 17.4, tried narcotics for the first time at 19.5, and began narcotics addiction careers at 20.8 years old. Differences due to race and gender are observed for a majority of the variables, but not for their interaction. In the case of ethnicity, compared to their Anglo counterparts, Chicano men and women were in general older when starting first daily use, attending treatment, and at interview; they also had longer addiction careers, lower educational achievement levels, lower family socioeconomic status, and less-skilled jobs, and were arrested at a younger age. More Chicanos than Anglos reported problems in school, gang membership, alcohol-related arrests, and incarceration before their first narcotics use. However, Chicano addicts reported fewer parental drinking problems than Anglos.

Regarding gender differences, women were, in general, older at first drunk and younger at MM entry and at interview. They had shorter addiction careers than their male counterparts. Women addicts also reported more problems in their families, more parental drinking problems, and an overall lower level of alcohol consumption. Women were also less likely to have been arrested or incarcerated.

3.2. Longitudinal Patterns of Use

The longitudinal patterns of heroin use, alcohol use, and other related activities before, during, and after the addiction career [defined as first addiction or first daily use (FDU) to last addiction or last daily use (LDU)] are listed in Tables V and VI for the CAP and the MM samples, respectively. Specifically, four major time periods are included: from 1 year prior to first narcotics use (PRE-FDU), the first half of the addiction career (FDU-MID), the second half of the addiction career (MID-LDU), and from termination of the addiction career to the time of the interview* (LDU-I). Dependent variables such as

---

*For the CAP sample, the interview time refers to the first interview; analysis of the longitudinal information has not been completed to the time of the second interview.

Table IV. Heroin Use, Alcohol Use, and Other Critical Events (MM Sample)[a]

Race (R) Gender (G)	Anglo (N = 534)		Chicano (N = 186)		Total	ANOVA[b]
	Male (N = 251)	Female (N = 283)	Male (N = 141)	Female (N = 45)	(N = 720)	
Age at MM entry	26.6	24.7	30.3	26.8	26.6	R, G
Age at interview	31.7	29.8	36.3	32.4	31.9	R, G
Narcotics use						
Age at FN	19.5	19.5	19.3	20.6	19.5	R
Age at FDU	20.8	20.4	21.3	21.5	20.8	R, G
Age at last daily use	29.2	27.3	33.6	30.7	29.4	R, G
Addiction career length (years)	8.4	6.9	12.3	9.2	8.6	
Alcohol use						
Age first drunk	14.1	14.9	13.7	15.2	14.0	G
Ever hospitalized for a drinking problem (%)	6.4	4.2	6.4	2.2	5.3	
Ever arrested due to drinking (%)	56.4	26.9	70.9	46.7	47.0	R, G
Parent drinking problem (%)	41.8	45.9	24.8	40.0	40.0	R, G
Drinking in the week before interview						
Ozs consumed	16.0	10.9	20.4	8.4	14.4	G
No. of times high	0.9	0.6	1.0	0.4	0.8	G
	(154)	(128)	(89)	(18)		
Marijuana use						
Ever used (%)	98	99	99	96	99	
Mean age first use	15.6	16.0	14.8	17.3	15.7	G, G*R
Ever daily use (%)	84	54	67	29	64	G, R
Mean age first daily use	16.4	17.2	16.6	18.5	16.7	G
School-related factors						
Education	11.4	11.2	9.4	10.0	10.9	R, R*G
Problem in school (%)	70.9	65.7	83.0	82.2	72.0	R, G
Family-related factors						
Socioeconomic status of family (%)						

(continued)

Table IV. *(Continued)*

Race (R)	Anglo (N = 534)		Chicano (N = 186)		Total	ANOVA[b]
Gender (G)	Male (N = 251)	Female (N = 283)	Male (N = 141)	Female (N = 45)	(N = 720)	
Poor	2.4	2.1	20.7	22.7	7.1	R, G
Working class	24.9	24.8	58.6	56.8	33.4	
Middle	55.8	54.6	17.9	15.9	45.5	
Upper-middle	16.9	18.4	2.9	4.6	13.9	
Problems in family	2.8	3.1	2.4	3.1	2.8	G
Age left home	18.0	17.2	18.2	16.8	17.7	G
	(246)	(279)	(137)	(44)		
Main occupation (%)						
Skilled	35.5	9.9	17.01	0	20.3	R, G
Semiskilled	54.6	58.0	56.0	46.7	57.6	
Unskilled/never worked	10.0	32.1	27.0	53.4	22.2	
Legal system involvement						
Gang membership (%)	17.6	5.3	40.4	25.0	17.7	R, G
Age at first arrest	16.9	18.6	16.0	17.8	17.4	R, G
	(233)	(263)	(134)	(41)		
Age at first legal supervision	22.0	22.4	23.2	22.6	22.4	
	(202)	(187)	(124)	(36)		
Incarcerated >30 days before FNU (%)	30.3	11.7	41.4	29.6		R, G
Status at interview (%)						
Incarcerated	13	7	13	16	11	
On MM	33	38	33	31	35	
Not on MM						
Using daily	7	6	11	13	8	
Irregular use	16	17	20	22	18	
No use in past 12 months	17	22	7	4	16	
Others	14	11	16	13	13	

[a] Numbers in parentheses represent total subjects reporting such behavior.
[b] * represents interaction between factors.

Table V. Longitudinal Pattern of Heroin Use, Alcohol Use, and Other Related Activities (Percent Time) (Information Collected at First Interview: CAP Sample)

Race (R)	Anglo (N = 150)						Chicano (N = 255)							
Parental alcohol problem (P)	Positive (N = 58)			Negative (N = 92)			Positve (N = 97)			Negative (N = 158)				
Relative onset sequence (S)	Alcohol first	Narcotics first	No alcohol	Alcohol first	Narcotics first	No alcohol	Alcohol first	Narcotics first	No alcohol	Alcohol first	Narcotics first	No alcohol	Total	Statistical[b] results
N	17	34	7	32	38	22	45	39	13	71	48	39	405	
Nonincarcerated months in period[a]														
Pre-FDU	27(17)	32(34)	28(7)	29(32)	26(38)	19(22)	29(45)	28(39)	17(13)	29(71)	29(48)	30(39)	28(405)	T, T*R, T*S
FDU-MID	28(15)	42(34)	24(7)	38(25)	44(38)	35(21)	38(44)	50(39)	54(13)	45(65)	55(48)	38(38)	43(387)	
MID-LDU	32(15)	35(34)	24(7)	39(25)	48(38)	34(21)	38(44)	44(39)	48(13)	46(65)	47(48)	34(39)	41(388)	
LDU-I1	42(13)	52(28)	99(6)	48(21)	56(26)	60(19)	44(29)	61(35)	60(11)	35(48)	51(41)	46(39)	50(316)	
Heroin, daily use														
Pre-FDU	0	0	0	0	0	0	0	0	0	0	0	0	0	
FDU-MID	67.9	79.8	65	77.3	72.0	80.5	79.9	72.4	78.0	75.2	71.4	82.6	75.8	
MID-LDU	48.0	68.0	48.1	55.3	58.3	73.6	71.4	73.1	65.9	66.9	60.8	71.6	65.5	
LDU-I1	0	0	0	0	0	0	0	0	0	0	0	0	0	
Heroin, no use														
Pre-FDU	68.2	66.3	67.1	71.2	70.2	70.3	62.4	63.6	81.1	69.8	63.9	67.9	67.6	T, R, T*R
FDU-MID	18.3	5.7	18.2	12.0	13.4	8.7	6.1	10.6	15.0	11.3	11.7	6.5	10.1	
MID-LDU	24.6	14.6	33.7	25.2	23.3	19.7	8.6	11.4	24.5	14.3	14.9	10.6	16.0	
LDU-I1	61.3	69.4	81.6	59.5	64.4	70.4	50.0	57.1	37.9	49.4	62.9	58.7	59.0	
Alcohol, heavy use														
Pre-FDU	69.1	45.2	19.5	65.0	45.5	0	76.1	51.5	22.4	72.7	44.0	16.0	50.1	T, S, T*S
FDU-MID	28.5	33.3	22.6	14.0	30.7	1.7	24.6	37.7	10.7	30.9	29.4	5.7	24.8	
MID-LDU	30.3	44.4	19.0	29.4	42.3	0	28.3	38.2	10.9	33.5	40.2	10.3	30.5	
LDU-I1	37.0	67.9	16.7	46.6	71.7	0	55.0	65.6	17.2	27.4	48.7	17.1	44.1	
Property crime														
Pre-FDU	38.2	43.0	40.7	41.3	31.6	46.8	38.9	39.8	24.1	25.9	34.3	38.4	35.9	T
FDU-MID	54.2	46.3	32.9	54.1	36.2	38.8	42.2	34.7	18.6	32.6	46.6	40.6	40.1	
MID-LDU	46.9	35.9	35.8	43.5	33.0	40.4	44.6	31.9	32.0	26.2	35.0	46.2	36.5	
LDU-I1	14.3	9.5	4.1	11.8	10.0	11.7	9.1	4.7	6.2	4.5	6.0	8.4	7.9	

(continued)

Table V. (Continued)

Race (R)	Anglo (N = 150)						Chicano (N = 255)							
Parental alcohol problem (P)	Positive (N = 58)			Negative (N = 92)			Positve (N = 97)			Negative (N = 158)				Statistical[b] results
Relative onset sequence (S)	Alcohol first	Narcotics first	No alcohol	Alcohol first	Narcotics first	No alcohol	Alcohol first	Narcotics first	No alcohol	Alcohol first	Narcotics first	No alcohol	Total	
Employment														
Pre-FDU	59.7	48.9	90.8	59.8	56.1	41.8	47.5	62.1	56.9	54.8	57.1	45.8	54.3	T
FDU-MID	52.2	53.9	56.1	46.0	49.9	39.6	41.1	51.9	52.2	44.8	53.8	41.3	47.7	
MID-LDU	42.8	50.1	59.0	52.0	55.3	39.9	42.3	47.9	59.1	41.2	50.2	39.1	46.7	
LDU-I1	68.2	65.0	77.0	70.3	66.7	74.2	58.0	67.3	66.1	56.2	61.9	65.2	64.4	
Methadone maintenance														
Pre-FDU	0	0	0	0	0	0	0	0	0	0	0	0	0	
FDU-MID	0	0	0	0	1.4	0	0.3	0	0	0	0	0	0.2	
MID-LDU	8.9	1.3	7.4	1.6	6.5	4.4	7.2	2.9	3.2	2.7	3.1	1.4	3.8	
LDU-I1	30.8	26.8	16.7	38.1	25.1	18.4	23.8	27.8	21.5	35.5	24.0	29.3	27.7	
Nonnarcotics drug use														
Pre-FDU	40.2	12.8	0	20.6	24.2	8.1	17.4	9.8	0	5.8	5.7	7.6	11.1	T,R,S,T*S,
FDU-MID	12.3	11.4	0	8.5	7.3	2.2	4.3	1.6	0	2.6	4.6	1.2	4.6	T*PTS,
MID-LDU	8.4	5.5	0	7.2	10.2	2.5	2.1	0.3	0	2.7	1.7	0.2	3.4	P*S
LDU-I1	7.4	2.6	11.5	2.6	1.6	0.1	2.7	0.8	0	6.0	2.8	2.2	2.0	
Marijuana														
Pre-FDU	48.6	43.6	42.2	49.4	40.1	39.6	45.6	36.3	21.8	38.9	44.5	42.5	40.6	T, R, T*R,
FDU-MID	16.2	29.5	19.0	33.2	11.4	24.6	10.0	8.9	1.2	4.2	8.6	5.8	12.6	T*R*P*S,
MID-LDU	26.4	24.3	23.8	31.8	14.5	14.8	2.0	5.0	0	1.8	3.8	8.1	10.2	P*S
LDU-I2	15.4	13.8	28.0	35.5	17.2	16.7	7.8	8.6	0	8.4	1.1	1.0	10.9	

[a] N for the various periods indicated in parentheses.
[b] Variables (between-subject variables include race, parental use, onset sequence, and repeated factor is time period) are significant at $p = 0.05$; * represents interaction.

Table VI. Longitudinal Patterns of Heroin Use, Alcohol Use, and Other Related Activities (MM Sample)

Race (R)	Anglo		Chicano			Statistical
Gender (G)	Men	Women	Men	Women	Total	results[b]
N	251	283	141	45	720	
Nonincarcerated months in period[a]						
Pre-FDU	26(249)	23(283)	29(138)	20(44)	25(714)	
FDU-MID	42(251)	38(283)	54(140)	45(45)	43(719)	
MID-LDU	44(251)	40(283)	60(140)	50(45)	46(719)	
LDU-I	32(212)	31(257)	35(112)	25(35)	32(616)	
Heroin, daily use						
Pre-FDU	0	0	0	0	0	T
FDU-MID	72.3	73.1	76.5	73.5	73.5	
MID-LDU	54.0	60.3	58.5	55.7	57.5	
LDU-I	0	0	0	0	0	
Heroin, abstinence						
Pre-FDU	67.6	73.6	63.5	75.8	69.7	T, R,
FDU-MID	13.7	13.5	10.8	12.0	13.0	G,
MID-LDU	19.3	19.7	16.4	23.5	19.1	T*R
LDU-I	57.0	56.7	41.2	46.0	53.4	
Alcohol, heavy use						
Pre-FDU	37.7	20.4	55.1	20.5	33.2	T, G,
FDU-MID	20.1	9.6	25.4	11.5	16.5	T*G
MID-LDU	24.4	12.9	30.2	11.7	20.2	
LDU-I	39.8	21.5	44.0	18.1	31.7	
Property crime						
Pre-FDU	18.7	13.2	22.0	19.0	17.2	T
FDU-MID	33.7	27.8	38.0	38.1	32.5	
MID-LDU	27.5	21.3	24.2	28.1	24.5	
LDU-I	6.7	6.1	8.2	15.8	7.2	
Employment						
Pre-FDU	56.4	39.4	60.5	26.4	48.6	T, R,
FDU-MID	49.4	23.9	47.2	14.2	36.8	G,
MID-LDU	59.9	26.9	50.8	13.1	42.2	R*G,
LDU-I	67.4	34.2	63.2	19.0	50.1	T*G
Methadone maintenance						
Pre-FDU	0.1	0.2	0.0	0.0	0.1	T
FDU-MID	7.7	9.3	5.0	7.4	7.8	
MID-LDU	36.3	35.0	38.5	41.7	36.6	
LDU-I	57.3	55.6	54.6	60.0	56.3	
Nonnarcotics drug use						
Pre-FDU	17.8	24.3	12.3	19.2	19.4	T, R, G
FDU-MID	7.1	9.6	4.2	6.4	7.5	
MID-LDU	4.2	6.1	2.7	2.0	4.5	
LDU-I	4.1	5.3	1.2	4.9	4.1	
Marijuana						
Pre-FDU	52.4	24.1	33.1	10.8	34.9	T, R,
FDU-MID	26.3	12.3	15.4	9.6	17.6	G,
MID-LDU	24.5	12.4	16.1	7.0	17.0	T*R,
LDU-I	27.2	15.4	16.4	8.4	19.3	T*G

[a] N for the various periods indicated in parentheses.
[b] Variables (between-subject variables include race, gender, and repeated factor is time period) are significant at $p = 0.05$; * represents interaction.

heroin use, alcohol consumption, marijuana use, other nonnarcotic drug use, and property crime activity are measured as mean percent time engaged in such activity during each of these four time periods. A repeated measures ANOVA was conducted for each measure, treating time—the four addiction career periods—as the repeated factor. For the CAP sample, the analysis continued the subdivision by race, parental alcohol history, and onset sequence; these three variables were treated as between-subject variables in the statistical analysis. For the MM sample, the between-subject variables were race and gender.

3.2.1. Overall Longitudinal Patterns.   For both the CAP and MM samples, the longitudinal patterns of behavior were predominantly affected by the time segmentations (T) spanning the addiction career. Overall, narcotics abstinence, alcohol consumption, and employment decreased during the two periods of the addiction career as compared with the preaddiction period, and levels of these behaviors increased after the addiction career terminated. Property crime activity followed the opposite pattern. Methadone maintenance participation increased over time, coinciding with a reduction in daily heroin use and an increase in abstinence. Consumption levels of both marijuana and other nonnarcotic drugs were high before narcotics addiction, decreased after addiction was initiated, and stayed at stable levels thereafter.

These patterns are consistent across both samples. The CAP sample did, however, show higher absolute levels of alcohol consumption and property crime involvement, while the MM sample had a higher level of MM involvement.

3.2.2. Effects of Ethnicity, Parental Alcohol Use, and Onset Sequence. Ethnic comparisons showed that, in both samples, Chicanos had lower levels of narcotics abstinence, nonnarcotics use, and marijuana use.[37] There was no significant difference in alcohol consumption between the two ethnic groups. Parental alcohol problem history did not seem to have much effect on the variables studied. Onset sequence was associated with the levels of alcohol consumption, and this relationship interacted with time. Most interestingly, when compared with the Narcotics-First Group, the Alcohol-First Group started with higher levels of alcohol consumption prior to addiction, but ended with lower levels of consumption after the addiction career terminated.

3.2.3. Effects of Gender.   Several major sex differences were observed, as well as significant interaction effects of gender with race and addiction career period. Women addicts, in general, showed typically higher levels of heroin abstinence and nonnarcotic drug use, as well as lower alcohol use, marijuana use, and employment.

3.3. Alcohol-Related Deaths

For the CAP sample, a special analysis of alcohol-related deaths among this group of narcotics addicts was possible because death certificates were obtained at each interview point. Comparisons were also made on selected variables collected at the first interview between those who died before the second interview and those who lived to be interviewed a second time.

Cumulative deaths and their causes in 1975 and 1986 are listed in Table VII. There were 85 deaths by 1975, and the total number increased to 160 by 1986. At both interview points, the major cause of death was drug overdose. However, the percentage of alcohol-related deaths increased considerably over the 10 years between interviews. Alcohol use was associated with 7.1% of deaths in 1975–1976 and 17.5% of deaths by 1986.

With this longitudinal sample, it was possible to compare the behavior patterns of addicts who died after the first interview ($N = 73$) with those of addicts who were still alive in 1985–1986. The results are presented in Table VIII. Overall, the death group were older by a year-and-a-half than the group who were alive at the time of the 1974–1975 interview. Analysis of the longitudinal patterns of behavior showed that the death group started both heavy drinking and narcotics addiction at significantly later ages than the alive group. The death group also had a slightly higher proportion of individuals who developed narcotics addiction prior to heavy alcohol use. Furthermore, they consumed higher levels of alcohol and narcotics; however, the former difference was not statistically significant.

Table VII. Comparisons of Causes of Death between 1975 and 1986 (CAP Sample)

| | Cumulative deaths as of: | | | |
| | 1975 | | 1986 | |
Cause of death	N	%	N	%
Natural causes, not drug-related	13	15.3	23	14.1
Drug-related disease	8	9.4	39	24.4
Alcohol-related[a]	6	7.1	28	17.5
Opiate-related	2	2.4	8	5.0
Other drug-related	0	0.0	3[b]	1.9
Violent deaths	24	28.2	46	28.8
Accidental	11	12.9	22	13.8
Homicide	10	11.8	18	11.2
Suicide	3	3.5	6	3.8
Drug overdose	36	42.4	52	32.5
Unknown[c]	4	4.7	0	0.0
Totals	85	100.1	160	100.1

[a]Four cases where both alcohol and opiates were implicated in death appear under alcohol-related.
[b]Includes two cases where death from lung cancer was attributed to addiction to tobacco by the physician in attendance.
[c]Death certificate not yet obtained.

Table VIII.   Comparisons on Selected Variables between Persons Alive and Dead in 1985/1986 Who Had Been Interviewed at 1974/1975 (CAP Sample)

	Alive (N = 332)	Dead (N = 73)	p
Ethnicity (%)			
Anglo	38	32	
Chicano	62	68	
Narcotics use			
Age at FN	18	19	
Age at FDU	20	21	<0.05
Alcohol use			
Age at first drunk	13.6	13.3	
Percent with heavy use period	79.5	82.0	
Age began heavy drinking	22.6(264)	25.5(60)	<0.05
Duration (months)	21.2	19.8	
Oz used/week	113.3	125	
Parental use history positive (%)	38.9	35.6	
Sequence of onset (%)			
Heavy alcohol first	41.9	35.6	
Narcotic addiction first	37.6	46.6	
No heavy alcohol	20.5	17.8	
Drinking in last 7 days			
Oz of alcohol	15.0	21.3	
No. times high	0.4	0.5	
Heroin overdose episodes (%)	68.0	66.0	
Hepatitis (%)	25.0	27.0	
Age at I_1	36.1	37.6	<0.05
Longitudinal patterns[a]			
Nonincarcerated months in period[b]			
Pre-FDU	27.4(332)	29.8(73)	T
FDU-MID	42.9(316)	43.1(71)	
MID-LDU	41.0(317)	40.9(71)	
LDU-I_1	50.3(257)	50.2(59)	
Alcohol, heavy use			
Pre-FDU	49.2	54.1	T
FDU-MID	24.5	26.1	
MID-LDU	29.5	35.0	
LDU-I_1	41.7	54.4	
Heroin, daily use			
FDU-MID	74.8	80.7	T, A ($p < 0.10$)
MID-LDU	64.4	70.5	
Heroin, no use			
Pre-FDU	68.7	62.8	T, A
FDU-MID	10.84	8.7	
MID-LDU	16.43	14.4	
LDU-I_1	60.44	52.8	

[a]T = time; A = alive vs. dead. Repeated measures ANOVA performed with T as repeated factor and A as between-subjects variable.
[b]N for the various periods indicated in parentheses.

4. Discussion

Results presented for two samples of narcotics addicts generally support research literature findings of high prevalence for polydrug use among addicts. Consumption data from both the CAP and MM samples demonstrated that, across the addiction career, most narcotics addicts have used multiple drugs, including heroin, alcohol, nonnarcotics, and marijuana. Heavy alcohol use seemed to be a persistent phenomenon; for some it led to arrest, hospitalization, or death. A discernible pattern of alcohol use occurred in relationship to narcotics use: after narcotics addiction began, alcohol use, as well as other substance use, decreased. However, alone among the substances studied, alcohol use increased again whenever narcotics use decreased. It should also be noted that, compared to the MM male sample, the CAP sample had an overall higher level of alcohol consumption both before and after the narcotics addiction career, even though the MM sample had overall higher levels of MM treatment participation. These results suggest that, as reported previously by Anglin et al.,[37] MM participation itself is unrelated to alcohol use.

There were, however, differences in these general patterns that related to onset sequence, parental alcohol problem history, race, and sex. In general, earlier development of heavy alcohol use relative to narcotics addiction was associated with positive parental alcohol use history; this pattern was more prevalent among Chicanos. Women addicts usually had a lower prevalence of alcohol use and related problems, but reported more family-related difficulties.

The CAP sample provided rich information that merits further discussion. For this sample, those who started heavy alcohol use prior to narcotics addiction had also used nonnarcotics and marijuana more heavily across the addiction career than the other two onset sequence groups. However, those whose addiction developed before heavy alcohol use had a higher alcohol consumption level after the addiction career ceased and were more likely to use alcohol as a coping strategy when under stress. These results seem to suggest that addicts with prenarcotic alcohol abuse are more likely to be heavy polydrug users, while even addicts without such developmental patterns still eventually used alcohol as a substitute for their narcotics use.

Status assessment at the second follow-up (see Table VI) showed that 34% of the CAP sample had not used narcotics during the year before the interview, while nearly two-thirds had either been incarcerated or in MM, or had used narcotics—a sobering long-term outcome finding. Drinking levels measured for the last 7 days at the second interview were higher than levels measured at the first interview. Also, about 10% of those who had not reported any heavy drinking during their mid-30s at the first interview subsequently reported above-average or out-of-control drinking during their mid-40s at the second interview. These findings suggest the persistence of both narcotics addiction and alcoholism as chronic disorders, as well as the progressive development of alcohol problems over time.[53]

Major ethnic differences in alcohol-related behavior were noted. More Chicanos developed heavy drinking before narcotics addiction and had alcohol-related arrests. Contrary to most research in cultural differences in alcohol use, no major ethnic differences were found in the longitudinal alcohol use patterns in either the CAP or the MM sample. Furthermore, Chicanos' alcohol consumption patterns were not different from those of Anglo women, even though both female addict groups had lower consumption levels than their male counterparts.

Death rates among the CAP sample increased at slightly more than 1% per year and accumulated to 27.5% by 1985–1986. Alcohol-related deaths accounted for 17.5% of the total. Differences between the alive and the dead in the few selected variables hypothesized to have contributed to the eventual death, however, did not show a discernible pattern.

Since alcohol abuse is frequently seen in patients coming into treatment for narcotics or other drug abuse, the diagnostic and prognostic implications of either active alcohol abuse or a past history of alcohol abuse merit close consideration. Most evaluation research has shown that the majority of drug treatment modalities achieved their primary goal of reducing illicit drug abuse, and better outcomes are most often associated with those who remain in treatment longer. For those with a history of problem drinking, premature discharge from treatment for alcohol-related violations is, unfortunately, all too common. These considerations point to the need for narcotics and other drug treatment programs to be aware of the potential for emerging or concurrent alcohol abuse problems in their patient populations and to address these problems, rather than simply terminating the patients. Although the major focus of such programs is on the presenting problem of drug abuse, problem drinking should be considered as complicating factor that must be incorporated in planning an individual's treatment.

Furthermore, the involvement of narcotics or other drug abusers with alcohol may be not only another aspect of their substance abuse, but also a possible indication of serious and pervasive underlying personal or social dysfunction. From this perspective, the problem drinking as such may not interfere so much with treatment, but may represent instead the underlying pathology that is responsible for both the problem drinking and the treatment difficulties. These considerations may, in particular, apply to the mentally ill substance abuser.

Unfortunately, the long-term course of alcoholism, whether concurrent with or subsequent to addiction, cannot be easily altered. Vaillant[53] pointed out that even prolonged hospital treatment does little to alter the natural history of alcoholism. A similar conclusion was also expressed by McCance and McCance[54] (p. 198): "The outcome in alcoholism depends very little on the treatment given, but largely upon individual factors relating to each patient and upon the natural history of the condition." These authors suggest that not only is the patient's social stability at the time of seeking treatment important to sustained abstinence, but so are four other factors. Namely, recovery is associated with the alcoholic discovering: (1) a substitute dependency, such as religion or support groups; (2) external reminders (such as disulfiram ingestion or a painful ulcer) that drinking is aversive, or supervision from employers or courts, or threat of divorce by spouses; (3) increased sources of unambivalently offered social support; and (4) a source of inspiration, hope, and enhanced self-esteem (such as religious activity). These factors should be considered for incorporation into any treatment for addicts or other drug abusers with drinking problems.

ACKNOWLEDGMENTS. Preparation of this chapter was supported in part by grant 87-IJ-CK-0042 from the National Institute of Justice and grant DA05544 from the National Institute on Drug Abuse. Dr. Hser is also supported by a Research Scientist Development Award (DA00139) from the National Institute on Drug Abuse. Further support was obtained from the California Department of Alcohol and Drug programs under state contract D-0001-8. Special thanks are due to Jungchi Wang for assistance in data analysis and Kean Mantius for editorial review.

References

1. Clayton RR: Multiple drug use: Epidemiology, correlates, and consequences, in Galanter M (ed): *Recent Developments in Alcoholism, Vol 4*. New York, Plenum Press, 1986, pp. 7–38.
2. Blum, K: *Handbook of Abusable Drugs*. New York and London, Gardner Press, 1984.
3. Hesselbrock MN: Alcoholic typologies: A review of empirical evaluations of common classification schemes, in Galanter M (ed): *Recent Developments in Alcoholism, Vol 4*. New York, Plenum Press, 1986.
4. Horton DJ: The functions of alcohol in primitive society: A cross-cultural study. *Q J Stud Alcohol* 4:199–320, 1945.
5. Gilbert MJ, Cervantes RC: Mexican Americans and alcohol. Monograph 11. Spanish Speaking Mental Health Research Center, UCLA, 1987.
6. Paine HJ: Attitudes and patterns of alcohol use among Mexican Americans. *J Stud Alcohol Use* 38:544–554, 1977.
7. Johnson LV, Matre M: Anomie and alcohol use. Drinking patterns in Mexican American and Anglo neighborhoods. *J Stud Alcohol* 39:894–902, 1978.
8. Belenko S, Kehrer B: Study of drinking patterns among adults and youth in Los Angeles County. (County Agreement No. 29550). Los Angeles, Los Angeles County Office on Alcohol Abuse and Alcoholism, 1978.
9. Clark WB, Midanik L: Alcohol use and alcohol problems among U.S. adults: Results of the 1979 National Survey, in *National Institute on Alcohol Abuse and Alcoholism Monograph No. 1, Alcohol Consumption and Related Problems*. DHHS Publication No. ADM 82-1190. Washington, DC: U.S. Government Printing Office, 1982, pp 3–52.
10. Fillmore KM: Prevalence, incidence and chronicity of drinking patterns and problems among men as a function of age: A longitudinal and cohort analysis. Berkeley, CA, Alcohol Research Group, 1984.
11. Caetano R: Self-reported intoxication among Hispanics in Northern California. *J Stud Alcohol* 45:349–354, 1984a.
12. Caetano R: Ethnicity and drinking in Northern California: A comparison among whites, blacks, and Hispanics. *Alcohol Alcoholism* 18(3):1–14, 1984b.
13. Lisansky ES: Alcoholism in women; social and psychological concomitants. 1. Social history data. *Q J Stud Alcohol* 18:588–623, 1957.

14. Bromet E, Moos R: Sex and marital status in relation to the characteristics of alcoholics. *J Stud Alcohol* 37:1302–1312, 1976.
15. Hesselbrock VM, Stabenau JR, Hesselbrock MN, et al.: The nature of alcoholism in patients with different family histories for alcoholism. *Prog Neural Psycho-pharmacol Psychiatry* 6:607–614, 1982.
16. Rimmer J, Pitts F, Reich T, et al: Alcoholism. II. Sex, socioeconomic status and race in two hospitalized samples. *Q J Stud Alcohol* 32:942–952, 1971.
17. Schuckit MA, Morrissey ER: Alcoholism in women, some clinical and social perspective with an emphasis on possible subtypes, in: Greenblatt M, Schuckit MA (eds): *Alcoholism Problems in Women and Children*, New York, Grune & Stratton, 1976.
18. Anglin MD, Hser Y, McGlothlin WH: Sex differences in addict careers. 2. Becoming addicted. *A J Drug Alcohol Abuse*, 13(1,&2), 59–71, 1987.
19. Robins LN, Murphy GE: Drug use in a normal population of young Negro men. *A J Public Health* 57:1580–1596, 1967.
20. Vaillant GE: The natural history of narcotic drug addiction. *Semin Psychiatry* 2:486–498, 1970.
21. Tennant FS, Detels R, Clark V: Some childhood antecedents of drug and alcohol abuse. *A J Epidemiol* 102:377–385, 1975.
22. Woody, RH: Therapeutic techniques for the adolescent marijuana user. *J School Health* 42:220–224, 1972.
23. Levy NJ: The use of drugs among teenagers. *Can Psychiatr Annu J* 17:31–36, 1972.
24. Kandel DB: Inter- and intragenerational influences on adolescent marijuana use. *J Soc Issues* 70:107–135, 1974.
25. Goodwin DM, Davis DH, Robins LN: Drinking amid abundant illicit drugs. *Arch Gen Psychiatry* 32:230–233, 1975.
26. Francis RJ, Timm S, Bucky S: Studies of familial and nonfamilial alcoholism. *Arch Gen Psychiatry* 37:564–566, 1980.
27. Schuckit MA: Relationship between the course of primary alcoholism and family history. *J Stud Alcohol* 45:334–338, 1984.
28. Penick EC, Powell BJ, Osthmer E, et al: Subtyping alcoholics by coexisting psychiatric syndromes; course, family history outcome, in: Goodwin DW, VanDusen KT, Mednick SA (eds): *Longitudinal Research in Alcoholism*. Boston, Kluwer-Nijhoff, 1984.
29. McCarthy W, Anglin MD: Narcotics addicts: Effect of family and parental risk factors on timing of emancipation and of drug use onset, on preaddiction incarcerations and on educational achievement, *J Drug Issues*, 19(4), 1989.
30. Carroll JFX, Malloy TE, Kendrick FM: Multiple substance abuse: A review of the literature, in Gardner SE (ed): *National Drug/Alcohol Collaborative Project: Issues in Multiple Substance Use*. Rockville, MD, National Institute on Drug Abuse, 1980, pp 9–24.
31. Single E, Kandel D, Faust R: Patterns of multiple drug use in high school. *J Health Soc Behav* 15:344–357, 1975.
32. Schut J, File K, Wohlmuth T: Alcohol use by narcotic addicts in methadone maintenance treatment. *Q J Stud Alcohol* 34:1356–1359, 1973.
33. Weppner R, Agar M: Immediate precursors to heroin addiction. *J Health Soc Behav* 12:10–18, 1971.
34. Rosen A, Ottenberg DJ, Barr HL: Patterns of previous abuse of alcohol in a group of hospitalized drug addicts. *Drug Forum* 4(3):261–272, 1975.
35. O'Donnell JA: A follow up of narcotic addicts. Mortality, relapse and abstinence. *Am J Orthopsychiatry* 34:948–954, 1964.
36. Vaillant GE: A twelve-year follow-up of New York narcotic addicts: IV. Some characteristics and determinants of abstinence. *Am J Psychiatry* 123:563–585, 1966.
37. Anglin MD, Almog IJ, Fisher DG, Peters KR: Alcohol use by heroin addicts: Evidence for an inverse relationship. *Am J Drug Alcohol Abuse* 15(2), 191–207, 1989.
38. Bihari B: Alcoholism and methadone maintenance. *Am J Drug Alcohol Abuse* 1(1)79–87, 1974.
39. Brown BS, Kozel NJ, Meyers MB, DuPont RL: Use of alcohol by addict and non-addict populations. *Am J Psychiatry* 130(5):599–601, 1973.

40. Maddux JF, Elliott B: Problem drinkers among patients on methadone. *Am J Drug Alcohol Abuse* 2(2):245–254, 1975.
41. Scott NR, Winslow WW, Gorman DG: Epidemiology of alcoholism in methadone a maintenance program, in DuPont RL, Freeman RS, co-chair: *Proceedings Fifth National Conference on Methadone Treatment*. New York, NAPAN, 1973.
42. Sells SB, Chatham LR, Retka RL: A study of differential death rates and causes of death among 9276 opiate addicts during 1970–1971. *Drug Problems* 1(4):665–706, 1972.
43. Barr HL, Rosen A, Antes DE, Ottenberg DJ: Two year follow-up study of 724 drug and alcohol addicts treated together in an abstinence therapeutic community. Paper presented at the Annual Conference of the American Psychological Association, Montreal, Canada, September 1973.
44. Watterson O, Simpson DD, Sells SB: Death rates and causes of death among opioid addicts in community drug treatment programs during 1970–1973. *Am J Drug Alcohol Abuse* 2(1):99–111, 1975.
45. Cohen S: The effects of combined alcohol/drug abuse on human behavior, in Gardner SE (ed): *Drug and Alcohol Abuse: Implications for Treatment*. Rockville, MD, National Institute on Drug Abuse, 1981, pp 5–20.
46. Cohen S. The substance abuse problems. New York, Haworth Press, 1981.
47. Barr HL, Cohen A: The problem drinking drug addict, in Gardner, SE (ed): *National Drug/Alcohol Collaborative Project: Issues in Multiple Substance Abuse*, DHEW Publication No. (ADM) 80–957, Washington, DC, U.S. Government Printing Office, 1980.
48. McGlothlin WH, Anglin MD, Wilson BD: *An Evaluation of the California Civil Addict Program*. NIDA Services Research Monograph Series. DHEW Publication No. (ADM)78–558. Washington, DC; U.S. Government Printing Office, 1977.
49. Anglin MD, Hser Y, Booth MW: The natural history of narcotics addicts: A 25-years follow-up study. Unpublished final report, 1988.
50. Hser Y, Anglin MD, Booth MW: Sex differences in addict careers. 3. Addiction. *Am J Drug Alcohol Abuse* 13(3):231–251, 1987.
51. Anglin MD, McGlothlin WH, Speckart G, Ryan TM: Shutting off methadone: The closure of the San Diego County Methadone Maintenance Program. Final report, NIDA Grant #DA02577, University of California, Los Angeles, 1983.
52. Anglin MD, Booth MW, Ryan TM, Hser Y: Ethnic differences in narcotics addiction: Part II. Chicano and Anglo addiction career patterns. *Int J Addictions* 23(4):1011–1027, 1988.
53. Vaillant GE: *The Natural History of Alcoholism*. Cambridge, MA, Harvard University Press, 1983.
54. McCane C, McCane PF: Alcoholism in Northeast Scotland: Its treatment and outcome. *Br J Psychiatry* 115:189–198, 1969.

8

Problem Drinking and Alcohol Problems

Widening the Circle of Covariation

Stanley W. Sadava

Abstract. This chapter reviews research pertaining to two basic premises regarding problem drinking: that a conceptual clarification is necessary, one which makes an explicit distinction between drinking behavior and alcohol-related problems or adverse consequences, and that an adequate theory of problem drinking must extend beyond the alcohol-specific theories to a broad matrix of biological, behavioral, psychological, and social variables. Both cross-sectional and longitudinal studies of drinking in nonclinical populations show that levels of alcohol consumption are only moderately related to alcohol-related adverse consequences, and that a broad array of variables mediate the extent to which normal-population drinkers will be vulnerable to alcohol problems. Factors contributing to differential vulnerability to alcohol problems include the concurrent use of other drugs, engaging in other problem behaviors, personality characteristics such as impulsivity, prior depression, and a lack of social conformity or conventionality, the lack of a protective family environment, stress, and being female. A model of problem drinking consisting of overlapping, but distinct sets of predictors for drinking behavior and alcohol-related adverse consequences is proposed.

1. Introduction

Many people experience significant problems with alcohol at some time in their lives. Drinking may have adverse consequences such as problems at work or school, injuries and health problems, financial problems, problems with the law such as through belligerence or drunken driving, and difficulties in relationships with spouses, children, family, friends, and neighbors. While most of these drinkers would not be diagnosed alcoholics in terms of generally accepted criteria, their patterns of drinking carry some heightened risk of a downward spiral which may culminate in alcohol addiction.[1-3] Even in the absence of alcoholism, significant problems with alcohol are not uncom-

Stanley W. Sadava • Department of Psychology, Brock University, St. Catharines, Ontario L25 3A1, Canada.

mon.[4-6] If we consider the spectrum of drinking patterns in our society, generally accepted estimates indicate that about 75% of adults are abstainers or drink without significant problems, and about 5% show symptoms of alcohol dependence.[7] Between these polarities, a substantial 20% of adults can be classified as "problem drinkers," those who do not manifest accepted clinical criteria of alcoholism, but who drink in ways that cause problems in their lives. Indeed, Room[8] estimates that significant problems with alcohol are experienced by about 20% of all *drinkers* at some point in their lives. While these problems may be transitory, they are far from trivial to the drinkers, those around them, and society as a whole.

This chapter focuses on the research on problem drinking in nonclinical populations, emphasizing two points. First, a conceptual clarification of problem drinking is necessary, one which makes an explicit distinction between drinking behavior and alcohol-related problems or adverse consequences. Second, an adequate theory of problem drinking must extend beyond the alcohol-specific theories to a broad matrix of biological, psychological, and social variables. Following a discussion of these two issues, evidence pertaining to the sources of differential vulnerability to alcohol problems among drinkers is reviewed, focusing on a set of longitudinal studies of problem drinking in adolescence and beyond, within a framework of psychosocial interactionism.[9,10]

2. Consumption and Consequences

2.1. Interrelationships and Causality

Most studies define problem drinking in terms of idiosyncratic criteria, often including both the pattern of behavior (quantity consumed, loss of control, binge drinking, frequent drunkenness) and adverse consequences (health, interpersonal, occupational, legal, etc.). It is interesting that DSM-III also defines "alcohol abuse" in terms of this combination of behavioral and consequential criteria.[11] Also, in terms of dose level, there is no clear consensus as to the boundaries that demarcate "safe" and "hazardous" drinking levels, whether one is referring to the acute effects of intoxication or accidents, aggressive behavior or pregnancy, or the chronic effects of drinking on physical and mental health or the onset of alcoholism.[12] One author in 1870[13] recommended 1.5 oz of absolute alcohol as a daily limit, and current epidemiologically based estimates range from 6 to 80 g. While this would appear to be a purely empirical question, it is important to consider that the consequences of any dose level or drinking pattern are determined by considerably more than the alcohol consumed.

Problem drinking is excessive drinking, and we know it is excessive because it is shown to cause problems. However, the link between behavior and its consequences is not as clear as the tautology implies. While abstinence will not lead to alcohol-related personal problems, and extremely heavy drinking would almost inevitably cause extremely high levels of problems for almost anyone, wide variations are found within the normal range of drinking patterns in the incidence and types of problems at given levels of consumption.

Table I presents evidence from a set of recent general-population studies. Measures of consumption include single and combined indices of frequency, quantity, and volume of intake, and rating scales, and measures of problems include loss of control, worrying about drinking, concern of others, specific drinking problems (e.g., with family, work, health), and diagnostic scales of alcohol misuse. The overall average correlation between consumption and problems is 0.40 (range = 0.16–0.59)—statistically significant, but surprisingly modest. When only about 16% of the variance in alcohol problems can be attributed directly to drinking behavior, it becomes reasonable to discuss the "correlative independence of consumption and problems,"[14] and much remains to be understood about alcohol-related problems.[20]

In our research, multiple measures of drinking behavior (quantity–frequency, frequency of drunkenness) and of alcohol problems (problem drinker status, adverse consequences) were administered to samples of Canadian working adults, students, and heavy-drinking, mostly unemployed adults. An average correlation coefficient of 0.41 was obtained, and factor analyses yielded remarkably consistent independent factors for consumption patterns

Table I.   Summary of Relationships between Measures of Consumption and Problems

Study	Consumption	Problem	Correlations
Calahan and Room[4]	Current heavy intake	Loss of control; symptomatic drinking problems: 8 areas	0.22 0.34 0.17–0.31
Orford et al.[15]	Weekly quantity	Concern over drinking; drinking complications; morning-after complication	0.47, 0.47.54 0.51, 0.53.56 0.46, 47
Roizen[14]	Current heavy intake	Problems with spouse	0.41
Wanberg et al.[16]	Quantity consumed	Social role maladaptation; loss of behavioral control; worry or guilt over drinking marital problems	0.53 0.44 0.20 0.16, 0.20
Celentano and McQueen[17]	Quantity-Frequency (Q-F)	Loss of control	0.29, 0.41
Jessor et al.[18]	Average intake	Negative consequences	0.38–0.53.
Glickman and Smythe[19]	Weekly intake	Drinking style; drinking effects	0.45 0.39
Skinner and Allen[7]	Daily quantity	Alcohol dependence scales	0.47
Hays et al.[21]	Intake (factor)	Negative consequences	0.59
Stein et al.[22]	Drug use	Problem drug use	0.21

and problems/consequences. Indeed, similar findings were reported for illicit drug use, and when analyses included both alcohol and drug use measures, the factors obtained represented the consumption vs. problem dimensions rather than the substances used (a third factor representing multiple drug use was obtained in some analyses).[23–26] Corroborating evidence has been obtained from a study of large samples of adolescents in the United States.[27] Four models of the structure of drinking measures were tested: (1) a *unidimensional model* incorporating measures of consumption, problems, and motivations for drinking, (2) a *three-factor model* for consumption, problems, and motives for drinking, (3) a *four-dimensional model* in which consumption, problems, intoxication, and motivation are factorially independent, and (4) a *two-dimensional model* of consumption (including intoxication) and problems, in which motivations load on both factors. A series of confirmatory factor analyses, replicated across two points in time and separately for males and females, clearly support the two-dimensional model.

Longitudinal evidence indicates that heavy intake at one time and even increasing intake over time are not strongly predictive of subsequent alcohol-related problems; indeed, intake may increase *after* the onset of problems.[4,14] Although both intrinsic drinking behavior problems (e.g., heavy intake, loss of control, binge drinking) and external consequences (e.g., with the law, marriage, work) remain relatively consistent over time, the correlations between behavior and external consequences are relatively low (range, −0.04 to +0.15).[3] Data covering a period of over 25 years reveal "extremely minor" to modest relationships between heavy intake and subsequent problems, and between problems in college and the type of problems, if any, experienced in later life.[1,28] In another 7-year follow-up of university students, 20–50% of those who experienced significant alcohol problems while at university were still experiencing such problems later, while 10–22% of those without alcohol problems in university developed such problems over the next 7 years.[2] Interestingly, it has been found that the early onset of adolescent drinking, of itself, tends to be followed by later problems with alcohol and other drugs.[2,29,30]

"Disruptive" drug use, defined in terms of inappropriate situations such as at work or school, is significantly related to problems with various drugs (including alcohol), driving while intoxicated and other legal problems, and attending treatment programs. As one would expect, disruptive use was significantly related to general levels of consumption of the various drugs and of overall drug consumption. However, these relationships are rather modest, accounting for an overall 40% of the variance over all drugs and less than 7% of alcohol use. That is, high levels of consumption of alcohol or any other drug did not necessarily imply disruptive use patterns. It is also interesting to note that, over a period of several years, levels of disruptive use were only moderately stable, considerably less so than overall levels of consumption; drinking patterns were particularly unstable over this time period.[31]

In summary, the evidence supports a two-dimensional structural model of problem drinking: drinking behavior (including high-risk patterns such as frequent drunkenness) and alcohol-related consequences or problems. Of course, drinking can lead to problems, and heavy drinking implies an increased risk of problems. It is equally evident that problems can cause changes in drinking behavior, particularly a self-correction or adjustment in drinking in response to adverse consequences. While the evolution of problem drinking cannot be described by metaphors such as a "slippery slope" or "boule de neige," it is possible that problems will generate increased drinking if the individual lacks access to other coping responses.

Thus, it is important to investigate factors that determine how *vulnerable* different individuals are to the consequences of their drinking. For example, the acute and chronic effects of alcohol are influenced by the state of the person, such as, physical health, mental health (e.g., depression), and the concurrent use of other drugs. Another source of differential vulnerability may be the beliefs and values of the drinker regarding drinking and his own definition of what constitutes a drinking problem. A third might be the response of others to the person's drinking, whether significant others approve, disapprove, or provide social supports that buffer the drinker against certain adverse consequences. For example, the incidence of adverse consequences, particularly those involving drunken behavior, tends to be higher in the "dry" regions of the United States in which alcohol is consumed the least and where drinking is frowned upon by most people.[4] Finally, the behavior of the person while drinking (or intoxicated) will have a profound effect on the development of alcohol problems.

In the literature review to follow, consumption and consequences are usually not disentangled, and thus it often becomes difficult to distinguish between direct causes of alcohol-problem vulnerability and indirect causes, those which predispose the person to high-risk drinking patterns. Also, the problem-drinking perspective is based on an adaptive, rather than exposure, orientation to addictions; that is, addictive behavior is motivated primarily by attempts to adapt to or cope with stress, distress, or simply the demands and norms of the situation, rather than being a direct result of acquired tolerance or fear of withdrawal symptoms.[32] Of course, a major source of adjustment demands faced by heavy drinkers may well be the consequences of their own drinking.[33]

2.2. Adolescent Consumption and Consequences in Adulthood

Recently, reports have appeared from longitudinal studies concerning the sequelae in early adulthood of adolescent involvement with alcohol and other drugs. Much of this research is based on a premise that behaviors such as drinking have symbolic meaning to people, signifying maturity, sophistication, and adult status, and that the meaning may well shift as one traverses the life course. For example, Jessor and Jessor[34] argue that adolescence is a period of transition from the conventionality of one's parents toward increasing tolerance of and engaging in problem, deviant, or transgressive behaviors, including certain patterns of drinking. Zucker[35] points out an important ambiguity in this conception, as to whether it is the deviant or transgressive quality of the behavior or the effect of producing independence from family and other conventional institutions that is crucial. In general, the studies indicate that problem drinking peaks in the 18–21 age group and then drops off, indicating a "maturing out" phenomenon.

Several possible outcomes of adolescent alcohol and other drug involvement have been suggested. One is that drug use may not directly cause problems but may contribute to the development of an avoidant or regressive manner of dealing with problems. For example, a relationship has been documented between heavy drinking in adolescence and increased self-derogation and dissatisfaction with life in later adolescence and early adulthood.[36] However, it is difficult to assume causality from such findings, as the same underlying personal and social factors may contribute both to early involvement with alcohol and to later dissatisfaction with oneself and one's life. It has also been argued that drug involvement impedes the normal psychosocial maturation of the adolescent, by reducing reality testing, reinforcing egocentric thinking, and consolidating adolescent negativism and rebelliousness.[37] Such effects would be subtle and difficult to demonstrate.

Certain forms or styles of drinking or other drug use in adolescence tend to be abandoned later as being inconsistent with the acquisition of normative adult roles. Indeed, heavy drug involvement, including heavy drinking and marijuana use, tends to be diminished or completely relinquished when the individual assumes adult role activities such as marriage and becoming a parent.[38] The dynamics involve both role selection and role socialization effects. That is, heavy drug users tend to delay entry into these roles and to discontinue or reduce drug involvement when adult roles are adopted. Other longitudinal data also show that alcohol use among graduating high-school students in the year after graduation tends to increase (as a marker of adult status[39]).

Newcomb[36,40] argues that early and relatively intensive involvement with drugs accelerates adolescent development, through the early acquisition of behaviors generally considered to be adult. This desire to "grow up fast" and enjoy the prerogatives of adulthood leads to the premature acquisition of adult roles such as jobs and marriage. However, the outcome is described as a "pseudomaturity", acquired without the necessary process of development and characterized by an inability to delay gratification. Adolescents who are heavily involved with multiple drugs tend to be married, have children, and get divorced at an early age. In early adulthood, they are also somewhat more likely than others to be involved in drug-related crime, have greater problems with social integration, and even may show symptoms of psychotic thinking. Significantly, teenage alcohol use alone, unaccompanied by other drug involvement, was not predictive of a troubled early adulthood. All of these findings held where "social conformity" during adolescence was controlled statistically, thus indicating that the consequences were specific to drug use and not to more general patterns of deviant behavior.

This does not augur well for the long term. Kandel et al.[41] report that adolescent alcohol involvement was a significant predictor of employment instability, marital disruption, involvement in theft, and the use of marijuana and other illicit drugs in adulthood. Cumulatively, extensive drug involvement in adolescence may be followed in adulthood by physical and mental health problems, delinquency, familial problems, and employment difficulties, as well as continued drug involvement in adulthood. The total percent of the variance accounted for, however, was in most cases quite modest, and the effects of continued drug use in adulthood on these outcomes was not partialed out. Indeed, analyses reveal that, if intervening drug use is accounted for, there is little relation between adolescent drug use and adult consequences; however, use reinforces further use, and if this pattern of use persists into adulthood, it is accompanied by problems. It is also possible that those who are heavily involved in drugs may be predisposed to choose unstable job situations or to behave in ways as to cause this instability.[40,42] In terms of the two-dimensional model, it is also instructive to note the importance of time in the assessment of problems. The immediate, short-term, or long-term consequences of drinking may differ considerably, and one may not be predictable from another.

3. Alcohol-Specific and Non-Alcohol-Specific Causes

A striking feature of problem drinking is the convergence of causal influences. The effects of alcohol as a drug, the genetic makeup of the person, the motives and expectancies for drinking and the prevalence of drinking around the person, characteristics of personality, the immediate social environment, and the larger sociocultural and historical context all contribute significantly to our understanding of the phenomenon. Nonetheless, the contemporary literature contains a number of highly influential models or minitheories, restricted to a small subset of variables. For the most part, these models are also restricted to alcohol-specific or proximal variables.

Let us briefly review several such examples:

1. The tension reduction theory states that alcohol relieves tension (fear, anxiety, frustration, conflict) and that drinking is reinforced by the tension-relieving properties of alcohol.[43] The research evidence is paradoxical; while epidemiological, clinical, and psychosocial research shows a relationship between tension (or stress) and drinking, experimental studies do not show that alcohol has consistent tension-relieving properties. Recent variations on this theme postulate that alcohol has a stress-response dampening effect, reducing physiological and emotional reactivity to stressors, and is used for that pur-

pose[44] or that drinking occurs in response to the depletion of endorphins following uncontrollable aversive events.[45]

2. Like all behaviors, drinking is determined by the consequences expected of it. A set of expectancies regarding drinking, such as the reduction of tension, diversion from worries, arousal and aggressive tendencies, feeling more powerful, enhanced pleasure, changing (disinhibiting) social behavior and emotional expressiveness, and the "magical transformation" of experience into a more effective present and a brighter future, have been derived empirically.[46] Overall, it appears that, with more experience, the expectancies of drinkers become more crystallized and that heavier drinkers have more positive expectancies, that is, more reasons for drinking. While some data relate specific subsets of expectancies to problem drinking or alcoholism, the findings are neither clear nor theoretically interpretable at this time.[47]

3. A family history of alcoholism or other drug abuse represents a significantly heightened risk for alcohol problems,[48,49] and the evidence reported thus far indicates that a genetic predisposition, in part, underlies the transmission of alcohol problems from one generation to the next. The offspring of alcoholics have differing expectancies about alcohol, tend to feel less intoxicated at moderate dose levels of alcohol, tend to experience a greater stress-attenuating effect from alcohol, and tend in temperament to be low in reward dependence, high in novelty seeking, and low in harm avoidance.[50–52] It is indicated that the sons of alcoholics have physiologically based difficulties in attributing meaning to stimuli, which becomes manifested as a hyperreactivity to stimulation.[53]

4. Several models deal with the impairment of cognitive and perceptual processes, such as that alcohol reduces psychological stress indirectly, by impairing stress-related information processing,[54] or that alcohol impairs the processing of self-relevant stimuli, thus reducing self-awareness or self-consciousness.[55] Another, related model proposes that alcohol is reinforcing because it impairs performance, particularly in achievement-related situations.[56] Individuals may thus drink in order to handicap themselves in advance of such situations in order to avoid personal responsibility for failure. Of course, these functionalist models imply that drinkers hold certain expectancies about how alcohol will affect them, and that their consumption is directed toward these purposes.

5. A large body of literature relates drinking and other drug use among adolescents to peer group modeling and pressures.[57] Indeed, several studies identify peer group behavior as the single most powerful predictor of adolescent drinking and drug use.[58]

All of these models have identified important subprocesses and represent some exciting advances toward an understanding of problem drinking. However, they all suffer from several important limitations. One problem is an ambiguity in disentangling the effects of alcohol from the causes or motives for drinking. For example, in tension-reduction models, it is stated both that alcohol reduces tension and that people drink for that reason. One might infer that heavier drinkers suffer from more tension (perhaps as a result of their life circumstances or their inability to tolerate stress), or that the tension-reducing effect of alcohol is greater for these people (perhaps for inherent constitutional reasons or perhaps because they lack effective coping strategies). Research has not clarified these ambiguities, and it has become evident that more variables will be required to link tension reduction and drinking behavior. Similarly, it is not clear whether adolescents who choose the wrong friends are then influenced into problem drinking, or whether those prone to problem drinking are attracted to the appropriate peer groups.

The research on familial transmission contains similar ambiguities. To be sure, a genetically transmitted predisposition has been established, but this must be seen as a risk factor, neither a necessary nor a sufficient condition for problem drinking. The offspring alcoholics constitute only a minority of the problem drinker or alcoholic populations. In addition to possible physiological differences that may predispose the person to alcohol problems, a parental modeling effect is evident; it has also been shown that when parental drinking is perceived as extreme, adolescents are less likely to imitate them than otherwise.[59] Again, it is apparent that other variables are necessary to explain how familial alcoholism and alcohol problems in the offspring are related.

Finally, the models offer an impoverished explanation of an exceedingly complex set of phenomena. Empirically this is shown in the multivariate studies in which more distal or non-alcohol-specific factors add to the variance accounted for by alcohol-specific factors.[34,60,61] For example, scores on alcohol expectancies increase prediction of problem drinking, but do not supplant ethnicity, sex, socioeconomic class and religiosity in regression equations.[62] Beyond the accounting function is the explanatory function. For example, in order to understand how tension-reducing or stress-response-dampening may contribute to problem drinking, we must understand the levels and sources of tension or stress in the environment, the sources of social support for the person, and the alternative coping strategies accessible to the person that may provide buffers against the stress. Mapping the behavioral choices and habits, personal characteristics, and environmental features of the drinker provides a context in which to understand how the drinker may acquire heavy-drinking friends or develop certain expectancies about drinking, and how they are linked to problem drinking.

In all of these models it is not clear whether the person is impelled to consume more or differently, or whether the person is more vulnerable to adverse consequences. For example, the tension-reduction hypothesis may be interpreted as leading to adverse consequences from drinking, perhaps as a result of ineffective coping strategies. Some evidence suggests that the genetically high-risk person may respond differently to alcohol, leading to different consequences.

4. Behavioral Specificity

4.1. Concurrent Use of Other Drugs

Perhaps one of the most firmly established findings in the literature is that substantial covariation exists among the patterns of use of various drugs.[63,64] Individuals who use one drug are more likely to be using another drug, and as one drug is used more heavily, a wider range of other drugs tends to be used concurrently. That is, those who drink heavily, and thus are at greater risk for adverse consequences, tend to be using other drugs as well. Thus, in this chapter, indicators of greater generalized drug involvement by adolescents are assumed to include problem drinking within that pattern.

An influential paper by Kandel[65] showed that adolescents initiate drug use in an invariant sequence: first beer and/or wine, then hard liquor, then marijuana, and finally the "hard" illicit drugs, such as, cocaine, heroin, psychedelics, amphetamines, and barbiturates. Subsequent research has corroborated this sequential pattern of initial use, at least during adolescence when most initial recreational use of any substance is likely to occur, although some inconsistencies have been reported regarding the place of cigarettes, prescribed tranquilizers and antidepressive medications, and various "hard drugs."[18,67–69] Note that this sequence represents a Guttman scale of intensified involvement with an expanding repertoire of drugs, not simply the stepping-stone substitution of an ostensibly more serious drug for one purported to be more benign.

Two findings are particularly relevant to a concern with problem drinking. Data from the UCLA study indicate that disruptive drinking (that which occurs at work) tends to be initiated after the person has begun to use illicit "hard" drugs at work.[31] Another study utilizing data from two large-scale national surveys of adolescents in the United States investigated where "problem drinking" (defined as frequent drunkenness and/or adverse consequences) would be placed relative to the use of various substances.[70] Current status as a problem drinker occupied a Guttman scale position after marijuana use and before the use of other illicit drugs. Therefore, problem drinking tends to occur after the initiation of illicit drug use and that problem drinking indicates greater involvement with drug use than does the use of an illicit drug, marijuana.

Do these sequences persist beyond adolescence? Research that followed adolescents over 8 years found that, while cannabis use peaked in late adolescence and then declined, the use of liquor, stimulants, hypnotics, and psychedelics increased or leveled off during that period.[71] While the sequence of alcohol–cannabis–hard drugs use is consistent throughout adolescence, alcohol use did not influence subsequent illicit drug use in early adulthood, reflecting the apparent independence of alcohol use in this period of life. Indeed, when cigarettes were added to the analyses, the role of drinking became even less important in predicting subsequent drug involvement.

Thus, alcohol does not seem to be a "gateway" drug which presages expanded polydrug involvement, but drinking seems to become a fairly stable and enduring behavior of itself in early adulthood.

In studies of established patterns of use, a relationship between heavy drinking and involvement with other drugs, including cigarettes, marijuana, and psychotherapeutic drugs, is reported.[63,64] Clinical studies show that alcoholics tend to abuse cigarettes, sedatives, and tranquilizers[72] and frequently are abusers of illicit drugs as well.[73] Particularly prone to the concurrent use of other drugs are those alcoholics described as being the heaviest drinkers, those who are functioning socially at a relatively effective level, and those having difficulty with attempted abstinence.[63] Female alcoholics are particularly likely to be using prescribed tranquilizers.[63] On the other hand, many heroin addicts, including those on methadone maintenance, also are heavy drinkers. One recent study of admissions to a drug treatment program identifies five clusters or groupings of subjects in terms of the substances used[74]: a group of primarily alcoholics who also tended to use tranquilizers; a second group of alcoholics who also were heavy users of cannabis, sedative hypnotics, and tranquilizers; a third group who combined alcohol, sedative hypnotics, tranquilizers, and stimulants; a fourth group who used cannabis and other recreational drugs (including alcohol); and a fifth group who used primarily solvents along with cannabis and alcohol. It is noteworthy that all five groups manifested alcohol use in addition to various combinations of other substances.

Why does heavy drinking tend to be associated with multiple drug use? In part, this question reflects a controversy between the "simplex" and "common factor" models which has emerged from the research on the stage–sequence phenomenon of drug use initiation. According to the simplex model, the sequence of drugs represent a series of discrete stages, and that involvement with beer/wine, liquor, marijuana, and "hard drugs" can best be predicted and explained by different variables. For example, one study identifies minor delinquency, beer drinking, and cigarette smoking as predicting liquor use; belief favorable to marijuana and peer group associations as predicting marijuana use; and depression, poor relationships with parents, and contact with drug-using peers as best predicting hard-drug use.[75] On the other hand, the "common factor" model indicates that the sequence of initiation depends, not on the intrinsic properties of the drugs, but on the support and availability of the drug in the social environment of the person, and that the same set of factors, rather than unique factors, will best predict patterns of use of various drugs. While unique predictor variables are not excluded, the common factor model best fits the data, thus indicating that the stages seem to represent a continuum of involvement with substance use, including alcohol, and that heavy drinking/multiple drug use represents one end of that continuum.[21,75]

Several explanations of multiple drug use are apparent. The use of one substance may act as a cue to elicit the use of another substance; for example, drinking may act as a conditioned cue to cigarette smoking. On the other hand, certain combinations of drugs may have desired antagonistic effects, and thus the mildly depressant effect of moderate-dose alcohol may be counteracted by the mildly stimulating effect of nicotine. Consider that the following interact significantly with alcohol is some way: barbiturates, benzodiazapine tranquilizers, phenothiazines, opiates, antidepressants, some anticoagulants, oral insulin, antihistamines, certain antibiotics, and marijuana.[76,77] In that these drug use patterns extend over time, chronic drug interactions must also be considered, in which cross-tolerance may develop or the prolonged exposure to one drug may affect reactions to another drug.

Does multiple drug use contribute to a vulnerability to the consequences of drinking? Our data indicate that, after controlling for the level of alcohol consumption and the frequency of drunkenness, the concurrent use of other drugs is significantly related to experienced adverse consequences or problems with alcohol.[26,27] Another study[78] of Scottish teenagers examined a set of "serious" consequences of alcohol consumption: frequent hangovers, morning drinking to steady the nerves, being advised by a physician to drink less, having an alcohol-related accident or injury, shaky hands due to drinking, and missing school. For males but not females, overall scores on the set of consequences of drinking were related to levels of consumption of tobacco and illicit drugs (cocaine, Librium, amphetamines). However, the level of alcohol consumption was not controlled in these analyses.

Clearly, as a covariate of heavy, high-risk drinking, concurrent multiple drug use may be an indicator of increased problems with alcohol. However, drug use that tends to accompany heavy drinking must also be seen as a direct cause of alcohol problems, based on pharmacological and psychosocial considerations. Problem drinking cannot be viewed in pharmacological isolation.

4.2. Other Problem Behaviors

The larger behavioral context of adolescent problem drinking is considered within Jessor and Jessor's problem behavior theory, in which problem behavior is defined as "behavior that is socially defined as a problem, a source of concern or as undesirable by the norms of conventional society and the institutions of adult authority, and its occurrence usually elicits some kind of social control response."[34] A variety of different adolescent behaviors are considered within this framework, including cigarette smoking, drinking, illicit drug use, certain forms of political activism, various illegal or delinquent behaviors, and precocious sexual involvement. In parallel studies of high-school and university students, it was found that the behaviors (with the exception of political activism) were positively correlated, and that a composite index representing levels of all of the component behaviors correlated negatively with measures of conventional behaviors such as church and school attendance. In further analyses of these data sets and another data set from a national sample of U.S. adolescents, consistent findings point to a single underlying factor representing a problem behavior syndrome.[79]

Other research also shows that increasing involvement with alcohol, marijuana, and tobacco is strongly associated with early and varied sexual involvement, delinquent behavior, and, to a lesser extent, social activities with peers.[80,81] Data from the UCLA study showed that teenage multiple drug use correlated highly with low law abidance, criminal activities, early sexual involvement, and low academic performance.[82] Another study examined alcohol and other drug use in relation to health, by including measures of exercise, meal regularity, and hours of sleep. Scores on alcohol use, illicit drug use, and cigarette smoking formed a coherent factor, but the other health-related behaviors fell outside the perimeter of this factor.[83]

The linkage between drug use and other types of delinquency is well established in the literature, as shown, for example, in relationships among drinking, illicit drug use, and law abidance in general.[82] However, the causal connections remains elusive. Apart from specific drug-related crime, the notion that drug effects cause delinquency has largely fallen into disfavor; indeed, delinquency often precedes drug involvement.[84,85] Recent longitudinal studies suggest a "common-cause model," in which variables related to impulse control and to differential peer associations appear to be central to both delinquency and drug involvement.[86,87] Yet, drug abuse and delinquency often do not coincide, suggesting a degree of causal independence between major forms of delinquency and the abuse of alcohol and other drugs.

While one set of analyses has shown a single common factor underlying the various behaviors among subjects in their mid- to late-twenties,[79] other data suggest that this pattern may not hold true in adulthood.[88] Age is a major determinant in the social definition of problem behavior; what may be considered as a problem behavior when performed by an adolescent (getting drunk) may not be so considered for a young adult. The UCLA study shows that the problem behavior syndrome of adolescence tends to differentiate into two deviant behavior clusters in early adulthood, one pertaining to drug-related crimes and the other to non-drug-related violence and property crimes.[40] Correlations between disruptive drug use and behaviors such as confrontational acts against authority, theft and property damage, dealing drugs, and sexual involvement were remarkably low, particularly in the case of drinking.[69] Indeed, while problem drinking may continue into adulthood, other deviant or problem behavior may be abandoned or may not be associated any longer with problem drinking.[89]

To the extent that drinking and other behaviors covary, they reflects both a common normative environment and common personal dispositions. It is interesting to note that the involvement of alcoholics in substitute, relatively benign activities, such as work, hobbies, meditation, or helping other people, is not only associated with recovery but is the factor to which alcoholics most often attribute their ability to remain abstinent.[90] While the causal linkages here remain ambiguous, the relationship between problem drinking and an entire repertoire of behaviors is clearly of major significance.

5. Psychosocial Variables and Vulnerability

In recent years, a set of longitudinal projects have been formulated within an interactionist framework, in the sense that both personality characteristics and aspects of the social environment are seen as important sources of prediction and explanation of problem drinking.[9,10] Thus, a broad set of variables are measured and tracked over time, necessitating the application of complex and, at times, innovative multivariate procedures. None of the projects are specifically devoted to problem drinking as such, and all of them investigate problem drinking within a matrix of related behaviors. While the projects were originally conceived as studying adolescent behavior, all of them have followed their subjects into early adulthood, providing a set of rich data sets.

For example, in problem behavior theory[34] a set of personal, environmental, and behavioral attributes is described as indicating proneness to problem behavior. The following set of predictors gives some flavor of the breadth of the theory: lower value on academic recognition, higher value on independence, lower expectations for academic recognition, greater attitudinal tolerance of deviance, lesser religiosity, lower perceived compatibility between parents' and friends' expectations, greater perceived influence from friends than parents, greater approval from friends for problem behavior, more peer models for problems behavior, greater involvement in minor "delinquent" behavior, less attendance at church. In total, the model has provided summated linear prediction over time (multiple regression) at better than 50% levels, and the findings have been replicated in a large national U.S. sample of adolescents.[18] Significantly, prediction was considerably less successful in the college student sample, suggesting that problem behavior theory may be specific to adolescence.

The DOMAIN model[60] concerns adolescent behavioral patterns or "styles," in which drinking behavior is embedded in a larger framework of behavioral tendencies or life-styles. The model includes biological factors such as reactivity to stress and genetic and developmental characteristics, intrapersonal factors such as cognitive and personality characteristics, socioeconomic resources accessible to the person, interpersonal factors such as perceived pressures and expectations of others and social supports, and sociocultural norms and other influences. An important feature of the research, particularly in a longitudinal study at UCLA, is a focus on subsystems of predictors and the use of sophisticated causal modeling procedures to determine "paths" by which variables may influence drinking directly or indirectly.

Are certain subsets of predictors specific to consumption or to consequences? One set of analyses is significant from that perspective in showing that different sets of variables, measured in adolescence, predicted consumption patterns and adverse consequences in early adulthood.[91] Adult multiple drug use (a latent variable including heavy drinking) was predicted by prior use in adolescence and continued use by adults in his or her environment, while the primary predictor of later drug-related problems was low scores on social conformity, a latent variable consisting of law abidance, liberalism, and religiosity. Another longitudinal study[92] examined psychosocial predictors of transitions from nondrinker to drinker status, and from drinker to "uncontrolled drinker" (defined as those who reported a typical drinking session's dose of more than 1.3 ml/kg alcohol, or about 5.7 drinks for a typical male). Of the 21 variables studied, nine demonstrated no relationship to either status change, nine showed a developmental relationship to both changes, and only three showed a relationship to one criterion but not the other; cigarette smoking, adults' approval of that adolescent's attitude toward drinking, and religiosity all predicted the onset of drinking but not the onset of heavy drinking. Other analyses have indicated that personality variables best distinguish between moderate and excessive drinkers, and perceived environment variables (parents, peers) between nondrinkers and moderate drinkers. Excessive drinkers were also characterized as drinking for both escapist and pleasure-enhancing reasons.[93]

6. Personality and Vulnerability

The research on personality and substance use has been extensive but not encouraging.[94–97] In the futile search for the "addictive personality," a wide assortment of single-trait or multifactor tests has been administered to addicted samples. Apart from the serious methodological problems, several metamethodological problems bedeviled this literature. One is the issue of causality; one cannot assume personality determines alcoholism from the study of clinical populations. While most personality research assumes relatively enduring and consistent traits that antedate behavior,[98] many of the characteristics may well be more subject to fluctuation within the person over time, suggesting a two-directional causal influence between personality and drinking and the possibility that personality may change after the onset of problem drinking.[90] That is, an "addicted personality" is not necessarily an "addictive personality."

It was also apparent that too much reliance was placed on personality trait measures, to the neglect of psychosocial and other factors. While some observers recommended that the entire enterprise be abandoned, it was obvious that problem drinking, alcoholism, and any other form of substance use or abuse are not randomly or uniformly distributed in any population, even after accounting for family history peer group behavior and the sociocultural environment. Thus, the study of individual differences that contribute to alcohol problems continues, albeit at a more sophisticated and realistic level.

Longitudinal studies that begin in childhood provide some important evidence regarding personal predispositions.[85,99–101] The following are shown to be indicators of high risk: childhood impulsivity, antisocial or aggressive behavior (particularly when accompanied by shyness), childhood achievement difficulties, perhaps related to "hyperactivity," problems in interpersonal attachment and estrangement from parents, inadequate parenting marked by a lack of both affectional expression and supervision. While not truly longitudinal in design or intent, these studies do support the notion that antecedent personality factors are significant.

Psychopathology

An important question is whether preexisting or concurrently developing psychopathology may contribute to a vulnerability to alcohol problems among drinkers. As discussed earlier, prospective studies reveal evidence of characteristics such as impulsivity, sex-role identity problems, nonconformity, problems both in parent–child relationships and in school adjustment and achievement, but no solid evidence of unusual psychological distress.[96] Scores on MMPI scales in a sample of university students also suggest characteristic patterns of impulsivity and nonconformity but not overt psychopathology among those who would become alcoholics over the next decade.[102] The research does not address the question of how these variables influenced the course of development of problem drinking and eventual alcoholism. Did they precipitate heavier drinking patterns, perhaps as a coping strategy or perhaps through peer group associations? Or did these factors contribute to a vulnerability to problems among heavy drinkers, perhaps related to how they reacted to alcohol, how they behaved while intoxicated, or how they were perceived by others?

Depression is common among alcoholics. Although there is little evidence of severe depression prior to the onset of major alcohol problems, the depression should not be seen solely as the result of the psychopharmacology of chronic alcohol abuse and the depressing life situation of the alcoholic. Indeed, longitudinal data show both drinking in response to depressed mood and changes in depression as a result of drinking.[103] It is also reported that there is no relationship between stress and depression among moderate drinkers, suggesting a stress-buffering effect of moderate levels of consumption.[104]

As noted earlier, personality variables seem to be more important in predicting the more serious, high-risk, or problem- prone patterns of drinking, while social factors such as peer group models and pressures account for more of the relatively benign forms of drinking. In the longitudinal study of disruptive drinking, rebelliousness and attitudes favorable to breaking the law were predictive of later disruptive drinking, while peer and adult models for substance use were predictive of general consumption levels but not disruptive use patterns.[69] Depression is reported to be related to hard drug use (representing a broad polydrug use pattern including problem drinking), while peer group behavior predicted earlier stages such as drinking.[75] Other data support a two-stage model, in which social variables determine alcohol intake patterns and personality relates more to alcohol problems; problem drinking is related to ego resiliency (somatization, anxiety, depression, guilt, and paranoia) and ego control (impulsivity, tolerance of deviance, sociability) while heavy consumption per se was related more strongly to social contexts, responses of others to the person's drinking, and attitudes toward drinking.[4] Among adolescents, peer group expectancies and support distinguish non-drinkers from moderate drinkers, while personality factors such as expectations for independence and values for academic recognition differentiate moderate drinkers from problem drinkers.[93]

7. Gender and Vulnerability

After years of neglect, gender has become a variable of interest in the addictions literature, and some long-lasting assumptions have been challenged.[105] Gender differences in the patterns of drinking, the use of both illicit drug and prescribed psychoactive medications, the impact of sex roles on the etiology of problems, physiological processes of absorption, distribution, and metabolization, all have been subject to intensive study in recent years. The most commonly reported findings show that males tend to drink and use illicit drugs more often, while females use prescribed psychoactive medications more often.

Several lines of evidence demonstrate that males and females differ, to an extent, in their vulnerability to alcohol problems. A review of general population studies concludes that, while the rates of drinking in general and of problem drinking are higher among men than women in Western societies, a higher proportion of female heavy drinkers than male heavy drinkers experience significant alcohol-related problems.[106] While heavy-drinking males tend to drink more rapidly, consume greater amounts, and are more likely to drive while intoxicated, they are less likely than females who drink heavily to report alcohol-related job loss, concern by family members, or fear of losing control.[107] One general-population survey showed that while men were more likely to report alcohol problems and women to report depressive symptoms, alcohol problems and symptoms of depression occurred together at about twice the rate for women as for men; that is, women with alcohol problems are also more likely to be depressed as well.[108] Among diagnosed alcoholics, women tend to have consumed less and abused alcohol for a shorter period of time, and yet their morbidity and mortality rates are equal to or higher than those of males in relation to conditions such as cirrhosis and cardiovascular diseases.[109] And women tend to reach significantly higher peak blood alcohol levels than males receiving the same dose levels, suggesting that acute alcohol effects may be quantitatively or qualitatively different for men and women.[110]

Thus, the effects of societal stigmatization of the intoxicated woman as a "fallen angel"[111] may be compounded by biological vulnerabilities.

In our data, as expected, males showed higher levels of intake of alcohol and of illicit drugs, while females consumed more prescribed psychoactives. However, on measures of alcohol problems, females scored only marginally lower, and their problem scores were much more highly correlated with consumption levels than they were with males. Of course, certain consequences tended to be male-typical (e.g., arrested drunk, sexual problems) and others female-typical (e.g., feeling guilty about drinking, neglect obligations).[111] Thus, it is not surprising that men are more likely to manifest disruptive (i.e., work-related) drinking patterns than are women.[66,112] Another clue is found in several longitudinal studies in which heavy/problem drinking in adolescence constitutes a greater risk of alcohol problems in adulthood for males than for females.[2,113] It is hypothesized that growing into adulthood may place greater constraints on their drinking than do the role situations of males of that age. If this is so, then the consequences of heavy drinking would be expected to be more severe for young women.

8. Family and Vulnerability

A substantial body of evidence links adolescent problem drinking to the family background.[114,115] Research has focused both on alcohol and other drug abuse and other deviant behavior by the parent and on the more distal characteristics of the family, particularly aspects of the relationship between parents and adolescent, such as the degree of intimacy, positive affect and expression of affection, and the limits and controls exercised by parents on the behavior of the child.[34] Unfortunately, most reports do not delineate the alcohol-related aspects of parental behavior in order to fully explore the role of more general characteristics of the family relevant to the care and feeding of adolescents. Also, some of the studies obtain measures of parental and familial variables directly from the parents, while others rely on reports of the child. Nonetheless, sufficient data of sufficient quality are reported to warrant an assertion that the family plays an important, although not decisive role in the genesis of adolescent problem drinking.

Brook and colleagues have conducted a series of studies that neatly address the causality question.[116,117] They define and measure three domains of variables: (1) personality of the adolescent (e.g., attitudes toward deviance, rebelliousness, impulsivity, sensation seeking, extraversion), (2) personality of the parent (e.g., attitudes toward deviance, impulsivity, masculinity/femininity), and (3) family socialization (e.g., communication, warmth and rejecting behavior, permissiveness, control, identification of child with same-sex parent). Then principally by hierarchical-entry multiple-regression analyses, alternative models of how these three variable sets interrelate to influence are tested: an interdependence model in which all three domains together influence behavior, an independent model in which each domain is related to behavior after controlling for the effects of the other two, and a mediational model in which one or two prepotent domains may directly influence behavior and one or two domains may influence behavior only indirectly through the other domain effects. Their findings, while complex and not entirely consistent, indicate that adolescent alcohol and drug use are directly related to both the personality of the adolescent and relationships within the family, which in turn are related to the personality of the parent. Protective factors such as identification of child with parent, conventional attitudes by both parent and child, and ego integration tend to ameliorate the effects of risk factors from other domains.

Data from the longitudinal UCLA study are instructive. The role of mothers' drug use, mothers' emotional distress, mothers' somatic complains, and family disruption (absence of at least one parent from the home) have been explored in relation to the attitudes and emotional stability of the child. Utilizing causal modeling procedure, it was found that family disruption did not lead directly to heavy drug involvement, but did lead to disenchantment with traditional values and the development of deviant attitudes, which in turn predispose the adolescent to drug involvement.[118]

The interplay of parental and peer group influences is complex. It seems that the parents' drug use has an indirect effect on the drug use of the teenager by influencing the deviant attitudes and emotional distress of the child.[119] and by influencing the choice of peer group,[120] rather than a direct effect on drug use by the teenager. More interesting, it seems that peer group and distal characteristics of the family relationships and socialization patterns have independent influences on substance involvement, along with the personality of the adolescent as well as parental factors determining the nature and impact of peer group influences.[116,117,120] Indeed, positive family characteristics can provide a protective function in regard to risky peer group influences. Jessor and Jessor's work shows a strong effect on problem drinking of a disjunction, a perceived incompatibility between parents and peers in what they expect of the adolescent.[34]

There is a connection between adolescent problem drinking and drug involvement, and the family milieu, but it is not at all clear how factors such as parental alcoholism, the personality of the adolescent, and peer group involvements may mediate between family and adolescent drug-related behavior. Familial factors may contribute to the development of high-risk drinking behavior by the adolescent and may also contribute directly to a vulnerability to alcohol problems, perhaps through the lack of a protected environment for early drinking experiences or by influencing the development of relevant characteristics of personality.

9. Stress, Drinking, and Vulnerability

The tension-reduction hypothesis, and its several variants, all imply a linkage between drinking and characteristics of the external situation that arouse tension. Thus, one would expect that increased drinking is related to situations that can be described as stressful. Let us examine this proposition and consider the possibility that stress may cause drinkers to become more vulnerable to adverse consequences of their drinking.

One important problem concerns the mechanism or process by which drinking is related to stress. Alcohol may intervene at the point of appraisal of the stressful situation, such as in causing a selective interference with the processing of threatening self-relevant information.[55] Alcohol may affect one's reaction to the situation, such as a stress-response dampening effect[44] or a relief of tension.[43] Finally, drinking behavior and the situations surrounding drinking may serve as a coping response to stress. All of these seem reasonable and supportable, but as yet we cannot distinguish among them on the basis of research evidence.

Another problem in the literature is a confusion over terms. Stress can be described in at least three different ways: the stress of major events such as severe illness, a major career failure, or the loss of a loved one; the stress of marital or work problems that persist over time and are not readily resolved; and the stresses of daily "hassles" which are usually resolved in time for the next one. In general, the research suggests that it is the second type, the chronic and persistent stress, that poses the greatest risk of substance abuse. The debilitating effects of such stressors may also contribute to a vulnerability to alcohol-related problems.

Marlatt's model[121] offers a useful framework for understanding the linkages between stress and drinking or other substance use. He proposes that drinking will vary according to the following factors: the perceived stress in the situation, the degree of perceived control in the situation, the availability of adequate coping resources to the person, the person's expectations regarding the tension-relieving properties of alcohol, and, of course, the availability of alcohol or any substance of choice. Crucial to the model is the proposition that stress-related drinking occurs when the individual's coping alternatives are so inadequate that any significant stress precipitates drinking, or when the stressors are so great to overwhelm the coping resources of the person.

One study based on the model illustrates the complexity and elusive nature of the stress–problem drinking relationships.[122] A large-scale survey included measures of substance use for coping reasons, the coping resources of the person, including coping styles and social supports, along with measures of economic, marital, and job stress. The results showed *both* that persons under high stress with few coping resources and persons under low stress with abundant coping resources tended to drink more. That is, people who cope poorly tend to drink more under stress and people who cope very well tend to drink more *unless* they are under stress. Another study suggests that people with high levels of stress (negative life events) and certain effective coping strategies tend to have unusually low rates of drinking.[123] Of course, stress–tension models cannot account for all high-risk drinking, and other high-risk situations, such as those involving associations with prior use and those involving social norms and pressures, must also be considered.[124]

Certainly there is ample evidence for the proposition that stressful life circumstances, with attendant discomfort, disequilibrium, and a loss of a sense of control, frequently result in greater consumption of alcohol and other psychoactive substances. The stressors may include the aftermath of war,[125] divorce or loss of a loved one,[126] economic hardship,[127] victimization by racism,[128] or being in stressful occupations such as urban law enforcement.[129] Drinking is related more to ongoing stress, such as heavy drinking by the spouse or a depressed affective state, than to specific events.[130] Several studies reported that heavy drinkers experience more major life changes or more undesirable life events,[104,127] but another reported no relationship between the two.[130] Another asked heavy-drinking males to keep a daily diary of drinking and mood states; no relationships were found between drinking and daily moods or between drinking and stressful life experiences.[131,132] Small relationships between job-related stress and problems or disruptive drinking have been reported.[36,47]

One important study used data from two extensive samples and applied causal modeling techniques to this problem. It was found that traumatic life events contributed to a loss of control and a sense of meaninglessness in life, lacking a sense of direction and plans for the future. These, in turn, led to increased generalized substance abuse, including heavy drinking. No support was found for alternative models, such as one in which stress led to drinking which, in turn, led to meaninglessness and a loss of control.[133] This study is important in providing rigorous evidence of one possible causal mechanism. However, a direct path between stress and substance abuse was also found, and the data accounted for only a "small to moderate" proportion of the variance in substance use.

It also appears that moderate drinking may have a beneficial stress-buffering effect. Two studies point in opposing directions. One found the correlation between stressful life events and depression to be higher among abstainers and heavy drinkers, and lower among moderate drinkers, suggesting that moderate levels of consumption attenuate the depressive effects of stress.[104] The other, using more sophisticated loglinear contingency analyses, found that the relationship over time between stresses in marriage, job, and the economic situation of the person and depression was not influenced at all by the level of alcohol consumption.[103] Of course, the latter study was longitudinal and the former was not, and the latter pertained to enduring, chronic stressors rather than the acute events assessed in the former. Thus, comparisons are difficult.

Can stress be linked to a vulnerability to adverse consequences of drinking? Clearly, excessive consumption can lead to adverse consequences which may, in themselves, constitute important sources of stress for the drinker. For example, longitudinal data show that heavy drinking and other substance sue lead to decreased social competence (and thus more stress in social situations) which, in turn, leads to heavier substance use.[133] Insofar as stress can have debilitating effects on the physical health, emotional state, and social functioning of the person, one can infer that such a person would be more vulnerable to the consequences of his or her drinking pattern. Our earlier research showed that, while life events and job stress scores were not related to measures of total intake of alcohol, small but significant relationships were found with the adverse consequences of drinking.[47]

10. Conclusions

Abundant epidemiological research shows that the incidence of alcohol problems is some function of the level of consumption. In this chapter, we have focused on the problem of variation among individuals in problems at given levels of consumption. The evidence presented shows that, among normal-population drinkers, the incidence and intensity of alcohol-related problems are only modestly related to the level of alcohol consumption, pointing toward the disaggregation of behavior and consequences. We then proceeded to an examination of factors that may contribute to differential vulnerability to problems among drinkers: the concurrent consumption of other psychoactive drugs, engaging in other problem behaviors, personality characteristics, aspects of the environment such as familial relationships and situational stress, and sex differences. Overall, the point was stressed that we must widen the circle of covariation beyond alcohol-specific factors in order to understand and predict both dimensions of problem drinking.

Time considerations are crucial to an understanding of alcohol problems. Adverse consequences or problems may flow from acute drinking episodes or chronic drinking patterns and may appear in a relatively short period of time or, as shown in research reviewed here, in the longer-term trajectory of development of the individual. Episodes of acute intoxication may lead to problems such as driving while intoxicated and violence, while chronic drinking patterns may lead to problems with physical and mental health, work, and family relationships, as well as with repeated episodes of acute intoxication and resultant drunken behavior. For example, the UCLA study investigates long-term consequences of adolescent drug involvement in the areas of family formation and stability, criminal and deviant behavior, sexual behavior, educational attainments, livelihood pursuits, mental health, and social integration.

Figure 1 presents the outline of a model of drinking derived from these premises. Drinking behavior and alcohol problems are seen in a relationship

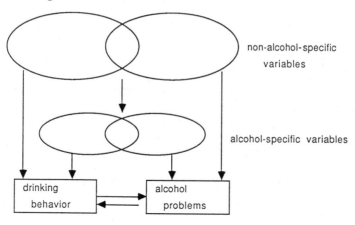

Figure 1. Two-dimensional model of problem drinking.

of mutual causality, in that behavior affects consequences and the development of alcohol problems will also affect the evolution of drinking behavior. We also make a distinction between alcohol-specific (or proximal) variables and non-alcohol-specific (or distal) variables, and postulate that the nonspecific factors will both affect the proximal variables and have some direct influence on the outcome variables. Thus, for example, the level of situational stress encountered by the individual may both influence proximal factors, such as the person's motives or reasons for drinking, and directly affect drinking and problems, apart from the influence or proximal factors. Finally, and most fundamental to our two-dimensional model of problem drinking, the psychosocial predictor variables are partitioned into those which affect alcohol-related problems directly (i.e., vulnerability to problems) and those which influence problems indirectly through their impact on drinking behavior. The model assumes some degree of overlap between the two sets of variables, in that some variables are expected to have direct effects on both behavior and problems.

As this is a model of problem drinking, the behavioral and problem variables are presented as outcomes of the antecedent and concomitant psychosocial influences. This must be seen as a convention, rather than as a full statement of causality. Indeed, notions of feedback or reciprocal causation are fundamental to the framework of psychosocial interactionism and to our understanding of problem drinking as a dynamic, temporally extended process. Certainly, drinking behavior can have influences on the person's subsequent personal characteristics and choices of environments. Clearly, alcohol-related problems will have an impact on the person's expectations about alcohol, choice of peer groups, personality characteristics, and environmental forces such as stress.

From this framework, an agenda for research becomes apparent. It will first become necessary to develop an understanding of which variables influence which (or both) of the two dimensions of problems drinking. That is, we want to know what causes people to drink in ways that may imply high risk, and why people who drink in a given way are at greater or lesser risk of experiencing alcohol-related problems. While a theory of vulnerability to alcohol-related problems would assist enormously in this task, the initial approximations are most likely to be based on empirical findings, and thus the model will be heuristic in nature. It will, of course, necessitate a different treatment of data commonly obtained in psychosocial research on problem drinking, one in which behavioral and problem measures are disaggregated, and in which direct and indirect causal paths to each dimension are explored at one point in time and over time. Equally important is the inclusion of distal variables, those not specific to alcohol, in order to broaden our understanding of the personal and social context of problem drinking. Again, one purpose of research will be to determine the direct and indirect influences of distal factors through appropriate analytical procedures.

ACKNOWLEDGMENT. This work was supported in part by the Alcoholic Beverages Medical Research Foundation.

References

1. Fillmore KM, Bacon SD, Hyman M: The 27 year longitudinal panel study for drinking by students in college, 1949–1976. Final report submitted to NIAAA, 1979.
2. Donovan JE, Jessor R, Jessor L: Problem drinking in adolescence and young adulthood: A follow-up study. *J Stud Alcohol* 44:109–137, 1983.
3. Clark W: Loss of control, heavy drinking and drinking problems in a longitudinal study. *J Stud Alcohol* 37:1256–1290, 1976.
4. Cahalan D, Room R: *Problem Drinking among American Men.* New Brunswick NJ, Rutgers Center for Alcohol Studies, 1974.
5. Cahalan D: *Problem Drinkers: A National Survey.* San Francisco, Jossey-Bass, 1970.
6. Cahalan D, Cisin I, Crossley H: *American Drinking Practices: A National Study of Drinking Behavior and Attitudes* (Rutgers Center for Alcohol Studies Monograph No.6). New Brunswick, NJ, Rutgers Center for Alcohol Studies, 1969.
7. Skinner H, Allen BA: Alcohol dependence syndrome: measurement and validation. *J Abnorm Psychol.* 91:199–209, 1982.
8. Room R: Measurement and distribution of drinking patterns and problems in general populations., in Edwards G, Gross MM Keller M, Moser J, Room R (eds): *Alcohol-Related Disabilities.* Geneva, World Health Organization, 1977.
9. Sadava SW: Interactional theory, in Blane HT, Leonard KE (eds): *Psychological Theories of Drinking and Alcoholism.* New York, Guilford Press, 1987, p 90.
10. Sadava SW: Psychosocial interactionism and substance use. *Drugs and Society* 2(1):1–30, 1987.
11. American Psychiatric Association, Committee on Nomenclature and Statistics: *Diagnostic and Statistical Manual of Mental Disorders,* 3rd edition, revised. Washington, DC, American Psychiatric Association, 1987.
12. Babor TF, Krantzler HR, Lauerman RJ: Social drinking as a health and psychosocial risk factor: Anstie's limit revisited, in Galanter M (ed.): *Recent Developments in Alcoholism, Vol 5.* New York, Plenum Press, 1987, p 373.
13. Anstie F: On the dietetic and medicinal use of wines, Part 1: On the place of wines in the diet of ordinary life. *Practitioner* 4:219–224, 1870.

14. Roizen R: Drinking and drinking problems: some notes on the ascription of problems to drinking. Paper presented at the Epidemiology Section meeting, 21st International Institute on the Prevention and Treatment of Alcoholism, Helsinki, Finland, 1975.
15. Orford J, Waller S, Peto J: Drinking behavior and attitudes and their correlates among university students in England. *Q J Stud Alcohol* 35:1316–1374, 1974.
16. Wanberg KW, Horn L, Epster FM: A differential assessment model for alcoholism: The scales of the Alcohol Use Inventory. *J Stud Alcohol* 38:512–543, 1977.
17. Celentano DD, McQueen DV: Reliability and validity of estimators of alcoholism prevalence. *J Stud Alcohol* 39:869–878, 1978.
18. Jessor R, Donovan JE, Widmer K: *Psychosocial Factors in Adolescent Alcohol and Drug Use: The 1978 National Sample Study and the 1974–1978 Panel Study.* Boulder, Institute of Behavioral Science, University of Colorado, 1980, pp 1–161.
19. Gliksman L, Smythe PC: Adolescent involvement with alcohol: A cross-sectional study. *J Stud Alcohol* 43:370–379, 1982.
20. Skinner H: Early detection of alcohol problems: Why? Unpublished manuscript, addiction Research Foundation, Toronto, 1988.
21. Hays RD, Widaman KF, DiMatteo MR, Stacy AW: Structural equation models of current drug use: Are appropriate models so simple(x)? *J Pers Social Psychol* 52:134–144, 1987.
22. Stein JA, Newcomb MD, Bentler PM: The structure of drug use behaviors and consequences among young adults: A multitrait-multimethod assessment of frequency, quantity, worksite and problem substance use. *J Appl Psychol,* 73:595–605, 1988.
23. Sadava SW, Forsyth R: Person–environment interaction and college student drug use: A multivariate longitudinal study. *Genetic Psychol Monogr* 96:211–245, 1977.
24. Forsyth R, Sadava SW: Criteria measures of drug-using behavior: Multivariate analyses. *Educational Psychol Measurement* 37:641–658, 1977.
25. Sadava SW: Problem behavior theory and consumption and consequences of alcohol use. *J Stud Alcohol* 46:392–397, 1985.
26. Sadava SW, Secord MJ: Problem drinking in context, in Sánchez-Sosa JJ (ed): *Health and Clinical Psychology.* Amsterdam, North-Holland Press, 1985, p 183.
27. White HR: Longitudinal stability and dimensional structure of problem drinking in adolescence. *J Stud Alcohol* 48:541–550, 1987.
28. Fillmore KM: Drinking and problem drinking in early adulthood and middle age. *Q J Stud Alcohol* 35:819–840, 1974.
29. Jessor R, Jessor SL: Adolescent development and the onset of drinking: A longitudinal study. *J Stud Alcohol* 36:27–51, 1975.
30. Yamaguchi K, Kandel D: Patterns of drug use from adolescence to young adulthood. III: Predictors of progression. *Am J Public Health* 74:673–681, 1984.
31. Newcomb MD: *Drug Use in the Workplace. Risk Factors for Substance Use among Young Adults.* Dover, MA, Auburn House, 1988.
32. Alexander BK, Hadaway PF: Opiate addiction: the case for an adaptive orientation. *Psychol Bull* 92:367–381, 1982.
33. Marlatt GA, Baer JS, Donovan DEM, Kivlahan DR: Addictive behaviors: Etiology and treatment. *Annu Rev Psychol* 39:232–252, 1988.
34. Jessor R, Jessor S: *Problem Behavior and Psychosocial Development.* New York, Academic Press, 1977.
35. Zucker R: Developmental aspects of drinking through the adult years, in Blane HT, Chafetz ME (eds): *Youth, Alcohol and Social Policy.* New York, Plenum Press, 1979, p 91.
36 Newcomb MD: Consequences of teenage drug use: The transition from adolescence to young adulthood. *Drugs Society* 4:25–60, 1987.
37. Baumrind D, Moselle KA: A developmental perspective on adolescent drug use. *Adv Alcohol Substance Abuse* 4(3/4):41–68, 1985.
38. Yamaguchi K, Kandel DB: On the resolution of role incompatibility: A life event history analysis of family roles and marijuana use. *Am J Sociol* 90:1284–1325, 1985.

39. Johnston LD: Drug use during and after high school: Results of a national longitudinal survey. *Am J Public Health* 64:29–43, 1974.
40. Newcomb MD, Bentler PM: *Consequences of Adolescent Drug Use.* Beverly Hills, CA, Sage, 1988.
41. Kandel DB, Davies M, Karus D, Yamaguchi K: The consequences in young adulthood of adolescent drug involvement. *Arch Gen Psychiatry* 43:746–754, 1986.
42. Kandel DB, Yamaguchi K: Job mobility and drug use: An event history analysis. *Am J Sociol* 92:836–878, 1987.
43. Cappell H, Greeley J: Alcohol and tension reduction: an update on research and theory, in Blane HT, Leonard KE (eds): *Psychological Theories of Drinking and Alcoholism.* New York, Guilford Press, 1987, p 15.
44. Sher KJ: Stress response dampening, in Blane HT, Leonard KE (eds): *Psychological Theories of Drinking and Alcoholism.* New York, Guilford Press, 1987, p 227.
45. Volpicelli JR: Uncontrollable events and alcohol drinking. *B J Addictions* 82:381–392, 1987.
46. Goldman MS, Brown SA, Christiansen BA: Expectancy theory: thinking about drinking., in Blane HT Leonard KE (eds): *Psychological Theories of Drinking and Alcoholism.* New York, Guilford Press, 1987, p 181.
47. Sadava SW, Thistle R, Forsyth R: Stress, escapism and patterns of alcohol and drug use. *J Stud Alcohol* 39:725–736, 1978.
48. Tarter RE: Are there inherited behavioral traits that predispose to substance abuse? *J Consul Clin Psychol* 56:189–196, 1988.
49. Goodwin DW: Alcoholism and genetics. *Arch Gen Psychiatry* 42:171–174, 1985.
50. Finn PR, Martin J, Pihl RO: Alexithymia in males at high genetic risk for alcoholism. *Psychother Psychosom* 47:18–21, 1987.
51. Levenson RW, Oyama ON, Meek PS: Greater reinforcement from alcohol for those at risk: parental risk, personality risk and sex. *J Abnorm Psychol* 96:242–253, 1987.
52. Cloninger CR: Neurogenetic adaptive mechanisms in alcoholism. *Science* 23:410–436, 1987.
53. Pihl RO, Peterson J, Finn P: An heuristic model for the inherited predisposition to alcoholism. *J Abnorm Psychol,* in press.
54. Steel DM, Joseph RA: Drinking your troubles away. II: An attention-allocation model of alcohol's effects on psychological stress. *J Abnorm Psychol* 97:196–205, 1988.
55. Hull JG: Self awareness model, in Blane HT, Leonard KE (ed): *Psychological Theories of Drinking and Alcoholism.* New York, Guilford Press, 1987, p 272.
56. Berglas S: Self-handicapping model., in Blane HT, Leonard KE (eds): *Psychological Theories of Drinking and Alcoholism.* New York, Guilford Press, 1987, p 305.
57. Braucht N: How environments and persons combine to influence problem drinking, in Galanter M (ed): *Recent Developments in Alcoholism, Vol 1.* New York, Plenum Press, 1983, p 237.
58. Kandel DB: Drug and drinking behavior among youth, *Annu Rev Sociol* 6:235–285, 1980.
59. Harburg E, Davis DR, Caplan R: Parent and offspring alcohol use. Imitative and aversive transmission. *J Stud Alcohol* 43:497–516, 1982.
60. Huba GJ, Bentler PM: A developmental theory of drug use: Derivation and assessment of a causal modeling approach, in Baltes PM, Brim OG (eds): *Life-span Development and Behavior, Vol 4.* New York, Academic Press, 1982, p 147.
61. Schlegel RP, Manske SR, d'Avernas JR: Alcohol and drug use in young adults: selected findings from a longitudinal study. *Bull Soc Psychol Addictive Behav* 4:213–225, 1985.
62. Brown SA: Expectancies versus background in the prediction of college drinking patterns. *J Consult Clin Psychol* 53:123–130, 1985.
63. Sadava SW: Concurrent multiple drug use: review and implications. *J Drug Issues* 4:623–636, 1984.
64. Istvan J, Matarazzo JD: Tobacco, alcohol and caffeine use: A review of their interrelationships. *Psychol Bull* 95:301–326, 1984.
65. Kandel DB: Stages in adolescent involvement in drug use. *Science* 190:912–914, 1975.

66. Yamaguchi K, Kandel DB: Patterns of drug use from adolescence to young adulthood. III Predictors of progression. *Am J Public Health* 74:673–681, 1984.
67. Kandel DB, Faust R: Sequence and stages in patterns of adolescent drug use. *Arch Gen Psychiatry* 32:923–932, 1975.
68. Gould LG, Berberian PM, Kasl SV, et al: Sequential patterns of multiple drug use among high school students *Arch Gen Psychiatry* 34:216–222, 1977.
69. Kessler RC, Paton SM, Kandel DB: Reconciling unidimensional and multidimensional models of patterns of drug use. *J Stud Alcohol* 37:632–647, 1976.
70. Donovan JE, Jessor R: Problem drinking and the dimension of involvement with drugs: A Guttman scalogram analysis of adolescent drug use. *Am J Public Health* 73:543–552, 1983.
71. Newcomb MD, Bentler PM: Frequency and sequence of drug use: a longitudinal study from early adolescence to young adulthood. *J Drug Education* 16:101–120, 1986.
72. Freed EX: Drug use by alcoholics: A review. *Int J Addictions* 8:451–473, 1973.
73. Sokolow L, Welte G, Hynes G, Lyones J: Multiples substance abuse by alcoholics. *Br J Addictions* 76:147–158, 1981.
74. Wilkinson DA, Leigh GM, Cordingley J, et al: Dimensions of multiple drug use and typology of drug use. *Br J Addictions* 82:259–273, 1987.
75. Kandel DB, Kessler RC, Margulies RZ: Antecedents of adolescent involvement into stages of drug use: A develop-mental analysis in DB Kandel (ed): *Longitudinal Research on Drug Use: Empirical Findings and Methodological Issues*. Washington, DC, Hemisphere Press, 1978, p 73.
76. Forney RB, Hughes FW: *Combined Effects of Alcohol and Other Drugs*. Springfield, IL, Charles Thomas, 1978.
77. Kissin H: Interactions of ethyl alcohol and other drugs in Kissin B, Begleiter H (eds): *The Biology of Alcoholism, Vol 3. Clinical Pathology*. New York, Plenum Press, 1974.
78. Plant MA, Beck DF, Stuart R: The correlates of serious alcohol-related consequences and illicit drug use amongst a cohort of Scottish teenagers. *Br J Addictions* 79:197–200, 1984.
79. Donovan JE, Jessor R: Structure of problem behavior in adolescence and young adulthood. *J Consult Clin Psychol* 53:890–904, 1985.
80. Hundleby J, Carpenter RA, Ross RAJ, Mercer GW: Adolescent drug use and other behaviors. *J Child Psychol Psychiatry* 23:61–68, 1982.
81. Hundleby J: Adolescent drug use in a behavioral matrix: A confirmation and comparison of the sexes. *Addictive Behav* 12:103–112, 1987.
82. Newcomb MD, Maddahian E, Bentler PM: Risk factors for drug use among adolescents: concurrent and longitudinal analyses. *Am J Public Health* 76:525–531, 1986.
83. Hays R, Stacy AW, DiMatteo MR: Covariation among health-related behaviors. *Addictive Behav* 9:315–318, 1984.
84. Huba GJ, Bentler PM: Causal models of the development of law abidance and its relationship to psychosocial factors and drug use, in Lanfer WS, Day JM (eds): *Personality Theory, Moral Development and Criminal Behavior*. Lexington, MA, Lexington Books, 1983, p 165.
85. Johnston LD, O'Malley PM, Eveland LK: Drugs and delinquency: a search for causal connections, in Kandel DB (ed): *Longitudinal Research on Drug Use: Empirical Findings and Methodological Issues*. Washington, DC, Hemisphere Press, 1978, p 137.
86. Elliott DS, Huizinga D, Ageton SS: *Explaining Delinquency and Drug Use*. Beverly Hills, Sage, 1985.
87. White HR, Pandina RJ, LeGrange RI: Longitudinal predictors of serious substance use and delinquency. *Criminology* 25:715–740, 1987.
88. Osgood DW: The drug-crime connection and the generality and stability of deviance. Paper presented at the annual meeting of the American Society of Criminology, 1985.
89. Newcomb MD, Bentler PM: Impact of adolescent drug use and social support on problems of young adults: A longitudinal study. *J Pers Soc Psychol* 97:64–75, 1988.
90. Vaillant GE: *The Natural History of Alcoholism*. Cambridge, MA, Harvard University Press, 1983.

91. Stein JA, Newcomb MD, Bentler PM: An 8-year study of multiple influences on drug use and drug use consequences. *J Pers Soc Psychol* 53:1094–1105, 1987.
92. Schlegel RP, d'Avernas JR, Manske SR: Longitudinal patterns of alcohol use: psychosocial predictors of transition, in Sánchez-Sosa JJ (ed): *Health and Clinical Psychology*. Amsterdam, North-Holland Press, 1985, p 201.
93. DiTecco D, Schlegel RP: Alcohol use among young males: an application of problem behavior theory, in Eiser JR (ed): *Social Psychology and Behavioral Medicine*. New York, Wiley, 1982, p 199.
94. Sadava SW: Personality, etiology and alcoholism. *Can Psychol Rev* 12:33–51, 1978.
95. Barnes GE: Clinical and prealcoholic personality characteristics, in Kissin B, Begleiter H (eds): *The Biology of Alcoholism: Vol 6. The Pathogenesis of Alcoholism*. New York, Plenum Press, 1987, pp 113–183.
96. Cox WM: Personality theory and research, in Blane HT, Leonard KE (eds): *Psychological Theories of Drinking and Alcoholism*. New York, Guilford Press, 1987, p 55.
97. Pihl RO, Spiers P: Individual characteristics in the etiology of drug abuse, in Maher B (ed): *Progress in Experimental Personality Research, Vol 8*. New York, Academic Press, 1978.
98. Labouvie EW, McGee CR: Relation of personality to alcohol and drug use in adolescence. *J Consul Clin Psychol* 54:289–293, 1986.
99. Kellam SG, Brown CH, Rubin BR, Ensminger ME: Paths leading to teenage psychiatric symptoms and substance use: Developmental epidemiological studies in Woodlawn, in Guse SB, Earls FJ, Barrett JE (eds): *Childhood Psychopathology and Development*. New York, Raven Press, 1983, p 17.
100. McCord W, McCord J: *Origins of Alcoholism*. Stanford, CA, Stanford University Press, 1960.
101. Jones MC: Personality correlates and antecedents of drinking patterns in adult males. *J Consul Clin Psychol* 32:2–12, 1968.
102. Loper RG, Kammeier ML, Hoffman H: MMPI characteristics of college freshmen who later become alcoholics. *J Abnorm Psychol* 82:159–162, 1973.
103. Aneshensel CS: An application of log-linear models: The stress-buffering effects of alcohol use. *J Drug Educ* 13:287–301, 1983.
104. Neff JA, Husaini BA: Life events, drinking patterns and depressive symptomatology: The stress-buffering effects of alcohol consumption. *J Stud Alcohol* 43:310–318, 1982.
105. Wilsnack SC, Beckman LJ (eds): *Alcohol Problems in Women. Antecedents, Consequences and Intervention*. New York, Guilford Press, 1984.
106. Wilsnack SC: Prevention of alcohol problems in women, in *Alcohol and Health Monograph No. 4: Special Population Issues*. D.H.H.S. Publication No. (ADM) 82–1193. Rockville, MD, National Institute on Alcohol Abuse and Alcoholism, 1982, p 71.
107. Knupfer G: Problems associated with drunkenness in women: Some research issues. *Alcohol and Health Monograph No. 4. Special Population Issues*. D.H.H.D. Publication No. (ADM) 82–1193. Rockville, MD, National Institute on Alcohol Abuse and Alcoholism, 1982, p 3.
108. Madanik L: Alcohol problems and depressive symptoms in a national survey. *Addictive Behav* 8:132–141, 1983.
109. Hill SY: Vulnerability to the biomedical consequences of alcoholism and alcohol-related problems in women, in Wilsnack SC, Beckman LJ (eds): *Alcohol Problems in Women: Antecedents, Consequences and Intervention*. New York, Guilford Press, 1984, p 121.
110. Sutker P, Libet JM, Allain AN, Randall CL: Alcohol, use, negative mood states and menstrual cycle changes. *Alcoholism: Clin Exp Res* 7:327–331, 1983.
111. Fillmore KM: "When angels fall": Women's drinking as a cultural preoccupation and as reality, in Wilsnack S, Beckman L (eds): *Alcohol Problems in Women*. New York, Guilford Press, 1984, p 7.
112. Sadava SW: Alcohol consumption and problems: gender differences. *Bull Soc Psychol Addictive Behav* 5:67–74, 1986.
113. Grant BF, Hartford TC, Grigson MB: Stability of alcohol consumption among youth: A national longitudinal survey. *J Stud Alcohol* 49:253–260, 1988.

114. Barnes GM: The development of adolescent drinking behavior: an evaluative review of the impact of the socialization process within the family. *Adolescence* 48:571–591, 1977.

115. Zucker R, Noll RB: Precursors and developmental influences on drinking and alcoholism: Etiology from a longitudinal perspective, in *Alcohol and Health, Monograph No. 1.* Rockville, MD, National Institute on Alcohol Abuse and Alcoholism, 1982.

116. Brook JS, Whiteman M, Gordon AS, Cohen P: Some models and mechanisms for explaining the impact of maternal and adolescent characteristics on adolescent stage of drug use. *Dev Psychol* 22:460–467, 1986.

117. Brook JS, Whiteman M, Gordon AS: Stages of drug use in adolescence: personality, peer and family correlates. *Dev Psychol* 19:269–277, 1983.

118. Newcomb MD, Bentler PM: The impact of family context, deviant attitudes and emotional distress on adolescent drug use: longitudinal latent-variable analyses of mothers and their children. *J Res Personality* 22:154–176, 1988.

119. Huba GJ, Wingard JA, Bentler PM: Beginning adolescent drug use and peer and adult interaction patterns. *J Consult Clin Psychol* 47:265–276, 1979.

120. Brook JS, Whiteman M, Gordon AS, Brook DW: Father's influence on his daughter's marijuana use viewed in a mother and peer context, in Brook JS, Lettieri DJ, Brook DW (eds): *Alcohol and Substance Abuse in Adolescence.* New York, Haworth Press, 1985, p 165.

121. Marlatt GA: Alcohol use and problems drinking: a cognitive-behavioral analysis, in Kendall PC, Hollon SD (eds): *Cognitive Behavioral Intervention: Theory, Research and Procedures.* New York, Academic Press, 1979.

122. Timmer SG, Veroff J, Colten ME: Life stress, helplessness and the use of alcohol and drugs to cope: An analysis of national survey data, in Shiffman S, Wills TA (eds): *Coping and Substance Use.* New York, Academic Press, 1985, p 171.

125. Wills TA: Stress, coping and tobacco and alcohol use in early adolescence, in Shiffman S, Wills TA (eds): *Coping and Substance Use.* New York, Academic Press, 1985, p 63).

124. Brennan A, Walfish S, AuBuchon P: Alcohol use and abuse in college students. II. Social/environmental correlates, methodological issues and implications for intervention. *Int J Addictions* 21:475–493, 1986.

125. Penk W, Robinowitz R, Roberts WR, et al: Adjustment differences among male substance abusers varying in degrees of combat experience in Vietnam. *J Consul Clin Psychol* 49:426–437, 1981.

126. Bruns C, Geist CS: Stressful life events and drug use among adolescents. *J Hum Stress* 10:135–139, 1984.

127. Pearlin L, Radabaugh C: Economic strains and the coping functions of alcohol. *Am J Sociol* 82:652–663, 1977.

128. Kleinman PH, Lukoff IF: Ethnic differences in factors related to drug use. *J Health Social Behav* 19:190–199, 1978.

129. Nordlicht S: Effects of stress on the police officer and family. *NY State J Med* 79:400–401, 1979.

130. Cronkite R, Moos R: The role of precipitation and moderating factors in the stress-illness relationship. *J Health Soc Behav* 25:372–393, 1984.

131. Stone AA, Lennox S, Neale JM: Daily coping and alcohol use in a sample of community adults., in Shiffman S, Wills TA (eds): *Coping and Substance Use.* New York, Academic Press, 1985, p 199.

132. Rohsenow D: Social anxiety, daily moods and alcohol use over time among heavy social drinkers. *Addict Behav* 7:311–315, 1982.

133. Newcomb MD, Harlow LL: Life events and substance use among adolescents: Mediating effects of perceived loss of control and meaninglessness in life. *J Personality Soc Psychol* 51:564–577, 1986.

III

Biological Issues: Ethanol–Drug Interactions

Richard A. Deitrich, Section Editor

In this section are reviewed only two of the many hundreds of ethanol–drug interactions known to occur. However, those discussed here are two of the most common and serious: the interactions of alcohol with nicotine and tobacco in general, and the interactions of alcohol with the benzodiazepines.

Zacny reviews the clinical and human research on smoking and drinking. In his chapter he documents what anyone who has ever been to a bar or to an Alcoholics Anonymous meeting has observed: there is a high correlation between smoking and drinking. The combined health hazard of this interaction is enormous and probably underestimated, if anything. There is a not-too-subtle message in the fact that the Federal government has an Alcohol, Tobacco and *Firearms* unit in the Treasury Department. The interaction of alcohol with either of the other two is deadly.

Collins then summarizes what little is known about the molecular aspects of the interaction between ethanol and nicotine. While a great deal is known about the nicotinic receptor at the molecular and molecular-genetic level, relatively little is known about how ethanol and nicotine interact at this level to give rise to the behavioral manifestations of the simultaneous intake of ethanol and nicotine. It is axiomatic, however, that given enough information at the molecular, cellular, and whole-animal level, behavior can eventually be understood in such a way that specific interventions can be designed on a rational basis. We are obviously a long way from this goal, but with the advent of highly sophisticated techniques in all scientific areas, it is only a question of time and money.

Hollister updates knowledge on the well-known ethanol–benzodiazepine interaction. With the recent cloning of the benzodiazepine–GABA–

Richard A. Deitrich • Alcohol Research Center, and Department of Pharmacology, University of Colorado School of Medicine, Denver, Colorado 80262.

chloride channel receptor from beef and human, along with the many studies of the interaction of benzodiazepines and alcohol at the function level, great strides should be forthcoming in the understanding of how these behavioral interactions are mediated at a molecular level as well.

9

Behavioral Aspects of Alcohol–Tobacco Interactions

James P. Zacny

Abstract. Alcohol and tobacco consumption are correlated—smokers consume more alcohol than do nonsmokers and alcohol consumers smoke more than do teetotalers. In addition, heavy drinking tends to be associated with heavy smoking. A large majority of alcoholics, who by definition are heavy drinkers, smoke. A number of studies examining the effects of ethanol pretreatment or availability on tobacco consumption have demonstrated that ethanol potentiates tobacco consumption. Whether smoking potentiates alcohol consumption is not known. Possible mechanisms underlying the alcohol/tobacco association, including cross-tolerance between the two drugs, are discussed. Tobacco appears to counteract the deleterious effects of alcohol on some measures of performance. The association between alcohol and tobacco consumption may have some relevance regarding the issue of relapse to either one of the drugs. Finally, combined use of alcohol and tobacco presents greater risk of certain diseases than the sum of the excess risks of alcohol and tobacco considered individually.

1. Introduction

Alcohol and tobacco cigarettes are two of the most frequently used psychoactive drugs in Western society. Approximately two-thirds of American adults consume alcohol[1] and approximately 30% smoke cigarettes.[2] The purpose of this chapter is to examine the association between use of these two drugs. First, correlational and experimental evidence are reviewed which document the association between drinking and smoking consumption. Second, possible mechanisms underlying the association are presented. Third, studies examining the behavioral effects of the joint administration of alcohol and tobacco are reviewed. Finally, two clinical issues are raised regarding the role of the alcohol/tobacco association in promoting relapse to drinking and/or smoking, and in potentiating risk of life-threatening diseases.

James P. Zacny • Drug Abuse Research Center, Department of Psychiatry, University of Chicago, Chicago, Illinois 60637.

2. Documenting the Relationship between Alcohol and Tobacco Consumption

2.1. Descriptive Studies

This section reviews several of the studies that have documented that alcohol and tobacco consumption are related; the reader is referred to a recent exhaustive review[3] for a more complete account of the many descriptive studies that have examined the association between the use of these two drugs. The finding that there is a moderately strong positive correlation between alcohol and tobacco consumption applies across various demographic variables (age, race, socioeconomic status) and has been replicated in different countries. Smokers are more likely to drink alcohol than nonsmokers, and they are likely to be heavier consumers of alcohol than nonsmokers. For example, in a study examining the drinking and smoking habits of over 36,000 American adults,[4] 89% of male smokers and 84% of female smokers currently drank alcohol, as opposed to 75% of male nonsmokers and 61% of female nonsmokers. The tendency for smokers to be heavier drinkers also held true in a younger age group: in a study of nearly 5000 American youths aged 12–17, 80% of the smokers in this sample had already reported using alcohol, whereas only 45% of the nonsmokers used alcohol by this age.[5] Not only are smokers more likely to be drinkers, they are likely to consume more alcohol than nonsmokers. In a study in which healthy American adults ($N = 471$) were asked to estimate the type and number of alcoholic drinks they consumed in a typical month, male and female smokers reported drinking an average of 58.9 and 23.8 drinks/month, respectively, while male and female nonsmokers reported drinking an average of 31.3 and 10.9 drinks/month. This study was particularly interesting because it also examined the response of exsmokers and found that their drinking consumption more closely resembled that of smokers than of nonsmokers.[6]

Looking at the alcohol/tobacco relationship from the other side, alcohol consumers are also more likely to smoke than are teetotalers. In a nationwide probability sample of 2411 adults, 47% of alcohol consumers were smokers, whereas only 27% of alcohol abstainers smoked.[7] The same relationship is evident with children and teenagers: In one study, for example, in which the smoking and drinking habits of American children and teenagers aged 9–17 ($N = 197$) were examined, 41% of alcohol consumers smoked, whereas only 3% of alcohol abstainers smoked.[8]

The alcohol/tobacco association is dose-related in that (1) heavy smokers drink more than light smokers and (2) heavy drinkers smoke more than light drinkers. In a study examining drinking and smoking habits of Swedish and Finnish adults, among men ($N = 9426$), 48% of heavy smokers (≥ 20 cigarettes/day) and 31% of light smokers (<20 cigarettes/day) fell in the highest alcohol consumption category (>500 g of absolute alcohol/month); in women ($N = 10,630$), 20% of heavy smokers and 7% of light smokers fell into this category.[9] Evidence that heavy drinkers smoke more than do light drinkers comes from a study of 7735 British males,[10] in which 39% of heavy drinkers (>6 drinks/day) were heavy smokers (>20 cigarettes/day) while only 15% of frequent light drinkers (1–2 drinks/day) were heavy smokers. In another study of 2000 American men, heavy drinkers (≥5 drinks/day) smoked more cigarettes (17.3 cigarettes/day) than lighter drinkers (10.2 cigarettes/day).[11]

The relationship between alcohol and tobacco is most apparent in alcoholics. A large majority of alcoholics smoke, and not surprisingly, they tend to smoke more heavily than alcohol abstainers or light drinkers. Most studies examining the incidence of smoking among alcoholics report that at least 80–90% of alcoholics smoke. For example, in a study examining the smoking status of 582 male and 83 female alcoholics,[12] 92% of the males and 95% of the females were current smokers. Obviously, this is a much higher percentage of smoking than that found in the general population. Kozlowski et al.[13] compared the pattern of smoking prevalence of alcoholic adults from Ontario presenting themselves for treatment to the Addiction Research Foundation Clinic in 1979 and 1980 ($N = 1142$) to the patterning of smoking prevalence of the general population of Ontario adults in 1979. Eighty-six percent of male alcoholics and 82% of female alcoholics smoked, compared to only 42% of males and 34% of females from the general Ontario population. Several studies have found that alcoholics smoke more heavily than do lighter drinkers or alcohol abstainers who smoke. For example, Ziener et al.[14] found that alcoholics smoked more cigarettes on a daily basis than did social drinkers (27.8 cigarettes/day vs. 12.8 cigarettes/day). When alcoholics were compared to a control group of substance abusers who were not alcoholics, alcoholics smoked more cigarettes on a daily basis (27.7) than did other-drug abusers (22.7).[15] Consistent with the higher cigarette consumption, alcoholics in the study were also more physically dependent on nicotine, as measured by the Fagerstrom Tolerance Questionnaire.

2.2. Experimental Studies

Given that alcohol and tobacco consumption are correlated, it is conceivable that consumption of one substance may have an effect on consumption of the other substance—i.e., alcohol consumption may increase tobacco consumption and tobacco consumption may potentiate alcohol consumption. This section examines the studies that have put these hypotheses to the empirical test.

In one of the first experimental investigations of the alcohol–tobacco interaction, Griffiths et al.[16] in a series of experiments examined the smoking behavior of alcoholics in an inpatient research ward setting. In one of the experiments, subjects were required to ingest a drink (alcohol or vehicle-only) every 30 min for a 6-hr period while the number of cigarettes smoked during that period was monitored. All five subjects increased their cigarette consumption during ethanol sessions, and the increase was directly related to the ethanol dose. In several control experiments, the increased cigarette consumption was observed even when opportunity to socialize or opportunity to drink and smoke concurrently were not allowed. In two subsequent studies by Griffiths and his associates, alcohol was administered as a pretreatment to a 90-min smoking session. In one study, subjects ($N = 5$) were alcoholics and in the other study, subjects ($N = 5$) were healthy normal volunteers. Number of puffs and cigarettes smoked by alcoholics increased after the alcohol pretreatment (89 or 134 g absolute ethanol), relative to a vehicle pretreatment.[17] In the study in which smoking behavior of healthy volunteers was monitored,[18] only the moderate drinkers (1 drink/day) smoked more in response to the ethanol pretreatment (1.0 g/kg of 95% ethanol)—lighter drinkers (< drink/day) did not alter their cigarette consumption. These findings prompted the authors to conclude that the effects of alcohol on smoking intake may be related to prior history of alcohol consumption. That is, potentiated tobacco consumption by alcohol may be more likely to occur in moderate and heavy drinkers than light drinkers. This conclusion appears to be consistent with the results from several descriptive studies in which light drinkers were no more likely than nondrinkers to be classified as heavy smokers.[10,19,20]

Two other alcohol pretreatment studies examined the effects of ethanol on smoking topography. Smoking topography refers to the precise manner in which people smoke and is described by measures such as duration and volume of the puff, postpuff inhalation, and postpuff exhalation. In one of the studies,[21] 0.7 g/kg of ethanol, but not 0.5 g/kg, induced increases in puff size (i.e., volume), as well as increases in total smoke volume per cigarette. A parallel increase in carbon monoxide exposure was also noted. In the second study,[22] ethanol pretreatment (designed to produce a peak blood alcohol level of 0.05%) increased puff volume in 10 of 14 smokers. Those individuals with the larger puff volumes during baseline sessions were less likely to increase their puff volumes during the ethanol pretreatment sessions, perhaps owing to a ceiling effect. Subjects in this study were narcotic addicts enrolled in a methadone maintenance program. In both studies, number of cigarettes smoked in the session was controlled by the experimenter, so it is unclear whether puff volume normally increases as a result of ethanol exposure in ad libitum smoking situations.

In the final two studies, healthy normal volunteers resided on a research ward for several weeks and were allowed to smoke ad libitum while alcohol availability was manipulated. In one of the studies,[23] daily cigarette consumption of six males did not increase when alcohol was made available. However, there was a positive relationship in the alcohol-available phase between number of drinks ingested per day and number of cigarettes smoked per day. That is, on days when subjects drank more, they smoked more, and on days when they drank less, they smoked less. This relationship was evident in light, moderate, and heavy smokers. Interestingly, with the light and moderate smokers, smoking tended to occur almost exclusively during drinking periods—with heavier smokers, smoking tended to occur throughout the entire day. In the other study, only women (N = 24) were used.[24] Heavy smokers ($\geq$25 cigarettes/day) consumed more cigarettes during the alcohol-available phase than during a no-alcohol phase. This relationship was not observed with lighter smokers. In the subgroup of heavy smokers, increased consumption was accomplished not by smoking over a longer period each day, but by decreasing intercigarette interval. Among the heavy smokers, there was a striking concordance between variations in alcohol intake and in cigarette smoking during the alcohol-available phase. When the data were analyzed based on alcohol consumption during the alcohol-available phase, those smokers who drank moderately (mean number of drinks/day = 4) or heavily (mean number of drinks/day = 8) increased their tobacco consumption, relative to a no-drinking baseline phase. Occasional drinkers during the alcohol-available phase (mean number of drinks/day = 1) did not increase their tobacco consumption, which is consistent with the study previously discussed in which subjects with a history of light drinking did not increase their tobacco intake after alcohol pretreatment.[18]

It appears that no studies to date have systematically examined the effects of cigarette dose or cigarette availability on alcohol intake. This is surprising, given the robustness of the alcohol/tobacco association found in both the descriptive and experimental studies reviewed here. It may be that cigarette smoking potentiates ethanol intake, in much the same way that ethanol potentiates cigarette smoking. If this were so, these results would be consistent with the descriptive studies discussed earlier which have documented that (1) smokers are more likely to drink than nonsmokers, (2) smokers consume more alcohol than nonsmokers, and (3) heavy smokers consume more alcohol than light smokers. While there are no experimental studies with humans demonstrating that smoking potentiates alcohol intake, there is a study with rats demonstrating that nicotine potentiates alcohol intake.[25] Rats acclimated to drinking both water and 10% v/v ethanol were implanted with slow-release nicotine pellets (3.4 mg/day). Rats doubled their ethanol intake (from 8.1 to 16.7 ml/day) and decreased their water intake (from 11.1 to 3.9 ml/day) after having been implanted with the pellets—a control group of rats implanted with an inert substance did not increase their ethanol intake. The increase in ethanol intake was not due to calorie-seeking behavior since intake of an isocaloric nonalcoholic liquid did not increase. A number of other drugs were implanted in animals (e.g., phencyclidine, secobarbital), but these drugs did not increase ethanol intake. The authors concluded that the results supported a self-medication model of ethanol intake—i.e., the chronic nicotine treatment induced chronic hyperactivity and the subjects drank more ethanol as a means of antagonizing this effect. This self-medication hypothesis is discussed in greater detail in the next section.

3. Possible Mechanisms Underlying the Relationship between Alcohol and Tobacco Consumption

While it is clear that a positive correlation exists between alcohol and cigarette consumption, and that drinking potentiates smoking, the mechanisms underlying the behavioral association between use of alcohol and tobacco are not well understood. This section outlines several mechanisms that might be involved.

One possible mechanism for the behavioral association between drinking and smoking is that chronic use of one substance may induce tolerance to the effects of the other substance. Tolerance to the effects of psychoactive drugs sometimes leads to an increase in use of those drugs.[26] Therefore, if chronic administration of ethanol confers cross-tolerance to the effects of smoking, smoking consumption might then increase. Similarly, if chronic smoking confers cross-tolerance to the effects of ethanol, then ethanol consumption might also increase. Two recent studies (discussed in more detail later in this volume by Collins) have documented that chronic infusion of nicotine resulted in the development of cross-tolerance to some of the effects of ethanol and chronic ethanol treatment resulted in the development of cross-tolerance to some of the effects of nicotine in mice.[27,28] In the first study,[28] DBA mice were treated with chronic nicotine (0.2–5 mg/kg per hr for 8–10 days), ethanol (liquid diet from which 20% of the calories came from ethanol for 8–10 days), or saline. Chronic ethanol-treated animals were cross-tolerant to the acute effects of nicotine (2 mg/kg, IP) on body temperature and heart rate but not to the effects of nicotine on rotarod performance (test of motor coordination). Chronic nicotine-infused animals were cross-tolerant to the acute effects of ethanol (2.5 g/kg, IP) on body temperature, but not to the effects of ethanol on rotarod performance or open field activity. In a second study employing more measures of tolerance, a longer chronic ethanol administration period (21 days), and a higher dose of chronically infused nicotine (8 mg/kg per hr),[27] chronic ethanol-treated animals were cross-tolerant to one out of six acute effects of nicotine. Nicotine-infused animals were cross-tolerant to two out of six acute effects of ethanol. Thus, partial cross-tolerance between alcohol and nicotine existed in both studies, which suggests that at least some of the effects of alcohol and nicotine may be mediated through similar mechanisms.[28] Indeed, both alcohol and nicotine have depressant and stimulant actions[29–31] and may act on common neural pathways.[27,28,32,33]

Another explanation for the alcohol/smoking association is based on drug metabolism and how one drug may affect rate of metabolism of the other. That is, smokers may drink more if smoking increases alcohol metabolism, and drinkers may smoke more if alcohol increases nicotine metabolism. Indeed, there are data suggesting that alcohol does increase nicotine metabolism. In a study in which rats were pretreated with ethanol (4 g/kg per day for 7 days and then 8 g/kg per day for 5.5 days) or with sucrose, and then injected with nicotine 36 hr later, ethanol-pretreated rats had significantly lowered plasma nicotine and cotinine levels and also increased volume of nicotine distribution and total plasma clearance of nicotine than sucrose-pre-treated rats.[34] However, in one of the cross-tolerance studies discussed earlier, chronic administration of either ethanol or nicotine in rats did not alter the elimination rates of these drugs when administered acutely.[28] In addition, ethanol pretreatment (0.5 or 1.0 g/kg) did not affect metabolic clearance of intravenous nicotine (1.5 g base/kg per min for 30 min) in healthy smokers,[35] prompting the authors to conclude that ethanol-induced increases in cigarette smoking observed in other studies were not due to an effect of ethanol on nicotine metabolism.

Another potential mechanism for the alcohol/tobacco association has been mentioned previously: The aversive effects of one drug may be counteracted by the other drug.[25] For example, if some effects of alcohol are aversive (e.g., sedation, behavioral impairment) and are counteracted by the effects of smoking, then it would be plausible that smoking would increase. Some studies from the following section on behavioral effects of the alcohol/tobacco interaction do provide some support for this possibility. Alternatively, the "positive" effects of one drug may be attenuated by the other drug and lead to an increase in drug taking. For example, if the "positive" effects of smoking (e.g., enhanced concentration) are attenuated by alcohol, then smoking might increase in much the same way that smoking increases in response to the nicotine antagonist mecamylamine.[36]

Finally, there are several studies indicating that the effects of alcohol can be potentiated by nicotine and tobacco. In a drug discrimination study,[37] rats were trained in a two-lever, food-motivated operant task to discriminate ethanol from vehicle. After dose–response functions for the ethanol discriminative stimulus (i.e., cue) were established, the dose–response functions were redetermined after pretreatment with nicotine. Dose–response functions for the ethanol discriminative stimulus were shifted to the left by nicotine, demonstrating that nicotine potentiated the discriminative stimulus properties of ethanol. In two other studies, ethanol-induced hypnosis in mice was potentiated by chronic administration of nicotine.[38,39] In humans, ethanol-induced increases in heart rate were enhanced by tobacco and nicotine.[31,35] Also in humans, ethanol-induced amplitude reduction of the contingent negative variation (a component of EEG associated with arousal and attentional processes) was potentiated by smoking.[40] Whether this potentiation of the effects of alcohol by smoking and nicotine is involved in mediating the association between alcohol and tobacco consumption is not well understood.[40]

4. Joint Effects of Alcohol and Tobacco on Behavior

Several studies have examined the joint effects of drinking and smoking on behavior in humans and are described in this section. Six of the seven experimental studies were conducted by J. E. Tong and/or his associates in Canada and have several methodological points in common: (1) all six studies employed within-subject designs, (2) alcohol dose was expressed as peak blood alcohol level (BAL), (3) cigarettes used in the studies were high yield (nicotine content: 1.2–1.3 mg), and (4) smokers were asked to abstain from smoking prior to attending the experimental session, usually for 12 hr.

Three of the studies examining the effects of alcohol/tobacco on behavior focused on sensory/perceptual effects. In the first study,[31] the effects of alcohol/tobacco on visual perception were assessed. Nonsmokers and smokers were given placebo or alcoholic drinks (0.02% and 0.08% BAL) prior to a visual discrimination task. Smokers were deprived of smoking for 12 hr prior to the session and were either allowed or not allowed to smoke two cigarettes during the session. The visual discrimination task measured the threshold at which subjects were able to detect two flashes of light as two flashes, rather than one flash, i.e., the two-flash fusion (TFF) threshold. The low dose of alcohol enhanced perceptual discrimination in smokers and had no effect in either nonsmokers or deprived smokers, relative to a baseline no-drug condition. The high dose of alcohol had no effect on perceptual discrimination in smokers, but worsened perceptual discrimination in nonsmokers and deprived smokers, relative to the baseline condition. The authors concluded that smoking altered the effects of alcohol, in some cases counteracting the deleterious effects of alcohol. This study was well designed in that it included a nonsmoker control group by which the effects of alcohol, per se, on visual discrimination could be assessed. In a second visual perception study, the effects of drinking/smoking on critical flicker frequency (CFF) was assessed.[41] The dependent measure in this task was the frequency at which the flickering of a light source could no longer be detected. Stimulants tend to increase CFF (increase ability to discriminate flicker) and depressant/sedatives tend to decrease CFF (decrease ability to discriminate flicker).[42] Although the results were complex, the basic finding was that in a long signal detection task, CFF was decreased by alcohol (0.88 ml/kg of 93% alcohol) but smoking cigarettes during the task partly antagonized this effect.

In the third perception study, the effect of drinking/smoking on time judgment (temporal discrimination) was examined.[43] When people are asked to estimate elapsed time under the influence of alcohol, they tend to overestimate the time interval—i.e., they produce a time interval longer than the actual interval.[44] Conversely, smoking tends to result in underestimation of a given time interval.[45] Subjects in the present study were deprived of smoking for 12 hr before performing a task in which they were to estimate time intervals (by activating an electric timer) of 1.5, 4.0, and 9.0 sec. Following one of four experimental conditions—No Alcohol, No Cigarette; No Alcohol, Cigarette; Alcohol (1.79 or 2.89 ml/kg 35% alcohol), No Cigarette; Alcohol, Cigarette—subjects performed the task again. Relative to scores obtained after 12 hr of cigarette deprivation, alcohol alone lengthened time-production scores, smoking alone shortened time-production scores, and, when given jointly, smoking tended to counteract the effects of alcohol.

The joint behavioral effects of alcohol/tobacco on psychomotor performance have been assessed.[46] In this study, subjects were to engage in three simple psychomotor tasks (finger and foot tapping, knob turning) and a complex psychomotor task (pursuit rotor). Both simple and complex psychomotor performance were decreased by alcohol (0.06% BAL) and these deleterious effects of alcohol were not counteracted by smoking two cigarettes prior to the tasks.

Three studies by Tong and his associates focused on the joint effects of alcohol/tobacco on cognitive processes. In one of the studies,[47] a conditional discrimination/reaction time task was employed in which under the presence of two stimuli, a given response was correct, and in the presence of another set of stimuli, another response was correct. The response was simply moving a finger from a center telegraph key to a right or left key. The time it took to do this was defined as reaction time (and was not affected by smoking and/or drinking). The latency between stimulus onset and removal of a finger from the center key was defined as decision time. Nonsmokers and smokers were given placebo or alcoholic drinks (0.01% and 0.055% BAL) before the task. Smokers were deprived of smoking for 12 hr before the session and then smoked two cigarettes before the task. Decision time was lengthened by alcohol in nonsmokers but not in smokers.

In a study examining the joint effects of alcohol and tobacco on divided attention,[48] subjects were instructed to attend simultaneously to two sets of auditory stimuli. Subjects were to detect the location of a tone in a segmented noise burst delivered to the left ear and report the number of clicks delivered to the right ear. Smokers were deprived of smoking for 12 hr prior to the session and were either allowed or not allowed to smoke a cigarette prior to the test. Deprived smokers had a higher error rate than smokers, suggesting that smoking deprivation had an adverse effect on performance. Alcohol (0.08% BAL) increased error rate in both smokers and deprived smokers.

In an auditory vigilance study,[49] smokers and deprived smokers performed an auditory task in which they were to pick out three consecutive odd digit "signals" from a string of digits recited to them, at the rate of 1 digit/sec, for six 12-min blocks. Smokers took three puffs from a cigarette during each of the 2-min interblock intervals. Deprived smokers did worse, i.e., were less vigilant over time, than smokers on this task. Alcohol (0.06% BAL) decreased vigilance in both deprived smokers and smokers, but less so in the latter group.

Several comments are in order concerning the preceding studies. First, in the studies that employed non-smoking control groups, it was clear that smokers were less affected by alcohol than were nonsmokers. Nicotine, then, appears to counteract or antagonize some effects of alcohol and indeed may be a mechanism that underlies the drinking/smoking association. Second, not all of the deleterious effects of alcohol are offset by smoking, including, it appears, psychomotor performance and some cognitive measures. Third, in those studies which did not employ nonsmoker control groups,[43,46,49,49] it was impossible to ascertain the effects of alcohol alone on behavior. The control condition in these experiments (i.e., no smoking, no drinking) involved smoke deprivation, but smoke deprivation by itself can impair performance.[50,51] Finally, smokers in most of these studies had been cigarette-deprived for 12 hr prior to the experimental session. Had they not been deprived, their physiological and/or behavioral response to smoking and/or smoking and drinking may have been different. In the only study that systematically examined the effects of presession smoking history, deprived smokers reacted differently than nondeprived smokers to the joint administration of tobacco and alcohol during the session.[40] The results obtained with smokers deprived before a session, then, may not be applicable to those conditions which typify a usual drinking situation of the smoker, i.e., smoking before and/or during alcohol consumption.

Finally, in a study examining the effects of alcohol and smoking on state-dependent learning (SDL),[52] subjects were required to learn a simple route map after having smoked two cigarettes (nicotine content: 1.4 mg) and ingested alcohol (0.66 g/kg). On the next day, subjects repeated the task under one of four conditions (alcohol + smoking; alcohol alone; tobacco alone; no alcohol or tobacco). Subjects had been deprived of smoking for 3 hr prior to the session. Recall impairment on Day 2 was negligible in the group of subjects who had smoked and ingested alcohol, and only slightly reduced in the group of subjects who had ingested alcohol alone. Recall impairment was the most severe in the other two groups. Alcohol appeared to have more impact on producing a state-dependent learning effect than did smoking.

Before closing, mention should be made that no studies were found that examined the joint effects of alcohol/tobacco on driving or simulated driving. Driving is a complex behavior involving perception, attention, psychomotor skills, and judgment. Alcohol impairs driving and many of the individual behavioral components that comprise the act of driving.[53] Smokers are more likely to be involved in motor vehicle accidents than nonsmokers, even when their drinking habits are factored out.[54] Further research is warranted to determine the extent to which cigarette smoking potentiates, counteracts, or has no effect on alcohol-induced driving impairment.

5. Alcohol/Tobacco Association and Drug Relapse

Given the association between consumption of alcohol and cigarettes that has been documented in both descriptive and experimental studies, what is the effect of attempting to abstain from one substance and continuing to use the other? Although there appear to be no studies that directly address this issue, there are at least two separate lines of reasoning which suggest that continued use of one of the substances would make it more difficult to abstain from the other. The first line of reasoning is based on data collected in animal drug reinstatement studies. Drug reinstatement is thought to be an animal model of drug relapse. In these studies, when self-administration of a drug such as heroin or cocaine has been extinguished in laboratory rats, lever pressing can be reinstated by a "priming" injection of the training drug.[55,56] To the extent that a different drug shares some pharmacological similarity to the training drug, it too may reinstate responding.[57] Because some of the behavioral effects of smoking and alcohol may be mediated by similar mechanisms of action,[27,28] it is possible that smoking might "reinstate," or trigger relapse to, drinking and/or drinking might trigger relapse to smoking.[58]

There is another reason why relapse to one of the drugs may be precipitated by continued use of the other drug. One of the behavioral principles frequently referred to in treatment programs dealing with weight reduction, smoking cessation, and substance abuse is the principle of stimulus control: Clients are advised to avoid stimuli or situations that are strongly paired with smoking, since these stimuli or situations are known to increase risk of relapse. It is possible, for example, that drinking may induce relapse to smoking in people who have habitually smoked while drinking. And, indeed, in a study in which exsmokers called a hot line designed to help them cope with temptations to smoke, alcohol was one of the reasons frequently given for a smoking lapse.[59] In another study in which smokers were paid for reducing their smoking or abstaining altogether, a strategy frequently mentioned by subjects to help them abstain from smoking was avoiding alcohol.[60]

Based on the preceding discussion, exsmokers might be advised to abstain from alcohol at least in the early phases of a smoking cessation attempt. Likewise, alcohol abusers might have better success abstaining from alcohol if they also quit smoking. Current alcohol abuse treatment programs do not usually encourage clients to quit smoking,[61] perhaps because of the untested allegation that trying to quit smoking and drinking at the same time would result in too much stress and eventually lead to relapse to both drinking and smoking. This approach of only focusing on the drinking problem has recently been called into question, though.[13,15,62,63] Very few data are available regarding whether successful treatment of smoking increases the chances of successful alcohol treatment in problem drinkers. In a descriptive study evaluating the impact of a behavioral self-control training intervention,[64] smokers who had entered treatment for problem drinking and quit smoking were more successful in the control or cessation of alcohol use than smokers who had not tried to quit smoking. Obviously, a great deal of further research is needed to explore such issues as (1) whether smoking cessation is a viable goal in recovering alcoholics, or whether smoking reduction is more realistic, (2) the appropriate timing of smoking cessation/reduction attempts in the context of an alcohol abuse treatment program, and (3) whether smoking cessation actually does reduce the probability of drinking relapse.

6. Alcohol/Tobacco Association and Disease

Alcoholics in alcohol abuse treatment programs should be encouraged to stop smoking, not only because smoking may lead to relapse to drinking, but because of the health consequences of smoking and the health consequences of the interaction between excessive alcohol use and smoking. Both smoking and excessive alcohol use are risk factors for cardiovascular disease, respiratory diseases, and some forms of cancer.[1] While the effects of these two drugs may be additive for some diseases, the effects are synergistic for diseases such as cancer of the mouth, pharynx, and larynx.[65–67] For example, the risk of laryngeal cancer for the smoking drinker is approximately 50% greater than the sum of the excess risks posed by smoking or drinking considered individually.[68] Alcoholics, then, are prime candidates for diseases associated with both excessive drinking and smoking.[69]

7. Summary

This chapter has focused both on reviewing those studies which document an association between use of alcohol and tobacco and on the consequences of the association. Smokers are more likely to drink than nonsmokers, and drinkers are more likely to smoke than nondrinkers. Heavy consumption of one drug tends to be associated with heavy consumption of the other. Experimental evidence demonstrates that alcohol potentiates tobacco consumption, but whether the reverse holds true is not known. The association between drinking and smoking may be mediated through one or more mechanisms. For example, chronic administration of one drug may induce cross-tolerance to the behavioral effects of another drug, leading to the probability of higher consumption of both drugs. In examining the joint effects of alcohol/tobacco on various measures of performance, the performance-impairing effects of alcohol in some cases appear to be counteracted by smoking. One interesting question that remains to be answered regarding the joint behavioral effects of alcohol/tobacco is whether alcohol-induced driving impairment is affected by cigarette smoking. There are at least two clinical ramifications of the association between alcohol and tobacco. Attempting to abstain from one of the drugs while still using the other drug may be difficult because the drug still being used may act either as a "primer" to reinstate administration of the other drug or as a discriminative stimulus which sets the occasion for use of the other drug. The other issue is that smoking and drinking in combination present greater risk of some diseases than the sum of the risks of ingesting each drug alone. The health consequences of the alcohol/tobacco association clearly justifies further research examining the behavioral and biological consequences of the alcohol/tobacco association.

ACKNOWLEDGMENTS. The preparation of this manuscript was supported by a grant from the National Institute on Drug Abuse DA 00250.

References

1. National Institute on Alcohol Abuse and Alcoholism: Fifth special report to the U.S. Congress on alcohol and health from the Secretary of Health and Human Services. DHHS Publication No. (ADM) 84–1291. Washington, DC, U.S. Government Printing Office, 1984.
2. Fielding JE: Smoking: health effects and control. N Engl J Med 313:491–498, 1985.
3. Istvan J, Matarazzo JD: Tobacco, alcohol, and caffeine use: A review of their interrelationships. Psychol Bull 95:301–326, 1984.
4. Friedman GD, Siegelaub AB, Seltzer CC: Cigarettes, alcohol, coffee and peptic ulcer. N Engl J Med 290:469–473, 1974.
5. Abelson H, Fishburne RM, Cisin I: National survey on drug abuse: 1977. Rockville, MD, National Institute on Drug Abuse, 1977.
6. Carmody TP, Brischetter CS, Matarazzo JD: Co-occurrent use of cigarettes, alcohol and coffee in healthy, community-living men and women. Health Psychol 4:323–335, 1985.
7. Abelson H, Cohen R, Schrayer D, Rappeport M: Drug experience, attitudes and related behavior among adolescents and adults, in: Drug Use in America: Problems in Perspective: Vol 1. The Technical Papers of the Second Report of the National Commission on Marijuana and Drug Use, 1973. Washington, DC, U.S. Government Printing Office, 1973, pp 488–871.
8. Coombs RH, Wellisch DK, Fawzy FI: Drinking patterns and problems among female children and adolescents: A comparison of abstainers, past users and current users. Am J Drug Alcohol Abuse 11:345–348, 1985.
9. Kaprio J, Hammar N, Koskenvuo M, Floderus-Myrhed B, Langinvainio H, Sarna S: Cigarette smoking and alcohol use in Finland and Sweden: A cross-national twin study. Int J Epidemiol 11:378–386, 1982.
10. Cummings RO, Shaper AG, Walker M, Wale CJ: Smoking and drinking by middle-aged British men: Effects of class and town of residence. Br Med J 283:1497–1502, 1981.
11. Dyer AR, Stamler J, Paul O, Berkson DM, Lepper MH, McKean MH, Shekelle RB, Lindberg HA, Garside D: Alcohol consumption, cardiovascular risk factors, and mortality in two Chicago epidemiologic studies. Circulation 56:1067–1074, 1977.
12. Ashley MJ, Olin JS, leRiche WH, Kornaczewski A, Schmidt W, Rankin JG: Morbidity patterns in hazardous drinkers: Relevance of demographic, sociologic, drinking, and drug use characteristics. Int J Addict 16:593–625, 1981.
13. Kozlowski LT, Jelinek LC, Pope MA: Cigarette smoking among alcohol abusers: a continuing and neglected problem. Can J Public Health 77:205–207, 1986.
14. Zeiner AR, Stanitis T, Spurgeon M: Treatment of alcoholism and concomitant drugs of abuse. Alcohol 2:555–559, 1985.
15. Burling TA, Ziff DC: Tobacco smoking: A comparison between alcohol and drug abuse in patients. Addict Behav 13:185–190, 1988.
16. Griffiths RR, Bigelow GE, Liebson I: Facilitation of human tobacco self-administration by ethanol: A behavioral analysis. J Exp Anal Behav 25:279–292, 1976.
17. Henningfield JE, Chait LD, Griffiths RR: Cigarette smoking and subjective response in alcoholics: Effects of pentobarbital. Clin Pharmacol Ther 33:806–812, 1983.
18. Henningfield, JE, Chait LD, Griffiths RR: Effects of ethanol on cigarette smoking by volunteers without histories of alcoholism. Psychopharmacology 82:1–5, 1984.
19. Parfrey PS: Factors associated with undergraduate alcohol use. Br J Prevent Soc Med 28:252–257, 1974.
20. Wechsler H, McFadden M: Drinking among college students in New England: Extent, social correlates and consequences of alcohol use. J Stud Alcohol 40:969–996, 1979.

21. Nil R, Buzzi R, Battig K; Effects of single doses of alcohol and caffeine on cigarette smoke puffing behavior. *Pharmacol Biochem Behav* 20:583–590, 1984.

22. Mintz J, Boyd G, Rose JE, Charuvastra VC, Jarvik ME: Alcohol increases cigarette smoking: A laboratory demonstration. *Addict Behav* 10:203–207, 1985.

23. Mello NK, Mendelson JH, Sellers ML, Kuehnle JC: Effect of alcohol and marijuana on tobacco smoking. *Clin Pharmacol Ther* 27:202–209, 1980.

24. Mello NK, Mendelson JH, Palmieri SL: Cigarette smoking by women: Interactions with alcohol use. *Psychopharmacology* 93:8–15, 1987.

25. Potthorf AD, Ellison G, Nelson L: Ethanol intake increases during continuous administration of amphetamine and nicotine, but not several other drugs. *Pharmacol Biochem Behav* 18:484–493, 1983.

26. Shuster CR: Theoretical basis of behavioral tolerance: Implications of the phenomenon for problems of drug abuse, in Krasnegor NA (ed): *Behavioral Tolerance: Research and Treatment Implications*. National Institute on Drug Abuse Monograph Series 18. DHHS publication no. (ADM) 78-551. Washington, DC, U.S. Government Printing Office, 1978, pp 4–17.

27. Burch JB, deFiebre CM, Marks MJ, Collins AC: Chronic ethanol or nicotine treatment results in partial cross-tolerance between these agents. *Psychopharmacology* 95:452–458, 1988.

28. Collins AC, Burch JB, deFiebre CM, Marks MJ: Tolerance to and cross-tolerance between ethanol and nicotine. *Pharmacol Biochem Behav* 29:365–373, 1988.

29. Gilbert DG: Paradoxical tranquilizing and emotion-reducing effects of nicotine. *Psychol Bull* 86:643–661, 1979.

30. Perrine MW: Alcohol influences on driving-related behavior. *J Safety Res* 5:165–184, 1973.

31. Tong JE, Knott VJ, McGraw DF, Leigh G: Ethanol, visual discrimination and heart rate: Effects of dose, activation and tobacco. *Q J Stud Alcohol* 35:1003–1022, 1974.

32. Hunt WA: Neurotransmitter function in the basal ganglia after acute and chronic ethanol treatment. *Fed Proc* 40:2077–2081, 1981.

33. Sakurai Y, Takamo Y, Kohjimoto Y, Honda K, Kamiya H: Enhancement of (3H) metabolites in rat striatum by nicotinic drugs. *Brain Res* 242:99–106, 1982.

34. Adir J, Wildfeuer W, Miller RP: Effect of ethanol pretreatment on the pharmacokinetics of nicotine in rats. *J Pharmacol Exp Ther* 212:274–279, 1980.

35. Benowitz NL, Jones RT, Jacob PJ: Additive cardiovascular effects of nicotine and ethanol. *Clin Pharmacol Ther* 40:420–424, 1986.

36. Nemeth-Coslett R, Henningfield JE, O'Keefe MK, Griffiths RR: Effects of mecamylamine on human cigarette smoking and subjective ratings. *Psychopharmacology* 88:420–425, 1986.

37. Signs SA, Schechter MD: Nicotine-induced potentiation of ethanol discrimination. *Pharmacol Biochem Behav* 24:769–771, 1986.

38. Bhagat B, Bayer T, Lind C: Effects of chronic administration of nicotine on drug-induced hypnosis in mice. *Psychopharmacologia* 21:287–293, 1971.

39. Joyce D, Steele J, Summerfield A: Chronic ingestion of nicotine modifies the behavior of mice after ethanol. *Br J Pharmacol* 45:164–165, 1972.

40. Knott VJ, Venables PH: Separate and combined effects of alcohol and tobacco on the amplitude of the contingent negative variation. *Psychopharmacology* 70:167–172, 1980.

41. Leigh G: The combined effects of alcohol consumption and cigarette smoking on critical flicker frequency. *Addict Behav* 7:251–259, 1982.

42. Smith JM, Misiak H: CFF and psychotropic drugs in normal human subjects: A review. *Psychopharmacology* 47:175–182, 1976.

43. Leigh G, Tong JE: Effects of ethanol and tobacco on time judgment. *Percept Motor Skills* 43:899–903, 1976.

44. Jones RT, Stone, GC: Psychological studies of marijuana and alcohol in man. *Psychopharmacologia* 18:108–117, 1970.

45. Ague C: Cardiovascular variables, skin conductance and time estimation: Changes after the administration of small doses of nicotine. *Psychopharmacologia* 37:109–125, 1974.

46. Valeriote C, Tong FE, Durding B: Ethanol, tobacco and laterality effects on simple and complex motor performance. *J Stud Alcohol* 40:823–830, 1979.

47. Lyon R, Tong JE, Leigh G, Claire G: The influence of ethanol and tobacco on the components of choice reaction time. *J Stud Alcohol* 36:587–596, 1975.
48. Leigh G, Tong JE, Campbell J: Effects of ethanol and tobacco on divided attention. *J Stud Alcohol* 38:1233–1239, 1977.
49. Tong JE, Henderson PR, Chipperfield BG: Effects of ethanol and tobacco on auditory vigilance performance. *Addict Behav* 5:153–158, 1980.
50. Ashton H, Savage RD, Telford R, Thompson JW, Watson DW: The effects of cigarette smoking on the response to stress in a driving simulator. *Br J Pharmacol* 45:546–556, 1972.
51. Heimstra NW, Bancroft NR, Dekock AR: Effects of smoking upon sustained performance in a simulated driving task. *Ann NY Acad Sci* 142:295–307, 1967.
52. Lowe G: State-dependent learning effects with a combination of alcohol and nicotine. *Psychopharmacology* 89: 105–107, 1986.
53. Mitchell MC: Alcohol induced impairment of central nervous system function: Behavioral skills involved in driving. *J Stud Alcohol* S10:109–115, 1985.
54. DiFranza JR, Winters TH, Goldberg RJ, Cirillo L, Biliouris T: The relationship of smoking to motor vehicle accidents and traffic violations. *NY State J Med* 86:464–467, 1986.
55. de Wit H, Stewart J: Drug reinstatement of heroin-reinforced responding in the rat. *Psychopharmacology* 79:29–31, 1983.
56. Stewart J, deWit H: Reinstatement of drug-taking behavior as a method of assessing incentive motivational properties of drugs, in Bozarth MA (ed): *Methods of Assessing the Reinforcing Properties of Abused Drugs*. New York, Springer-Verlag, 1987, pp 211–227.
57. Stewart J: Reinstatement of heroin and cocaine self-administration behavior in the rat by intracerebral application of morphine in the ventral tegmental area. *Pharmacol Biochem Behav* 20:917–923, 1984.
58. Wise RA: The neurobiology of craving: Implications for the understanding and treatment of addiction. *J Abnormal Psychol* 97:118–132, 1988.
59. Shiffman S, Read L, Jarvik ME: Smoking-relapse situations: A preliminary typology. *Int J Addict* 20:311–318, 1985.
60. Burling TA, Stitzer ML, Bigelow GE, Russ NW: Techniques used by smokers during contingency motivated smoking reduction. *Addict Behav* 7:397–401, 1982.
61. Bobo JK, Gilchrist LD: Urging the alcoholic client to quit smoking cigarettes. *Addict Behav* 8:297–305, 1983.
62. Battjes RJ: Smoking as an issue in alcohol and drug abuse treatment. *Addict Behav* 13:225–230, 1988.
63. Bobo JK, Gilchrist LD, Schilling RF, Noach B, Schinke SP: Cigarette smoking cessation attempts by recovering alcoholics. *Addict Behav* 12:209–215, 1987.
64. Miller WR, Hedrick KE, Taylor CA: Addictive behaviors and life problems before and after behavioral treatment of problem drinkers. *Addict Behav* 8:403–412, 1983.
65. Brownson RC, Chang JC: Exposure to alcohol and tobacco and the risk of laryngeal canser. *Arch Environ Health* 42:192–196, 1987.
66. Saxe TG: Drug-alcohol interactions. *Am Fam Physician* 33:159–162, 1986.
67. U.S. Public Health Service: *The Health Consequences of Smoking: Cancer, a Report of the Surgeon General*. DHEW Publication No. DHHS PHS 82-50179. Washington DC, U.S. Government Printing Office, 1982.
68. Flanders WW, Rothman KJ: Interaction of alcohol and tobacco in laryngeal cancer. *Am J Epidemiol* 115:371–379, 1982.
69. Rosengren A, Wilhelmsen L, Wedel H: Separate and combined effects of smoking and alcohol abuse in middle-aged men. *Acta Med Scand* 223:111–118, 1988.

10

Interactions of Ethanol and Nicotine at the Receptor Level

Allan C. Collins

Abstract. Several studies have demonstrated that alcohol use is generally accompanied by an increase in smoking in humans. In rats, nicotine administration increases alcohol consumption. Genetic evidence from animal studies also suggests ethanol–nicotine interactions in that mouse lines that were selectively bred for differential sensitivity to ethanol also differ in sensitivity to nicotine. In addition, animals that have been chronically treated with alcohol are cross-tolerant to some of the actions of nicotine and chronic nicotine-treated animals are cross-tolerant to alcohol. This review summarizes the data which indicate that lipids and lipid membranes modify the binding of nicotinic agonists and antagonists to non-neuronal nicotinic receptors as well as modifying the function of these well characterized receptors. These results suggest that studies of ethanol disruption of membrane lipid regulation of brain nicotinic receptor binding, structure, and function may provide insights into why humans frequently use and abuse alcohol and tobacco together.

1. Introduction

The 20th Report of the Surgeon General on the Health Consequences of Smoking presents data indicating that over 50 million Americans used tobacco on a daily basis in 1986; this represents approximately 26% of the adult population. As many or more Americans use alcoholic beverages on a daily basis, and many people use these substances together. This chapter discusses the available literature which suggests that ethanol and nicotine are used together, at least in part, because both substances affect brain nicotinic cholinergic receptors.

Allan C. Collins • School of Pharmacy, and Institute for Behavioral Genetics, University of Colorado, Boulder, Colorado 80309.

2. Behavioral Interactions between Alcohol and Nicotine

2.1. Ethanol–Nicotine Self-Administration

As outlined in detail in other chapters of this volume, a considerable literature demonstrates that an association exists between the consumption of alcohol and cigarette smoking. For example, a higher fraction of alcoholics smoke than do nonalcoholics[1-3] and cigarette smokers who are also diagnosed alcoholics smoke more cigarettes per day than do nonalcoholic cigarette smokers.[4] Laboratory studies utilizing alcoholic subjects indicate that ethanol administration increases the number of cigarettes smoked as well as the number of puffs per cigarette.[5,6] These findings in male alcoholics have been extended to male[7] and female[8] social drinkers. The increased use of tobacco accompanying alcohol use does not seem to be due to an effect of ethanol on the rate of metabolism of nicotine.[9] Thus, it is clear that as alcohol consumption increases, so does tobacco use and this increased use is not due to an effect of ethanol on the rate of elimination of the most important psychoactive substance in tobacco, nicotine.

The potential influence of tobacco use on alcohol consumption has not received nearly as much attention. It has been reported that exsmokers drink more alcohol than do either smokers or nonsmokers,[10] but laboratory studies of the effects of tobacco use on alcohol consumption by humans are lacking. An effect of tobacco on alcohol consumption by humans seems possible since rats that are implanted with a slow-release nicotine pellet exhibit a significant increase in ethanol (10% v/v) consumption.[11] Interestingly, the chronic administration of other drugs with abuse potential, such as caffeine, phencyclidine, secobarbital, LSD, and mescaline, did not alter ethanol consumption; amphetamine treatment resulted in a modest increase in alcohol consumption. These observations suggest that ethanol–tobacco interactions are specific.

2.2. Physiological and Behavioral Interactions

A few studies have investigated interactions between alcohol and smoking, as manifested by altered behavioral or physiological effects of alcohol in subjects who were also allowed to smoke. For example, as little as two cigarettes enhance alcohol-induced improvement in tone/click discrimination. These effects are seen at low doses of alcohol (blood ethanol concentrations up to 0.02%) whereas at higher blood alcohol levels the same smoking dose counteracted the impaired performance found after alcohol.[12] Benowitz et al.[9] examined the effects of ethanol given orally and nicotine given intravenously on cardiovascular function and skin temperature. Ethanol (0.5 or 1.9 g/kg) increased heart rate, systolic blood pressure, and pressure–rate product in a dose-dependent manner. Nicotine had additive effects on heart rate and pressure–rate product. On the other hand, ethanol antagonized the depressant effects of nicotine on skin temperature. These results indicate an interaction between ethanol and nicotine, but they also suggest that the interaction may be dose and test specific.

2.3. Cross-Tolerance between Ethanol and Nicotine

Very few investigators have attempted to investigate whether coadministration of nicotine with ethanol alters the behavioral effects elicited by ethanol in animals, perhaps because experiments of this sort are often difficult to interpret. However, there is evidence which suggests that ethanol and nicotine affect similar systems. The author's research group has been investigating potential ethanol–nicotine interactions by assessing cross-tolerance. These studies have involved two approaches. In the first, we measured nicotine effects in two mouse lines that have been selectively bred for differences in duration of ethanol-induced anesthesia (sleep time). We have determined that these two mouse lines, designated long-sleep (LS) and short-sleep (SS), also differ dramatically in sensitivity to nicotine as measured by a battery of behavioral and physiological tests.[13,14] Because the two mouse lines do not differ in rates of nicotine metabolism or in brain nicotine concentrations at the time of behavioral testing, we concluded that the two mouse lines differ in central nervous system sensitivity to nicotine. Thus, the LS and SS mouse lines differ in acute sensitivity or initial tolerance to ethanol and they also differ in acute sensitivity or initial tolerance to nicotine. This implies that gene products that regulate sensitivity to ethanol also regulate sensitivity to nicotine.

The second approach that we have been taking is to ascertain whether chronic treatment with ethanol and nicotine results in cross-tolerance between these two drugs. Our studies have involved treating DBA/2 mice with nicotine or ethanol, assessing whether tolerance to the chronic treatment drug had developed, and then determining whether the mice were cross-tolerant.[15] Ethanol was administered in ethanol-containing liquid diets and nicotine was administered by intravenous infusion. Tolerance and cross-tolerance were measured using several tests for each drug. Although tolerance was seen for both drugs for virtually every test, cross-tolerance was seen only for the body temperature test. Both ethanol- and nicotine-treated animals were tolerant to the hypothermic effects elicited by the drug that had been used for chronic treatment and cross-tolerant to the hypothermic effects elicited by the challenge drug. Thus, cross-tolerance was seen for some, but not all, measures. Because chronic ethanol and nicotine treatment did not alter the rate of metabolism of either drug, we concluded that cross-tolerance arose from changes in central nervous system sensitivity to ethanol and nicotine. These results are consistent with the suggestion that ethanol and nicotine interact at the behavioral level and suggest that alcoholics smoke more cigarettes than do nonalcoholics because they are cross-tolerant to the effects of nicotine.

3. Mechanisms of Ethanol–Nicotine Interactions

Although alcohol and tobacco, or nicotine, are used together by literally millions of people, we know surprisingly little about the potential mechanisms that might underlie this interaction. Nicotine acts by binding to and, at least initially, activating a protein complex that is usually referred to as the nicotinic cholinergic receptor. Ethanol's mechanism of action is less well defined, but the most likely mechanism seems to involve dissolution in neuronal membranes and "fluidizing" the membrane. Presumably, this fluidization process results in the disruption of one or more critical membrane functions, such as ion flux, neurotransmitter uptake and/or release, or neurotransmitter receptor activation. Indeed, there is ample evidence which suggests that ethanol may alter all of these processes. In the remainder of this chapter, the data which suggest that ethanol may elicit some of its actions by disrupting nicotinic receptor function are discussed.

3.1. Structure of the Nicotinic Receptors

The nicotinic receptors found in the electric organs of animals such as the marine elasmobranch *Torpedo californica* and those found at the neuromuscular junction are probably the most thoroughly characterized neurotransmitter receptors. The primary sequence of each of the four polypeptide subunits has been determined, as has the subunit stoichiometry ($\alpha_2\beta\gamma\delta$). In addition, tremendous strides have been made toward understanding the tertiary and quaternary structure of the receptor complex. Current thinking indicates that each of the polypeptides that make up the receptor complex has four hydrophobic alpha helical sequences, labeled M1–M4, that cross the lipid bilayer. A fifth alpha-helical sequence may also exist. This sequence, labeled M5, is amphipathic and may form the lining of the ion channel and the amphipathic sequences of each of the five polypeptides that make up the receptor combine to form the ion channel in a fashion that resembles the staves of a barrel. The interested reader is referred to the article by McCarthy et al.[16] for a recent review of the structure and function of the *Torpedo* and neuromuscular junction nicotinic receptors.

Despite the fact that we know a great deal about the structure and function of nicotinic receptors in *Torpedo* and at the myoneural junction, we know very little about the brain nicotinic receptors. Until recently, all that was known was that the brain contains a minimum of two different classes of nicotinic receptors that could be detected via the binding of iodinated α-bungarotoxin (BTX), the snake venom that binds with high affinity to the myoneural nicotinic receptor, and via the binding of tritiated nicotine. BTX and nicotine bind to different receptor populations as defined by biochemical criteria[17] and anatomical distribution in brain.[18] The BTX binding site has been studied extensively, but questions remain regarding both its structure and function. The structure of the brain BTX binding site is probably very similar to the myoneural junction nicotinic receptor,[19] but its function remains unknown primarily because BTX fails to block cholinergic activities, as measured by electrophysiological techniques, in several systems.[20–22]

The nicotinic receptor measured with high-affinity L-[^{3}H]-nicotine binding has received only minimal attention, but remarkable progress has been made toward understanding its structure. Molecular genetic strategies have allowed the sequencing of a family of genes that probably code for polypeptide subunits of high-affinity nicotinic receptors. The strategy used to isolate several of these genes involved making the cDNA probe for the α subunit of the mouse muscle receptor and carrying out low stringency DNA/DNA hybridization. To date, three different genes that code for polypeptides that resemble the subunit of the muscle nicotinic receptor have been sequenced,[23–25] and a sequence that codes for a second type of subunit, called β-2, has been reported.[26,27] The three α subunits that have been described to date are called α-2, α-3, and α-4. These peptides differ from one another, but all contain sequences that are highly homologous to those found in the muscle receptor. For example, all of the α subunits have sequences that are very similar to the agonist binding site of the muscle polypeptide, and the brain receptor α peptides have sequences that are highly homologous to the M1–M4 transmembrane regions found in the *Torpedo* and muscle nicotinic receptors. The major differences between the brain nicotinic receptors and the muscle receptor are found at sites that are outside the membrane. In particular, the α-4 polypeptide has a very large loop that is probably found on the inner side of the cell membrane.

The β-2, peptide does not have an agonist binding site associated with it, but does seem to have four hydrophobic, alpha-helical sequences that are highly homologous to those found in the α sequences. The β peptide has been referred to as the structural subunit. Genes corresponding to the muscle γ and δ peptides have not been described, and the stoichiometry that has been proposed for the brain nicotinic receptor is α_2-β_3.[28]

3.2. Effect of Lipids on Nicotinic Receptor Function

The structure and function of the nicotinic receptor from *Torpedo* is clearly regulated by lipids, as is indicated by the observation that solubilization of the receptor by detergent extraction results in partial or total loss of the associated lipids as well as stabilizing the receptor in a low-affinity state that cannot be converted to a high-affinity state by agonists. However, if the lipids are retained during solubilization, agonists will elicit a conformational change in the receptor which is detectable by an increase in affinity.[29] This high-affinity state is believed to be a desensitized form of the nicotinic receptor. Thus, membrane lipids seem to play a role in receptor desensitization.

Studies of solubilized receptor reconstituted into liposomes made up of pure synthetic lipids have demonstrated that chain length and degree of unsaturation influence both the affinity of agonists for the receptor and magnitude of ion flux elicited by the agonists.[30] Increasing the chain length of saturated lipids results in a decrease in agonist affinity. On the other hand, increasing lipid unsaturation increases the ion flux elicited by nicotinic agonists. Similarly, if cholesterol content is increased in reconstitution experiments, agonist affinity decreases.[31] Thus, increasing chain lengths of fatty acids and increasing membrane cholesterol, which both decrease membrane fluidity, result in a decrease in the affinity of agonists for the receptor. Changes in cholesterol also affect ion flux; flux is optimal when cholesterol content of the membranes approximates that found in natural membranes.[31]

Several studies suggest that membrane fluidity affects nicotinic receptor function. Fong and McNamee[32] measured the effects of various lipids and lipid mixtures on membrane fluidity as well as low to high agonist affinity state transition and ion-gating activity of reconstituted receptors. Both receptor functions were affected by changes in fluidity. Reconstitution experiments have also demonstrated that fatty acids will inhibit agonist-induced ion flux above the melting point of the fatty acids, but not below the melting point.[33] These effects of lipids may be explained by the observation that altering membrane fatty acid and cholesterol content alters the structure of the receptor.[34] Increasing sterol content, for example, results in an increase in the amount of receptor that is in the α-helical configuration, and increasing negatively charged lipids increase the fraction of the receptor that is in the β-pleated sheet configuration.

While the structures of the brain α and β peptides that make up the brain nicotinic receptors are well described, relatively little is known about the interactions of these receptors with their surrounding lipid matrix. However, because the brain α and β peptides are very similar to the muscle receptors in the transmembrane regions, it seems reasonable to expect that many of the same effects of lipids on receptor function will be found when adequate methods for detecting these properties are developed.

3.3. Ethanol's Effects on Nicotinic Receptor Binding

Consistent with the suggestion that membrane fluidity affects low to high affinity transitions, several studies have demonstrated that high concentrations of ethanol will alter the binding properties of the *Torpedo* nicotinic receptor. Ethanol, other aliphatic alcohols, and several other anesthetic agents increase the rate of agonist-induced conversion of BTX binding to the high-affinity state.[35] Very large concentrations of ethanol (approximately 0.5 M) are required to elicit this effect, but this effect may be important since the relative effectiveness of the various anesthetic agents tested in converting the receptor to the high-affinity state paralleled the relative potencies of the agents as anesthetics. Incubation of the *Torpedo* receptor with ethanol and other anesthetic agents also retards the rate of association of BTX to one of the binding sites on the high-affinity form of the receptor, and the kinetics of BTX binding become biphasic after incubation with ethanol and other anesthetics.[36] These results suggest that ethanol and other anesthetics alter the tertiary structure of the high-affinity, desensitized, conformer of the receptor as well as stabilizing it relative to the low-affinity conformer. Thus, it would be expected that under certain circumstances ethanol would inhibit nicotinic receptor function.

This reviewer is unaware of any studies that have attempted to investigate whether ethanol alters binding to brain nicotinic receptors in a fashion that mimics the effects seen on *Torpedo* binding. However, there may be reason to investigate this issue. Yoshida et al.[37] have reported that long-term (5 months) treatment of rats with ethanol, given in the drinking water, results in significant increases in [^{3}H]-nicotine binding in hypothalamus and thalamus; hippocampal binding was decreased by this treatment regimen. We[15] have failed to replicate this effect, but our studies used a different treatment protocol; ethanol was given in a liquid diet for a maximum of 28 days. Thus, we treated our animals with a higher dose for a much shorter time period. In this same study we demonstrated that chronic nicotine treatment resulted in a dose-dependent increase in [^{3}H]-nicotine binding and that animals that exhibit this increased nicotine binding are tolerant to nicotine and cross-tolerant to some of ethanol's effects, particularly hypothermia. We have suggested that chronic nicotine treatment results in receptor up-regulation because chronic treatment results in chronic desensitization of the receptor which is equivalent to chronic blockade. If ethanol stabilizes the nicotine binding site in a high-affinity, desensitized state as it does the *Torpedo* receptor, chronic treatment with ethanol would also be equivalent to chronic receptor blockade and could, therefore, result in up-regulation of receptor numbers.

3.4. Effects of Ethanol on Nicotinic Receptor Function

One of the best ways of assessing receptor function is to measure the electrophysiological actions of receptor agonists and antagonists. As might be expected, several investigations of the actions of ethanol on the neuromuscular junction nicotinic receptor have been described. These studies have demonstrated that low concentrations of ethanol may augment cholinergic receptor function and high concentrations may inhibit receptor function. Ethanol apparently increases the lifetime of channel opening elicited by acetylcholine (ACh) at the toad, frog, and mouse neuromuscular junctions.[38–40] Ethanol-induced increases in ACh effects have been interpreted as arising from promotion of channel opening and increasing the tendency of ACh to act more than once in opening ion channels.[40] These actions may explain the observation that low concentrations of ethanol shift the dose–response curves for ACh-induced activation of the frog muscle endplate to the left.[41] This effect would occur if ethanol decreases the dissociation constant for ACh at the neuromuscular junction nicotinic receptor. Higher concentrations of ethanol (>1 M) result in a shift to the right of the ACh dose–response curves.[42] Other alcohols also shift the ACh dose–response curves to the right and potency increased with increase in the chain length of the alcohol. Thus, low concentrations of ethanol may increase nicotinic receptor function whereas high concentrations may decrease receptor function. In addition, chronic ethanol treatment results in tolerance to the effects of ethanol on neuromuscular junction function.[43]

The electrophysiological effects of ACh in the brain may also be modified by ethanol. Ethanol, given systemically, enhances the excitation of hippocampal pyramidal cells which is elicited by ACh.[44] Unfortunately, these investigations did not determine whether the cholinergic effects being measured were regulated by nicotinic or muscarinic receptor systems, but the effects of ethanol on ACh actions are apparently specific since ethanol did not alter the activities of several other neurotransmitter substances (glutamate, GABA, norepinephrine, serotonin) as measured on rat hippocampal pyramidal cells.

4. Conclusions

Alcohol use seems to be highly correlated with the use of tobacco, but potential mechanisms that may explain this interaction have not been investigated intensively. Ethanol effects on the nicotinic receptor may be a prime candidate for a site of ethanol actions since these receptors are membrane-associated proteins that are regulated by the lipids that surround them. In particular, the lipids associated with the *Torpedo* receptor appear to alter the rate of desensitization of the receptor as well as the receptor's capacity for transporting ions across the membrane. Although high concentrations of ethanol are required to affect these same processes, the observation that effects on these processes correlate with anesthetic potency for a series of straight-chain alcohols suggests that investigations of ethanol–brain nicotinic receptor interactions may be fruitful. However, as is often the case with alcohol-related research, further studies must demonstrate that important effects are detectable at physiologically relevant concentrations of ethanol.

Determining whether ethanol facilitates the desensitization of brain nicotinic receptors may be a critical step in furthering our understanding of why people increase their tobacco use when ethanol is consumed. Available evidence indicates that nicotinic receptor blockade affects tobacco use. Pretreatment with mecamylamine, the centrally acting nicotinic receptor antagonist, results in an increase in smoking.[45,46] This has been interpreted as indicating that the smoker increases his/her nicotine intake to overcome the receptor blockade. By analogy, if ethanol increases, by whatever mechanism, the fraction of nicotinic receptors in the desensitized state, smokers may increase their tobacco intake following ethanol for the same reason as they do following mecamylamine: to overcome the receptor blockade.

Obviously, ethanol has many actions on other systems, and many of these actions are likely to be important in determining alcohol actions and consequently alcohol use. Nonetheless, it seems reasonable to suggest that determining those mechanisms that underlie alcohol–nicotine interactions will be especially useful in understanding those mechanisms that underlie alcohol abuse.

ACKNOWLEDGMENTS. Studies from the author's laboratory described in this review were supported by a grant from the National Institute on Alcohol Abuse and Alcoholism (AA-06391). Dr. Collins is supported, in part, by a Research Scientist Development Award from the National Institute on Drug Abuse (DA-00116).

References

1. Walton RG: Smoking and alcoholism: A brief report. *Am J Psychiatry* 128:1455–1456, 1972.
2. Maletzky BM, Klotter J: Smoking and alcoholism. *Am J Psychiatry* 131:445–447, 1974.
3. Moody PM: Drinking and smoking behavior of hospitalized medical patients. *J Stud Alcohol* 37:1316–1319, 1976.
4. Ayers J, Ruff CF, Templer DI: Alcoholism, cigarette smoking, coffee drinking and extraversion. *J Stud Alcohol* 37:983–985, 1976.
5. Griffiths RR, Bigelow GE, Liebson I: Facilitation of human tobacco self-administration by ethanol: A behavioral analysis. *J Exp Anal Behav* 25:279–292, 1976.
6. Henningfield JE, Chait LD, Griffiths RR: Cigarette smoking and subjective responses in alcoholics: Effects of pentobarbital. *Clin Pharmacol Ther* 33:806–812, 1983.
7. Henningfield JE, Chait LD, Griffiths RR: Effects of ethanol on cigarette smoking by volunteers without histories of alcoholism. *Psychopharmacology* 82:1–5, 1984.
8. Mello NK, Mendelson JH, Palmieri SL: Cigarette smoking by women: Interactions with alcohol use. *Psychopharmacology* 93:8–15, 1987.
9. Benowitz NL, Jones RT, Jacob III P: Additive cardiovascular effects of nicotine and ethanol. *Clin Pharmacol Ther* 40:420–424, 1986.
10. Carmody TP, Brischetto CS, Matarazzo JD, O'Donnel RP, Conner WE: Co-occurrent use of cigarettes, alcohol, and coffee in healthy, community-living men and women. *Health Psychol* 4:323–335, 1985.
11. Potthoff AD, Ellison G, Nelson L: Ethanol intake increases during continuous administration of amphetamine and nicotine, but not several other drugs. *Pharmacol Biochem Behav* 18:489–493, 1983.
12. Leigh G, Tong JE, Campbell JA: Effects of ethanol and tobacco on divided attention. *J Stud Alcohol* 38:1233–1239, 1977.
13. de Fiebre CM, Medhurst LJ, Collins AC: Nicotine response and nicotinic receptors in long-sleep and short-sleep mice. *Alcohol* 4:493–501, 1987.
14. de Fiebre CM, Collins AC: Decreased sensitivity to nicotine-induced seizures as a consequence of nicotine pretreatment in long-sleep and short-sleep mice. *Alcohol* 5:55–61, 1988.
15. Collins AC, Burch JB, de Fiebre CM, Marks MJ: Tolerance to and cross tolerance between ethanol and nicotine. *Pharmacol Biochem Behav* 29:365–373, 1988.
16. McCarthy MP, Earnest JP, Young EF, Choe S, Stroud RM: The molecular neurobiology of the acetylcholine receptor. *Annu Rev Neurosci* 9:383–413, 1986.
17. Marks MJ, Collins AC: Characterization of nicotine binding in mouse brain and comparison with binding of α-bungarotoxin and quinuclidinyl benzilate. *Mol Pharmacol* 22:554–564, 1982.
18. Clarke PBS, Schwartz RD, Paul SM, Pert CB, Pert A: Nicotinic binding in rat brain: Autoradiographic comparison of [^{3}H]acetylcholine, [^{3}H]nicotine, and [^{135}I]-α-bungarotoxin. *J Neurosci* 5:1307–1315, 1985.

19. Conti-Tronconi BM, Dunn SM, Barnard EA, Dolly JO, Lai FA, Ray N, Raftery MA: Brain and muscle nicotinic acetylcholine receptors are different but homologous proteins. *Proc Natl Acad Sci USA* 82:5208–5212, 1985.
20. Chou TC, Lee CY: Effect of whole and fractionated cobra venom on sympathetic ganglion transmission. *Eur J Pharmacol* 8:326–330, 1969.
21. Miledi R, Szczepaniak AC: Effect of dendroaspis neurotoxins on synaptic transmission in the spinal cord of the frog. *Proc Roy Soc Lond B Biol Sci* 190:267–274, 1974.
22. Duggan AW, Hall JG, Lee CY: Alpha-bungarotoxin, cobra neurotoxin and excitation of Renshaw cells by acetylcholine. *Brain Res* 107:166–170, 1976.
23. Boulter J, Evans K, Goldman D, Martin G, Treco D, Heinemann S, Patrick J: Isolation of a cDNA clone for a possible neural nicotinic acetylcholine receptor α-subunit. *Nature* 319:368–374, 1986.
24. Boulter J, Connolly J. Deneris E, Goldman D, Heinemann S, Patrick J: Functional expression of two neuronal nicotinic acetylcholine receptors from cDNA clones identifies a gene family. *Proc Natl Acad Sci USA* 84:7763–7767, 1987.
25. Nef P, Oneyser C, Alliod C, Courturier S, Ballivet M: Genes expressed in the brain define three distinct neuronal nicotinic acetylcholine receptors. *EMBO J* 7:595–601, 1988.
26. Deneris E, Connolly J, Boulter J, Wada E, Wada J, Swanson LW, Patrick J, Heinemann S: Primary structure and expression of β2: A novel subunit of neuronal nicotinic acetylcholine receptors. *Neuron* 1:45–54, 1988.
27. Schoepfer R, Whiting P, Esch F, Blacher R, Shimasaki S, Lindstrom J: cDNA clones coding for the structural subunit of a chicken brain nicotinic acetylcholine receptor. *Neuron* 1:241–248, 1988.
28. Whiting P, Esch F, Shimasaki S, Lindstrom J: Neuronal nicotinic acetylcholine receptor β-subunit is coded for by the cDNA clone α4. *FEBS Lett* 219:459–463, 1987.
29. Heidmann T, Sobel A, Popot J-L, Changeux J-P: Reconstitution of a functional acetylcholine receptor. Conservation of the conformational and allosteric transitions and recovery of the permeability response; Role of lipids. *Eur J Biochem* 110:35–55, 1980.
30. Criado M, Eibl H, Barrantes FJ: Functional properties of the acetylcholine receptor incorporated in model lipid membranes. *J Biol Chem* 259:9188–9198, 1984.
31. Zabrecky JR, Raftery MA: The role of lipids in the function of the acetylcholine receptor. *J. Receptor Res* 5:397–417, 1985.
32. Fong TM, McNamee MG: Correlation between acetylcholine receptor function and structural properties of membranes. *Biochemistry* 25:830–840, 1986.
33. Andreasen TJ, McNamee MG: Inhibition of ion permeability control properties of acetylcholine receptor from *Torpedo californica* by long-chain fatty acids. *Biochemistry* 19:4719–4726, 1980.
34. Fong TM, McNamee MG: Stabilization of acetylcholine receptor secondary structure by cholesterol and negatively charged phospholipids. *Biochemistry* 26:3871–3880, 1987.
35. Young AP, Sigman DS: Allosteric effects of volatile anesthetics on the membrane-bound acetylcholine receptor protein. I. Stabilization of the high-affinity state. *Mol Pharmacol* 20:498–505, 1981.
36. Young AP, Oshiki JR, Sigman DS: Allosteric effects of volatile anesthetics on the membrane-bound acetylcholine receptor protein. II. Alteration of α-bungarotoxin binding kinetics. *Mol Pharmacol* 20:506–510, 1981.
37. Yoshida K, Engel J, Liljequist S: The effect of chronic ethanol administration on high affinity ³H-nicotine binding in rat brain. *Naun-Schmied Arch Pharmacol* 321:74–76, 1982.
38. Gage PW, McBurney RN, Scheider GT: Effects of some aliphatic alcohols on the conductance change by a quantum of acetylcholine at the toad endplate. *J Physiol (London)* 244:409–429, 1975.
39. Quastel DMJ, Linder TM: Pre- and postsynaptic actions of central depressants at the mammalian neuromuscular junction. *Prog Anesthesiol* 1:157–168, 1975.
40. Linder TM, Pennefeather P, Quastel DMJ: The time course of miniature endplate currents and its modification by receptor blockade and ethanol. *J Gen Physiol* 83:435–468, 1984.

41. Bradley RJ, Peper K, Sterz R: Effects of ethanol at the frog end plate. *Nature (London)* 284:60–62, 1980.
42. Bradley RJ, Sterz R, Peper K: The effects of alcohols and diols at the nicotinic acetylcholine receptor of the neuromuscular junction. *Brain Res* 295:101–112, 1984.
43. Borges R, Feria M, Diaz E, Rodriguez Mendez SA, Boada J: Effect of ethanol on neuromuscular function in rats. Its interaction with alcuronium. *Gen Pharmacol* 17:569–572, 1986.
44. Mancillas JR, Siggins GR, Bloom F: Systemic ethanol: selective enhancement of responses to acetylcholine and somatostatin in hippocampus. *Science* 231:161–163, 1986.
45. Stolerman IP, Goldfarb T, Fink R, Jarvik ME: Influencing cigarette smoking with nicotine antagonists. *Psychopharmacologia* 28:247–259, 1973.
46. Pomerleau CS, Pomerleau OF, Majchrzak MJ: Mecamylamine pretreatment increases subsequent nicotine self-administration as indicated by changes in plasma nicotine level. *Psychopharmacology* 91:391–393, 1987.

Interactions between Alcohol and Benzodiazepines

Leo E. Hollister

Abstract. Because alcohol is so widely used as a social drug and benzodiazepines are so widely used as therapeutic agents, the number of persons who may be using both drugs concurrently is high. Despite this frequent concurrent use, interactions of major consequence are not common. Major interactions are pharmacodynamic, involving common actions of both drugs as sedatives. Excessive sedation from a combination of both drugs is a most important consideration when driving an automobile. However, it is well known that tolerance develops quickly to the sedative effects of benzodiazepines when used in anxiolytic doses. Also, one must balance the benefit from relief of anxiety versus possible impairment of function from oversedation. Abuse of benzodiazepines is almost exclusively among subjects who also abuse alcohol, doubtless due to the fact that the two drugs show cross-dependence. The clinical practice of avoiding use of benzodiazepines (or other sedative-hypnotics) in known alcoholics is sound and should avoid many potential problems.

1. Introduction

Benzodiazepines are the most widely prescribed drugs having an effect on the central nervous system. Alcohol is one of the most widely used social drugs. Purely by chance, if for no other reason, the concurrent use of both drugs should be common. The most important question about such combined use is whether it produces unexpected effects more harmful than the effects of either drug alone.

This subject has been reviewed recently from rather different perspectives. One review focused primarily on the effects of combined use of benzodiazepines and alcohol in the context of abuse of these drugs.[1] Another focused on both pharmacokinetic and pharmacodynamic interactions, largely in humans.[2] A third review focused primarily on the lack of any significant interactions between alcohol and a representative of a new class of antianxiety

Leo E. Hollister • Department of Psychiatry and Pharmacology, University of Texas Medical School at Houston, Houston, Texas 77025-0249.

medications, buspirone.[3] The general conclusions of these reviews were that interactions between benzodiazepines and alcohol are far less important than with other centrally acting drugs. No additional information has been developed that would change this conclusion.

2. Clinical Considerations of Interactions

2.1. Concurrent Abuse

Alcohol is second only to tobacco in being the most widely abused drug in the United States and creating the most serious health problems of all abused drugs. As the clinical actions of alcohol are predominantly sedative, one would assume that alcoholics might be especially prone to develop dependence on or abuse of other types of sedatives. Such a relationship has long been known. It is sometimes all too easy to convert an alcoholic into one dependent on sedatives, although usually not for long. More often, one finds a pattern of concurrent abuse.

Estimates of the prevalence of combined use of alcohol and benzodiazepines are uncertain because the latter drugs, rather than being specified in various surveys, are usually lumped together under the rubric of tranquilizers, which may involve a number of different drug classes. One survey suggested that 20% of alcoholics used other addictive drugs conjointly while another estimated the prevalence as 60–80%.[4,5] Our own experience suggests that even the higher estimate may be somewhat conservative. Because of this tendency of alcoholics to substitute sedative–hypnotic drugs, the usual clinical dictum has been to use such drugs very cautiously in the treatment of alcoholics, lest one foster dual abuse. The judicious use of benzodiazepines in alcoholics, if carefully monitored, may be beneficial. Indeed, were it possible to substitute benzodiazepines entirely for alcohol, most authorities would consider the tradeoff to be advantageous.

2.2. Cross-Tolerance

Benzodiazepines are generally thought to be cross-tolerant with alcohol, which provides the basis for their use in treating alcohol withdrawal syndromes. Clinical evidence of cross-tolerance is obvious by the unusually large doses (600–800 mg/day of chlordiazepoxide or 200–300 mg/day of diazepam) required to sedate chronic alcoholics during withdrawal.[6] Although it is conceivable that cross-tolerance between the two drugs is not complete, it is difficult to demonstrate more than one type of cross-tolerance experimentally. Mice made dependent on alcohol by a liquid diet showed significantly less hypothermia induced by chlordiazepoxide compared with mice fed an isocaloric diet. This cross-tolerance dissipated after 1 week.[1] The implication of such cross-tolerance between benzodiazepines and alcohol is that alcoholics who abuse benzodiazepines require large doses of the latter drugs. The withdrawal syndrome from both alcohol and benzodiazepines is quite similar except for differences in time course depending on the somewhat longer plasma half-lives of most benzodiazepines.[7] In the animal model of alcohol withdrawal, diazepam reduced overall withdrawal intensity but failed to suppress completely all symptoms. Tremor, piloerection, abnormal posture, and bizarre behavior were diazepam-resistant.[8] While it is known that benzodiazepines do not totally control alcohol withdrawal in the clinic, they show enough cross-tolerance to be highly acceptable.

2.3. Driving Ability

That alcohol, taken in large amounts, can impair driving ability is not at all questioned. Surveys of the various drugs found in the blood of traffic fatalities, either passengers or pedestrians, show alcohol to be by far the most frequent drug found in significant amounts. Only 2.1% of traffic fatalities in a California survey showed both alcohol and diazepam in the blood.[9] Considering that most benzodiazepines can be detected in either blood or urine much longer following the last dose than alcohol, it seems clear that the major contribution to fatal accidents comes from alcohol. In this survey, barbiturates were far more often encountered in association with alcohol.

Laboratory experiments, even those which use simulated driving, are minimally pertinent to the real world. Depending on the dose of either alcohol or benzodiazepines as well as the time interval following which they are tested, one can hardly fail to demonstrate impairment from either drug, with even greater impairment from the combination.[10] The situation in the real world is quite different. Benzodiazepines are usually prescribed for patients who suffer from enough anxiety to be distressing or disabling. It is impossible to determine the relative contributions to accidents of the emotional state of the anxious driver vs. possible impairment from drug. The usual clinical experience, with some support from the laboratory, is that tolerance develops to the overt sedative effects of benzodiazepines while the anxiolytic effects are retained. Indeed, even single doses of diazepam in mice produced long-lived tolerance to neurological impairment.[11] Consequently, one can never be sure about whether the relief of anxiety, on the one hand, or impairment from anxiolytic drugs, on the other, results in more or less accidents. Experiments in which alcohol has been administered following subacute exposure to benzodiazepines indicate greater impairment than from alcohol alone, confirming the conventional wisdom that the combination may still be deleterious.[2] The usual clinical practice has been to warn patients being treated with benzodiazepines about possibly greater impairment from additional alcohol as well as not attempting to drive close to the last dose of benzodiazepine.

2.4. Overdoses

The additive respiratory depressant effects of alcohol and barbiturates are dangerous. It has long been observed clinically that known alcoholics may be found dead with sublethal amounts of both alcohol and barbiturates aboard. The additive respiratory depressant effects of both drugs taken acutely in large doses were enough to be lethal. Such unintentional suicides seem to be less frequent now that benzodiazepines have supplanted the barbiturates as the preferred group of sedative–hypnotics. However, even though they may have less respiratory depressant effects than the barbiturates, occasional instances of such deaths have been reported. For instance, a survey of deaths studied in medical examiners' offices found diazepam to be present on toxicological analysis in 1239 cases. However, drugs alone were thought to cause death in 914 cases; only two had taken diazepam alone. Among those with other drugs aboard, the combination of alcohol and benzodiazepines contributed to only a small percentage of these deaths.[12] Another survey of overdoses from a major teaching hospital during the years 1962–1975 indicated that only 99 of 773 patients (13%) involved benzodiazepines. Only 12 were with these drugs alone; none needed respiratory assistance. The addition of alcohol led to a more serious intoxication with increased need for respiratory assistance.[13] Thus, it appears that overdoses of benzodiazepines alone are remarkably safe and that problems due to their combination with alcohol derive largely from the amount of the latter drug that is present

3. Experimental Studies of Interactions

3.1. Pharmacokinetics

The pharmacokinetics of benzodiazepines has been exhaustively studied. Such studies usually involve single doses of drugs, which is obviously different from the way these drugs are used in the clinic. When single doses of alcohol and benzodiazepines given close together have been studied, effects have varied. Disposition of benzodiazepines metabolized by demethylation or hydroxylation (diazepam, chlordiazepoxide, clorazepate dipotassium, flurazepam) is usually decreased. No effects have been noted on the disposition of drugs that immediately form glucuronides (oxazepam, lorazepam, and temazepam). Concentration of alcohol following acute administration may inactivate enzymes necessary for the former type of metabolism. Following chronic administration of alcohol, enzymes may be induced so that the converse applies; drugs metabolized by demethylation and hydroxylation have an increased clearance. Once again, glucuronidation is not affected. The kinetics of ethanol, owing to its short half-life, are essentially unchanged by prior exposure to benzodiazepines.[2]

Sometimes results are contradictory, even in studies by related groups of investigators. The hypnotic benzodiazepine triazolam, which has a short (2–6 hr) half-life, showed a 21% greater bioavailability following alcohol. The impairment on psychomotor tests from the combination was far greater than could be accounted for by this relatively small change in availability, suggesting the major interaction was pharmacodynamic.[14] An earlier study failed to demonstrate any kinetic interaction between triazolam and alcohol.[15]

The significance of any pharmacokinetic interaction of benzodiazepines is probably minor. Clinical efficacy of these drugs has never been clearly related to their plasma concentrations. While it is probable that sedative side effects, which could impair performance, might be expected from major changes in plasma concentrations, at steady-state concentrations such changes are likely to be minimal.

3.2. Pharmacodynamics

Because both alcohol and benzodiazepines share sedative actions, one might anticipate additive effects when both drugs are used together. In general, combined use leads to greater impairment than use of either drug alone in a variety of tests. Such results occur when both drugs are given close together in single doses as well as when alcohol follows subacute administration of benzodiazepines.[2] Usually, the effect of alcohol contributes most to the impairments.

Human beings are notably capricious. Although sedative effects were additive when both drugs were given together, the combination of the drugs made normal volunteers more anxious.[16] Such an experience provides another example of what has long been axiomatic; drugs affecting the mind operate in a complex interplay between their pharmacological effect, the personality of the human taking the drug, and the environment in which the drug is given. Both alcohol and benzodiazepines disinhibit behavior in certain personality types, but thus far no enhanced disinhibition from the combination has been reported.

Another problem with experimental studies is that results can often be difficult to interpret. The 1,4-benzodiazepine lorprazolam given alone impaired manual dexterity, mental arithmetic, tracking, and memory tasks. Alcohol given alone impaired simple reaction time and tracking; a memory task and choice reaction time were improved. Although both drugs impaired the ability to track when given alone, the combination showed no such effect. Alcohol also mitigated the impairment of manual dexterity from lorprazolam.[17] The notion that alcohol might actually mitigate some of the effects of a benzodiazepine seems counterintuitive. One must await further studies.

It has long been assumed that alcohol and benzodiazepines exert their sedative actions through different mechanisms, alcohol by disordering cell membranes and benzodiazepines through the GABA–benzodiazepine receptor. This view has been challenged by some recent experiments. For instance, ethanol has been found to increase diazepam binding at the GABA–benzodiazepine receptor complex. It was thought that this action might be responsible for the antianxiety, muscle relaxant, and sedative effects of alcohol.[18] However, as the binding is not enhanced directly at the benzodiazepine site but rather at the picrotoxin-sensitive site, such conclusions might be premature. Cortical cerebral blood flow and metabolism were studied in rats following the short-acting anesthetic benzodiazepine midazolam and alcohol, either given alone or together. The decrease in blood flow and metabolism was greater from the combined drugs than from either alone. However, it was reversed by 3-carbo-t-butoxy-b-carboline, a putative benzodiazepine antagonist. Thus, the effects of the combination might not be merely additive but related to facilitation of receptor binding of benzodiazepines by alcohol.[19]

Another line of evidence suggested an interaction between alcohol and the benzodiazepine receptor. The increased uptake of chloride ion in brain vesicles induced by ethanol was antagonized by the putative benzodiazepine antagonist Ro 15-4513. The latter material given as a pretreatment blocked the anticonflict and behavioral intoxication of ethanol but not that of pentobarbital. This action was reversed by Ro 15-4513. Other inverse benzodiazepine agonists had no such effect. Thus, it appeared that a benzodiazepine antagonist might also block the effects of ethanol.[20] This interpretation has been challenged. The same antagonist, Ro 15-4513, failed to block the sedative effects of high doses of ethanol in mice. In fact, it appeared to have intrinsic depressant effects itself, which could have explained the earlier findings.[21] Like other inverse agonists, the benzodiazepine antagonist Ro 15-1788 may also be anxiogenic, which might account for its apparent antagonism of alcohol effects.[22] Obviously, the issue of whether benzodiazepines and alcohol may share some common mechanism of action remains unsettled. Were this to be the case, it might afford another interpretation of the pharmacodynamic interactions between these two drugs.

4. Conclusions

Based on abundant clinical experience as well as experimental data, the conclusion that interactions between alcohol and benzodiazepines are far less important than those with other psychotropic drugs remains true. More specifically, one can conclude:

1. Both benzodiazepines and alcohol are cross-tolerant. The advantage is that the former drugs may be used to treat withdrawal syndromes from alcohol. On the other hand, benzodiazepines may be used interchangeably with alcohol by alcoholics.
2. Both drugs produce additive sedative effects which might be important in impairing the ability to operate a motor vehicle. The tradeoff between mitigating anxiety and possible drug-induced impairment might still favor use of benzodiazepines for treating anxious drivers.
3. Pharmacodynamic interactions are of greater importance than pharmacokinetic interactions; the latter are relatively trivial.
4. The question of whether some pharmacodynamic interactions may be explained by a common site of action at the GABA–benzodiazepine receptor is presently unsettled.

Common clinical practice in regard to the combined use of these drugs is well advised and need not be changed.

References

1. Chan AWK: Effects of combined alcohol and benzodiazepine: A review. *Drug Alcohol Dependence* 13:316–341, 1984.
2. Sellers EM, Busto U: Benzodiazepines and ethanol. Assessment of the effects and consequences of psychotropic drug interaction. *J Clin Psychopharmacol* 2:249–262, 1982.
3. Schuckit MA: Alcohol and drug interactions with antianxiety medications. *Am J Med* 82 (suppl 5A):27–33, 1987.
4. Freed EX: Drug abuse by alcoholics. *Int J Addict* 8:451–473, 1973.
5. Carroll JFX, Malloy TE, Kenrick FM: Drug abuse by alcoholics and problem drinkers: A literature review and evaluation. *Am J Drug Alcohol Abuse* 4:317–341, 1977.
6. Linnoila M: Benzodiazepines and alcoholism, in Trimble MR (ed): *Benzodiazepines Divided—A Multidisciplinary Review.* New York, Wiley, 1983, pp 291–308.
7. Hollister LE, Motzenbecker FP, Degan RO: Withdrawal reactions from chlordiazepoxide ("Librium"). *Psychopharmacologia* 2:63–68, 1961.
8. Aaronson LM, Hinman DJ, Okamoto M: Effects of diazepam on ethanol withdrawal. *J. Pharmacol Exp Ther* 221:319–325, 1982.
9. Lundberg GD, White JM, Hoffman KI: Drugs (other than or in addition to ethylalcohol) and driving behavior: A collaborative study of the California Association of Toxicologists. *J Forensic Sci* 24:207–215, 1979.
10. Linnoila M, Mattila MJ: Drug interaction on psychomotor skills related to driving: diazepam and alcohol. *Eur J Clin Pharmacol* 5:186–194, 1973.
11. Henauer SA, Gallaher EJ, Hollister LE: Long-lasting single-dose tolerance to neurological deficits induced by diazepam. *Psychopharmacology* 82:161–163, 1984.
12. Finkle BS, McCloskey KL, Goodman LS: Diazepam and drug associated deaths in a United States and Canada survey. *JAMA* 242:429–434, 1980.
13. Greenblatt DJ, Allen MD, Noel BSN, Shader RI: Special article: Acute overdosage with benzodiazepine derivatives. *Clin Pharmacol Ther* 21:497–514, 1977.
14. Dorian P, Sellers EM, Kaplan HC, Hamilton C, Greenblatt DJ, Abernethy D: Triazolam and ethanol interactions: Kinetic and dynamic consequences. *Clin Pharmacol Ther* 37:558–562, 1985.
15. Ochs HR, Greenblatt DJ, Arendt RM, Hubbel W, Shader RI: Pharmacokinetics noninteraction of triazolam and ethanol. *J Clin Psychopharmacol* 4:106–107, 1984.
16. Lister RG, File SE: Performance impairment and increased anxiety resulting from the combination of alcohol and lorazepam. *J Clin Psychopharmacol* 3:66–71, 1983.
17. McManus JC, Ankier SI, Norfolk J, Phillips M, Priest RG: Effects on psychological performance of the benzodiazepine, lorprazolam, alone and with alcohol. *Br J Clin Pharmacol* 16:291–300, 1983.
18. Davis WC, Ticku MK: Ethanol enhances ^{3}H-diazepam binding at the benzodiazepine–gamma-aminobutyric acid receptor ionophore complex. *Mol Pharmacol* 20:287–294, 1981.
19. Van Gorder P, Hoffman WE, Baughman V, Albrecht RF, Miletich DJ, Guzman F, Cook JM: Midazolam-ethanol interaction and reversal with benzodiazepine antagonist. *Anesth Analg* 64:129–135, 1985.
20. Sudzak PD, Glowa JR, Crawley JN, Schwartz RD, Skolnick P, Paul SM: A selective imidazobenzodiazepine antagonist of ethanol in the rat. *Science* 234:1234–1247, 1986.
21. Misslin R, Belzung C, Vogel E: Interaction of Ro 15-4513 and ethanol on the behavior of mice: antagonistic or additive effects? *Psychopharmacology* 94:392–396, 1988.
22. Belzung C, Vogel E. Misslin R: Benzodiazepine antagonist Ro 15-1788 partly reverses some anxiolytic effects of ethanol in the mouse. *Psychopharmacology* 95:516–519, 1988.

Emerging Clinical Issues in the Treatment of Alcohol and/or Other Drugs of Abuse

Edward Gottheil, Section Editor

Studies of biological, psychological, and sociocultural similarities and differences between alcoholism and other drug dependencies are reviewed in other sections of this volume. The chapters in this section are concerned with the implications of these findings for the delivery of effective treatment.

In general, the kinds of issues that concern us in treating alcoholism are very much the same as those involved in treating drug abuse. These include (1) assessment—development of better methods for subtyping, treatment planning, outcome predictions, etc.; (2) detoxification—selection of appropriate medical and/or psychosocial techniques; (3) setting—specification of criteria for admission to inpatient hospital, residential nonhospital, day treatment, night treatment, intensive outpatient, or outpatient care; (4) modality—determination of criteria for individual, couple, family, group, network therapies; (5) approach—proper selection of psychodynamic, behavioral, pharmacological, combined techniques; (6) therapists—professional, recovering, self-help groups; (7) combined disorders—multiple drug dependencies, other psychiatric disorders; (8) matching—patient characteristics, treatment methods; (9) cost-effectiveness—length of treatment, cost per unit of treatment, follow-up, outcome evaluation. This list is anything but comprehensive, and each item on it could be subdivided and further subdivided, but it is still a long list. Moreover, the issues represent problems that are very familiar to anyone currently involved in providing or planning clinical services for patients with substance use disorders.

What is perhaps most noteworthy about the list is that only several decades ago these issues were nonissues. Except for treating the medical consequences of alcohol/drug use (skin abscesses, septicemia, cirrhosis, delir-

Edward Gottheil • Division of Substance Abuse, Department of Psychiatry and Human Behavior, Thomas Jefferson University, Philadelphia, Pennsylvania 19107.

ium tremens), health care professionals were not interested in thinking about or providing care for "drunks" and "addicts." In the absence of programs there was little need to become concerned about issues relating to assessments, settings, and modalities.

The demonstration that alcoholics could indeed be helped by Alcoholics anonymous (AA), the emergence of the "disease concept," the founding, growth, and lobbying efforts of the National Council on Alcoholism (NCA) in the 1940s, and the recognition of alcoholism by the American Medical Association in the 1950s resulted finally in focusing public and professional attention on the need for clinical services and research in the field of alcoholism. Following the establishment of the National Institute on Alcoholism and Alcohol Abuse (NIAAA), the field developed rapidly in the 1970s and 1980s. In contrast, the field of drug abuse developed much more suddenly. It came about in response to the explosion in the number of drug abusers in the late 1960s and the spread of the problem from the inner city to the suburbs, leading then to the establishment of a separate National Institute on Drug Abuse (NIDA).

As the fields of alcoholism and drug abuse developed and grew, fashions changed with respect to whether the similarities or the differences between them were emphasized. For a period, clinical formulations focused on the common elements in the backgrounds of patients with these conditions. Drinking and drug taking as well as smoking, overeating, and gambling were seen as related impulse disorders characterized by similar psychodynamic structures, oral traits, compulsivity, and behavioral problems.

These views were not embraced by AA, NCA, or the new clinical programs starting up to treat alcoholism in the 1950s. When cases of drug addiction began presenting themselves for treatment in the 1960s, they appeared quite different from the alcoholic patients and were generally treated by different individuals in different programs. The patients themselves did not wish to be mixed. The drug abusers looked down on the older, more dependent, more compliant "winos," and the alcoholic patients objected to associating with the younger, aggressive, delinquent "junkies." The establishment of NIAAA and NIDA served to institutionalize the differences between the fields. Separate funding streams led to separate clinical, teaching, training, and research programs. Each field had its own constituency and developed its own professional organizations, journals, controversies, researchers, and clinical experts.

But the pendulum began to swing again toward a more generic approach. The Eagleville experiment[1] demonstrated that alcohol and drug abusers could be treated together in the same program; research studies were revealing more biological, social, and psychological similarities between them[2]; and more and more patients were being seen who, instead of paying attention to our discrete diagnostic classifications, were using multiple drugs, including opiates, uppers, and downers, and alcohol as well as whatever else came to hand. Dual diagnoses and combined disorders were recognized and treated, first in special units designed to treat patients using both alcohol and other drugs, but now more and more commonly in general alcohol and drug programs that are treating alcoholism, or drug abuse, or alcoholism and drug abuse. The current influx of cocaine users, who generally use many drugs in addition to cocaine, merely accelerated the trend.

The changes in drug usage and in clinical practice have given rise to other changes, such as the increased number of journals accepting articles on both alcohol and drug abuse and the concept of chemical dependency, which has come to refer to alcohol and/or drug dependence. The American Society on Alcoholism has become the American Society on Alcoholism and Other Drug Dependencies, and DSM-III-R has now adopted a single set of criteria for all of the psychoactive substance use disorders.

Our question is not really whether the various substance use disorders are similar or not, for there are many similarities among them as well as many differences, but whether a generic or a drug-specific approach is likely to be more fruitful. This is not merely an academic issue. It relates to the organization of treatment delivery systems, policies regarding research and teaching, and the debate about whether NIAAA and NIDA should continue operating separately or be combined. It also underlies the practical issues listed at the beginning of this overview. Should we be treating individuals who use different chemicals with the same techniques, in the same programs, for similar lengths of time? Is total abstinence from all addictive behaviors a requirement including nicotine, caffeine, and gambling? Is the particular substance used important for matching purposes and what do we do when we consider that only five drugs taken either singly or two at a time provide us with 15 different matching alternatives? Do we need phencyclidine (PCP)-recovering individuals to treat individuals with problems with PCP?

The questions have a familiar ring and to some it may appear that we are not making a great deal of progress. But the questions are now more specific and more complex. We do not ask whether treatment works any more, but what type of treatment for what type of patient, delivered by whom under what conditions. Instead of asking whether alcoholism and drug abuse are similar or not, we are focusing on which biological, psychological, and sociocultural similarities and differences have theoretical and clinical relevance.

The major concern, as I see it, is not that we do not as yet have definitive answers to our questions and need further research in these areas, but that we fail to recognize the limits of our knowledge base and, under the pressure of the current "cost-effectiveness" movement, foreclose too quickly on our options. The field continues to change. Combined disorders,[3] matching [4] and cost-effectiveness[5] have become prominent issues only within the last decade. Even as we attempt to evaluate whether particular matching parameters result in more effective treatment outcomes for alcoholics and drug abusers, "pure" alcoholics and drug abusers are becoming more and more rare. As suggested in the following chapters, it may be that in the 1990s combined alcohol and drug problems will be the normative problem and may require different treatment approaches.

We have actually come a long way in a short time. In the five chapters that follow, observations, experience, data, ideas, and suggestions relevant to the clinical issues previously mentioned are reviewed and there are thoughtful discussions of the contributions of the generic and drug-specific approaches to the treatment of substance use disorders.

References

1. Ottenberg DJ, Carroll JFX: Combined treatment of alcoholism and drug addiction, in Solomon J, Keeley KA (eds): *Perspectives in Alcohol and Drug Abuse: Similarities and Differences.* Boston, John Wright, PSG, 1982, pp 117–144.
2. Gottheil E, Evans BD, Verebey K: Research relating to alcohol and opiate dependence, in Solomon J, Keeley KA (eds): *Perspectives in Alcohol and Drug Abuse: Similarities and Differences.* Boston, John Wright, PSG, 1982, pp 179–206.
3. Gottheil E, McLellan AT, Druley KA (eds): *Substance Abuse and Psychiatric Illness.* Elmsford, NY, Pergamon Press, 1980.
4. Gottheil E, McLellan AT, Druley KA (eds): *Matching Patient Needs and Treatment Methods in Alcoholism and Drug Abuse.* Springfield, IL, Charles C Thomas, 1981.
5. Gottheil E: Evaluating alcoholism treatment research, in Lettieri D, Sayers MA, Nelson JE (eds): NIAAA Research Report on Treatment Assessment. Washington, DC, ADAMHA, 1985, pp 1–8.

Cultural Factors in the Choice of Drugs

Dwight B. Heath

Abstract. The human animal has discovered a wide range of drugs, some of which are readily available products of nature, and has invented others by means of manufacture or processing. The meanings, uses, and associations that are attached to such drugs vary from one population to another and are often different for subgroups within a given population. Even the effects of drugs vary, demonstrating that they are not inherent in the substances or in the biochemical impact they have on the human organism. Meanings, uses, and associations often change over time as well. These facts, briefly illustrated with selected examples, demonstrate that culture is an important aspect of the environment—interacting with biological and psychological factors—in relation to choices individuals make about drugs, their uses, and the outcomes of use.

The concept of culture has heuristic value in describing and analyzing beliefs and behavior, but it should not be construed as an etiologically powerful entity. Culture can be viewed as a metaphor, reflecting and incorporating social consensus and controls. Any serious attempt to change patterns of drug use must involve changes in the culture, and education promises to be the most likely way of altering both individual choices and cultural patterns. Whereas "the control model" of prevention unrealistically relies on formal legislative and regulatory controls, "the sociocultural model" emphasizes more powerful informal social controls.

1. Introduction

It is remarkable that the majority of human cultures throughout history have included rules about the use of at least some drug or some disciplined activity that has psychoactive effects on perception and behavior. Only during the last two decades have "polydrug use" or "multiple addictions" been reported with any regularity in the medical or sociological literature, and even now they tend to occur mostly among small segments of urban industrial societies. Furthermore, it is apparent that most of these polydrug users have a strong preference for one drug and use others primarily to modulate the effects of that "drug of choice."[1] A brief overview of cultural variations with respect to

Dwight B. Heath • Department of Anthropology, Brown University, Providence, Rhode Island 02912-1921.

drug use and abstention may help shed light on the choices that individuals make in this connection.

2. Psychoactive Drugs and the Human Animal

Whatever else *Homo sapiens* may be, the animal substrate cannot be ignored. During recent years we have learned in increasing detail about biological aspects of the interaction of humankind with psychoactive drugs, even at the level of neurons and their component parts. But relatively little attention has been paid to some of the distinctively human factors, namely drug–human interactions at the level of social groups and cultures.

We have no record of the earliest use of drugs by humankind, but it is commonplace to see birds and insects acting intoxicated after having drunk ethanol that occurs naturally during the process of fermentation in overripe fruits or berries. It has recently been suggested that agriculture may have developed in the ancient Near East more to assure a steady supply of beer than of bread.[2] In parts of Mexico, stones carved in the shape of mushrooms suggest the importance of those fungi more than 2 millennia ago, often in regions where they still play an important religious role in inducing hallucinations. Such use may be even older; it is widespread across Siberia,[3] and a bewildering variety of naturally occurring psychoactive drugs are used in other native cultures on all continents.[4]

The spread of coffee, tea, and chocolate around the world was rapid, although each traveled a different route at different times. The spread of tobacco around the globe in less than a century is well documented; its prompt acceptance and integration into diverse cultures is unusual. The story of opium's having been introduced from India to China by the English is well known, if only because the Opium Wars focused world attention on some of the political and economic repercussions. Although its use had been well known long before, opium become popular in the West only a century ago, with English refinement of laudanum and American production of morphine for medical purposes. Coca has been used by Andean Indians for millennia in a variety of ways that appear to have caused little harm to anyone's health and to have been positively integrative in social terms. Cocaine, by contrast, is viewed as harmful and socially disruptive in many industrialized nations, especially in the newly refined form of "crack." Amphetamines, barbiturates, and other drugs that have been synthesized in recent years for medical purposes have quickly been adopted for a variety of unanticipated uses, just as solvents, glues, paint, and many other commercial and industrial substances are used for psychoactive effects. Throughout much of tropical America, a wide variety of snuffs, enemas, and teas concocted from various plants are commonly used, often in strictly ritualized contexts and for religious purposes. Peyote is similarly important to some Indian tribes in northern Mexico and to the Native American Church for its hallucinogenic qualities, very unlike the faddish use of mescaline and LSD derivatives by others in a secular context. The many meanings and uses of alcohol, and the diametrically contrasting evaluations of drunkenness that can be found among populations throughout the world, seem to have a closer relationship to the nature and extent of alcohol-related problems than does sheer volume of consumption.

It is remarkable that so many naturally occurring substances have strongly psychoactive properties, some with minimal processing, but in other cases, only after elaborate preparation.[5] One of the striking curiosities is the fact that the Western Hemisphere is home to hundreds of such plants, whereas there are only about a dozen elsewhere in the world. Another unresolved question has to do with how anyone ever discovered the special properties of plants of which only selected portions induce the desired states while other portions are highly toxic, some must be boiled to dispel toxicity whereas other become dangerous when so treated, and so forth. The often sophisticated and elaborate technology of dealing with psychedelics must represent the distillation of an enormous amount of trial-and-error learning on the part of peoples around the world.

3. The "Drug-of-Choice" Phenomenon at a Cultural Level

Within most societies, there tends to be a preferred or focal drug—or a strong sentiment against the use of any drug. Those societies that have opted against drug use often allow, or even encourage, some stylized pattern of behavior that results in altered states of consciousness that are at least analogous to those that result from drug use. Examples of such behaviors are meditation, exercise, rhythmical dancing, possession, prolonged hunger, and isolation.

Although it is obvious that no group could emphasize a drug that was not available to them, availability alone seems to play only a minor role in such selection. In fact, a drug that is enthusiastically embraced by people far away is often ignored or neglected by those to whom it is easily accessible and relatively inexpensive. One example of this is the well-known fact that producers of opium have rarely been consumers of it, all through history. Similarly, those who grow and harvest *khat* in the Near East do not use it, although urban consumers in Yemen are estimated to spend as much as 20% of their monthly household budget on it.[6]

There is wide variation in the meanings, uses, and values that are attached to the same drug by various populations. An array of patterned attitudes, beliefs, and norms tends to grow up around each drug, and those patterns vary for different drugs within a given culture. The use of peyote for religious purposes by the Huichol Indians of Mexico is inextricably embedded in a dense matrix of ritual activity, mythology, and religious belief; the Huichols appear to use no other drug.[7] In a village in northern India, Brahmans who esteem their cannabis tea deplore the locally distilled liquor that is enjoyed by their similarly high-caste Rajput neighbors—and vice versa.[8] Despite the shrill clamor against "hard drugs" that is sweeping the United States these days, alcohol is still widely enjoyed in moderate quantities as a healthful relaxant and accompaniment to sociability. Members of the Native American Church, who use peyote as a sacrament, decline to drink. Swedes, for whom coffee plays an important role, tend to have little patience with Britons, who favor tea, or the French, who drink wine throughout the day; each group similarly considers its preference to be "natural" and "fitting."

3.1. Changing Patterns of Drug Use

Even when a drug is introduced from one population to another, the patterns of use and associated meanings are not necessarily diffused at the same time. And even when that does occur, a process of evolution can result in gradual and often significant differences over time. A few examples will illustrate the reality and depth of cultural variation in this connection. Although carrying few of the overtones that are associated with it in China, Japan, or southern Asia, tea has permeated the fabric of British society, affecting patterns of eating, sociability, and the whole chronology of daily activities, in ways that are not replicated elsewhere. When alcohol was first adopted by the Iroquois of North America, they used it for religious purposes as an adjunct to a young man's vision quest. Among the same population, a half-century of widespread boisterous and brawling drunkenness ensued, which ended in the late 17th century when the Handsome Lake Religion emerged, combining abstinence as an article of faith with its own special blend of indigenous and Christian morality. In many regions of Africa, Oceania, and North America, where alcoholic beverages were banned to native populations, drinking has become associated with high social status, and alcoholic beverages are important items for securing social credit among people who have little and irregular access to money. While a few notorious opium dens in Victorian England replicated the Oriental pattern of smoking, intravenous injection and ingestion in liquid tonics were more common. Expatriates from many nations have converged on the Mazatec region of Mexico to enjoy secular recreational use of the hallucinogenic mushroom that is a sacrament and aid to divination for the Indians.

Even as embedded as a drug may become in the context of a society's way of life, the nature of its linkages with other aspects of culture is still subject to change. Rum, beer, and cider were the most common beverages in colonial North America, but whiskey soon displaced the first when domestic production was permitted, and cider virtually dropped out over time. The average per capital annual consumption of alcoholic beverages in the early 19th century was over three times as large as today's,[9] with a period of widespread temperance (and even prohibition in many states) in the middle of that century, followed by a new abrupt rise, culminating in nationwide prohibition in 1919. With repeal in 1933, consumption again climbed steadily for many years, but leveled off and dropped in the 1980s. Marijuana was an exotic recreational drug among small counterculture groups until the 1960s, when its use become widespread, despite continuing illegality. Cocaine, once thought to be a last resort of hard-core down-and-outers, is now fashionable among wealthy professionals, although it too remains illegal. Cigarette smoking was not popular in the United States until World War I, but spread rapidly thereafter. No social scientist or student of drugs appears to have predicted, as recently as 1970, that the use of tobacco would be so widely banned in public places, and that nonsmokers would find broad support in asking smokers to refrain. LSD, mescaline, phencyclidine (PCP or "angel dust"), and a host of minor tranquilizers, all of which were popular in the 1960s and 1970s, were little used at the end of the 1980s. There can be no doubt that "drugs of choice" change over time, and the attitudes and values that are associated with them similarly vary within a given society. One might almost say that there are fads and fashions in drug use, as there are in hair styling, clothing, music, and many others aspects of culture. Although the rate of change may be unusually rapid in the United States, such changes also occur in other nations and in other cultures around the world.

3.2. Intracultural Variation

Within a given population, there is almost never universal use of any drug, no matter how favorably it may be valued and how esteemed its effects may be. Usually there is a minimum age for initiation into use, and often very different rules apply to people at various stages in the life cycle. Even so widespread a drink as beer in Austria or wine in Italy is permitted in only small amounts to infants, allowed in slightly larger amounts to young children, and in larger amounts to adolescents, expected and sometimes even pressed on young adults, and then allowed in diminishing quantities to the aged. The agaric mushroom tends to be monopolized by older men among various Siberian tribes, after which younger men may drink the urine of their elders in order to get a diluted but still strong drug experience.

In the "golden triangle" of southeast Asia where much of the world's opium is produced, its use is generally restricted to the aged, just as Zapotec "magic mushrooms" used to be reserved to a few shaman–curers and the powerful hallucinogenic snuff of the Yanomamo of Venezuela is primarily an adjunct to divination by sorcerers. Women tend to drink less than men in all societies that have been studied, and the differential persists even when adjusted to compensate for differences in weight and body fat. By contrast, in many societies women use more barbiturates and amphetamines than do men. In the United States drinking is heaviest among young men, most of whom moderate their consumption markedly before 30; the opposite is true in much of Latin America and elsewhere. Solvent sniffing seems to be popular only with adolescent and younger people, except among Australian Aborigines.

Religious groups vary in the rates of use of different drugs, and they also vary in rates of different drug-related problems. It is noteworthy that the occurrence of problems is not always directly proportional to consumption. A familiar illustration of the independent variation of consumption and problems is the comparison of Catholic and Jewish immigrants to the United States. In the former population, few other than adult males customarily drink alcoholic beverages, whereas in the latter, people of both sexes and all ages drink at least weekly. The relatively few Catholic users suffer psychological and social complications out of proportion to the overall population, however, whereas it is relatively rare for a Jew to suffer alcohol-related problems. Social surveys confirm the popular stereotype that lower-class Americans drink more beer, while wine tends to be drunk by people with more income and education.

Occupational groups also differ, with sailors, cowboys, and lumberjacks notorious as heavy drinkers during respites between jobs. Jazz and swing musicians appear to have pioneered disproportionately in marijuana use in the United States, and students were notorious for experimentation with LSD in the 1960s, just as heroin tends, rightly or wrongly, to be viewed as a drug primarily used by pimps, hustlers, and others who are already on the fringe of the law. In Costa Rica, longshoremen and others engaged in work that requires great expenditure of effort use marijuana in large quantities as an energizer,[10] much as Jamaican peasants do while harvesting sugarcane.[11,12] In both countries, the same drug is used in much smaller amounts by university students and other young people who do little physical work but who enjoy the psychotropic effects for recreation and relaxation. The amotivational syndrome as an outcome of marijuana smoking is clearly not so much a reflection of pharmacological action on human physiology as it is a reflection of psychosocial expectations.

As we have gained increasing insights into the natural history of drugs, including the ways in which people interact with them in everyday life (and not only under laboratory conditions), it has become increasingly evident that there is not a single unitary deviant way of life that can appropriately be labeled "the drug subculture," but rather there are several diverse "drug subcultures," each involving mostly members of a drug-specific interpersonal network.

4. Implications for Culture and Choice

Even so cursory an overview of drug use patterns as this allows for some generalizations about both the nature of culture and the choices that individuals make, as well as guiding us to education as the best means of preventing any related problems.

4.1. Culture as Metaphor

"Culture" is not a remote thing that manipulates people, nor is it a mysterious "black box" that makes pronouncements about what is and what ought to be. "Culture" (or "the sociocultural system") is a convenient shorthand label that subsumes broad patterns of thinking and behaving that are manifested in daily life by individuals. To be sure, a major portion of every culture is a precipitate of history, but when we are talking about "drinking patterns," "styles of drug use," "cultural norms," and so forth, we are usually talking about generalizations of everyday behavior. To refer to "culture" is simply to say, in a sense, "what most of the people in this society say (or do) is such-and-such." It's sometimes helpful to distinguish between *real* culture— what people actually *do*—and *ideal* culture—what people say *ought* to be done. (A somewhat outdated example in the United States may be premarital chastity, highly praised but little practiced; perhaps more enduring is the norm against lying—a general rule but one everyone recognizes should be violated in special circumstances: such as occasionally declining an invitation, accepting a tasteless gift, and so forth.)

The very fact that the norm about premarital chastity has changed significantly in our lifetime is clear evidence that culture is not so monolithic, but rather it reflects what individuals do, exerting their own choices, sometimes in direct opposition to the cultural norm. This is not nihilism, nor is it a counsel of despair, to the effect that whatever people want to do is acceptable. It is a realistic recognition that social constructions regulate our thinking and our behavior at least as much as anything else, and social constructions are notoriously subject to being changed. Rewards, punishments, promises, threats, new information—all of these are forces that can change what we think is right or wrong. It is not so much that culture determines what people do. Quite the contrary: In a very real sense, what people do determines culture. Culture does not "cause" behavior; it defines the range of alternatives that are more (or less) acceptable and the reactions that individuals can expect when they make choices among those alternatives.

A person who did not drink at a party in the United States was considered "odd" as recently as a decade ago, and hosts often teased or cajoled in a thinly disguised effort to push drinks on him or her. Nowadays deciding not to drink is viewed as anyone's right, even in a context where most others are drinking fairly heavily. There is even a major advertising campaign favoring such behavior by a "designated driver" for each carload of people. We have witnessed the emergence of a new cultural norm, with no clear indication of who planned it (if indeed anyone did) and with no fanfare before or when it happened. For that matter, it may not even be possible to pinpoint when such a change occurred—shifting consensus is almost always gradual rather than abrupt, and there may be a significant delay (what sociologists call "culture lag") between a shift in what is normal behavior and what is viewed as the prescriptive norm.

Cultures evolve, and the rapidity with which they do so is one of the reasons why the human animal has been able to adapt to so many different environments. It is also why so many different cultures have emerged among the populations of the world. Beyond that, the fact that cultures change can be a cause for hope—or for alarm—as we comment on the beliefs and behaviors of people around us today. The fact that we make value judgments about norms and their violations shows that these norms have a certain degree of inertia, tending to be accepted as a result of enculturation. In general, people do learn to do what they ought to do, and to want what they ought to want. But not in perpetuity, and sometimes not for long at all.

4.2. Education as Prevention

Even the most outspoken opponents of drug use are careful to point out that their concern is primarily to prevent the myriad problems (in the realms of health, familial relations, employment, public safety, and so forth) that tend to be associated with such use. The most widely known and increasingly used strategy for prevention is the so-called "control model," emphasizing a combination of legislative and regulative changes that would supposedly make drugs less readily available. Large-scale interdiction, harassment of dealers and consumers, varied and disproportionately severe penalties for violations, and so forth are invoked with relation to illegal drugs; the system of physicians' prescription limits access to others, whereas heavy taxes, warning labels, increasing restrictions on sales and advertising, and so forth are proposed for the most popular licit substances such as tobacco and alcohol.

There is a vast literature on the efficacy and inefficacy of some of these measures, but the experience of failed prohibitions on alcohol in many jurisdictions, and of repeatedly ineffectual "wars against drugs,"[13] demonstrates that popular norms often are so strong as to defy legislative and regulatory controls.

An alternative approach to prevention that emphasizes norms is "the sociocultural model," which recognizes that people tend to make sense of the world around them through reference to the attitudes, values, and actions of people they know and care about.[14,15] In short, sociocultural norms give meaning to experience.

Comparing numerous ethnographic reports from around the world suggests that problems seem likely to ensure in a context of ambivalence about drugs: for example, an environment in which drug use is viewed as "fun" or "grownup," but also as "dangerous" or risky. Similarly with the "forbidden fruit syndrome," whereby young people are exhorted to abstain but adults are then expected, with no preparation, to use drugs wisely. By contrast, sociocultural factors that are associated with fewer problems include, for example, the custom of drinking with meals, drug-use embedded in a ritual or religious context, socially accepted periods of "time out," when selected restrictions on behavior are lifted, recognition that an individual is responsible for him or herself and his or her actions, and so forth.[16,17]

Some might say that "the sociocultural model" is all very well for analysis and interpretation of a particular pattern in sociological or anthropological terms, but useless when it comes to offering practical suggestions for confronting and reducing actual problems in the real world. Such a view is naïve and incorrect. "The sociocultural model" can and should be applied for the prevention of drug-related problems through education.

It is unfortunate that, in recent years, education has often been discredited as a means of prevention. When proponents of "the control model" say that education does not work, they are generally referring to superficial efforts, limited to the classroom, often emphasizing unrealistic scare tactics and taught by people who have little interest in or special knowledge about drugs.

However, there is a very real sense in which education has not yet been given a fair trial. Certainly that is the case if we use education in the broad sense of health promotion, addressed to all ages and levels of society, and using a variety of approaches in addition to realistic classroom teaching. The heart-health program that has been going on in Framingham, Massachusetts, for several decades is one good example; a similar program in Pawtucket, Rhode Island, has a shorter track record but is similarly broad-based and has already had considerable impact, measurable in epidemiological terms. "The control model" holds out the empty promise of a quick solution; it lets politicians "talk tough" and reassures the public at large that "those bad people" will be duly punished.[18] "The control model" has to do exclusively with legal and regulatory controls that are imposed by formal agencies of various levels of government, and those are the only kinds of control that most people think of when any mention is made of the need to control drugs.

But every society throughout the world has other controls over drug use and other behaviors; this is true even of isolated, nonliterate societies that have no written laws or regulations and no formal legislative or administrative agencies.[19] The rules about what is permissible to whom, where, when, how, how much, and so forth—whether they be called norms, or mores, or values—are as much controls as are laws about minimum purchase, age, a ban on possession, death penalty for drug dealing near schools, taxation, regulations about advertising, and so forth. In fact, as repeatedly evidenced throughout the world, informal controls are even more meaningful and effective than those other kinds of formal controls, largely because they are internalized and deeply felt by the people whose behavior is to be affected.

What all this adds up to is that "the sociocultural model" is not at all opposed to controls. It is misleading that some people presume that to be the case because of its being so often contrasted with "the control model." "The sociocultural model" is, in fact, premised on self-control as the cornerstone of harmonious social living. And that kind of self-control, in turn, grows out of social controls, be they peer pressure, parental example and exhortation, friends' and co-workers' ideas about what is acceptable behavior and what is not—in short, the many and varied informal controls that constitute so large a part of any cultural system.

References

1. Khantzian EJ, Schneider RJ: Addiction, adaptation and the "drug-of-choice" phenomenon: Clinical perspectives, in Milkman HB, Shaffer HJ (eds): *The Addictions: Multidisciplinary Perspectives and Treatments.* Lexington, MA, DC Heath, 1985, pp 121–129.
2. Katz SH, Voigt MM: Bread and beer: The early use of cereals in the human diet. *Expedition* 28(2):23–34, 1987.
3. Wasson RG, Wasson VP: *Mushrooms, Russia and History.* New York, Pantheon, 1957.
4. Furst, PT: *Hallucinogens and Culture.* San Francisco, Chandler & Sharp, 1976.
5. Rios, MD de: *Hallucinogens: Cross-Cultural Perspectives.* Albuquerque, University of New Mexico Press, 1984.
6. Kennedy JG: *The Flower of Paradise.* Hingham, MA, Kluwer Academic, 1987.
7. Myerhoff BG: *Peyote Hunt: The Sacred Journey of the Huichol Indians.* Ithaca, NY, Cornell University Press, 1974.
8. Carstairs GM: *Daru* and *bhang:* Cultural factors in the choice of an intoxicant. *Q J Stud Alcohol* 15:220–237, 1954.
9. Rorabaugh WJ: *The Alcoholic Republic: An American Tradition.* New York, Oxford University Press, 1979.
10. Carter WE (ed): *Cannabis in Costa Rica: A Study of Chronic Marihuana Use.* Philadelphia, ISHI Publications, 1980.
11. Rubin V, Comitas L: *Ganja in Jamaica.* The Hague, Mouton, 1975.
12. Dreher MC: *Working Men and Ganja: Marihuana Use in Rural Jamaica.* Philadelphia, ISHI Publications, 1982.
13. Brecher EM: Drug laws and drug law enforcement: A review and evaluation based on 111 years of experience. *Drugs Society* 1:1–27, 1986.
14. Heath DB: A critical review of the sociocultural model of alcohol use, in Harford TC, Parker DA, Light L (eds): *Normative Approaches to the Prevention of Alcohol Abuse and Alcoholism.* Rockville, MD, National Institute on Alcohol Abuse and Alcoholism Research Monograph 3, 1979, pp 1–18.
15. Heath DB: Emerging anthropological theory and models of alcohol use and alcoholism, in Chaudren CD, Wilkinson DA (eds): *Theories on Alcoholism.* Toronto, Addiction Research Foundation, 1988, pp 354–410.
16. Heath DB: A critical review of ethnographic studies of alcohol use, in Gibbins RJ, Israel Y, Kalant H, et al (eds): *Research Advances in Drug and Alcohol Problems 2.* New York, Wiley, 1975, pp 1–92.
17. Heath DB: Drinking and drunkenness in transcultural perspective: an overview. *Transcultural Psychiatr Res Rev* 21:7–42, 103–126, 1986.
18. Heath DB: Alcohol control policies and drinking patterns: An international game of politics against science. *J Substance Abuse* 1:109–115, 1988.
19. Westermeyer J: Cultural patterns of drug and alcohol use: an analysis of host and agent in the cultural environment. *Bull Narcotics* 34(2):11–27, 1987.

Self-Regulation and Self-Medication Factors in Alcoholism and the Addictions

Similarities and Differences

E. J. Khantzian

Abstract. Addicts and alcoholics suffer vulnerabilities and deficits in self-regulation. A principal manifestation of their self-regulation disturbances is evident in the way they attempt to self-medicate painful affect states and related psychiatric problems. Individuals select a particular drug based on its ability to relieve or augment emotions unique to an individual which they cannot achieve or maintain on their own. Addicts and alcoholics usually experiment with all classes of drugs, but discover that a particular drug suits them best. Usually, painful affect states interact with other problems in self-regulation involving self-esteem, relationships, self-care, and related characterological defenses, making it more likely that addicts will experiment with and find the action of a particular drug appealing or compelling. Stimulants have their appeal because their energizing properties relieve distress associated with depression, hypomania, and hyperactivity; opiates are compelling because they mute and contain disorganizing affects of rage and aggression; and sedative hypnotics, including alcohol, permit the experience of affection, aggression, and closeness in individuals who are otherwise cut off from their feelings and relationships.

1. Introduction

It is probably not insignificant that the widespread misuse and abuse of addictive drugs in our society emerged approximately one decade after the introduction of modern psychopharmacological agents. When these drugs were first introduced in the 1950s, they were called "major" (for major mental illness, i.e., psychosis) or "minor" (for minor mental illness, i.e., neurosis) "tranquilizers," and as the terms imply, it was believed they worked simply by tranquilizing or attenuating emotional distress. However, with the subsequent advent of the antidepressants in the early 1960s and the identification and clarification of the role of neuroreceptors and neurotransmitters, re-

E. J. Khantzian • Department of Psychiatry, Harvard Medical School at The Cambridge Hospital, Cambridge, Massachusetts 02139.

searchers and clinicians began to appreciate that psychoactive drugs had different sites and modes of action. Consequently, this appreciation modified our designation of these drugs to more precisely describe their action—i.e., antipsychotic, antianxiety, antidepressant, and antimanic agents.

As the original and subsequent names of these drugs implied, these agents promised to reduce or counter emotional suffering associated with mental illness. It should not be surprising, then, that some of these drugs (especially antianxiety drugs) and other illicit substances were adopted and used increasingly in the 1960s and 1970s by individuals who were not necessarily patients to relieve and remove emotional distress.

However, for the most part, and until recently, few investigators, clinicians, or theoreticians have considered drugs of abuse to have appeal or addictive potential because of their ability to reduce emotional pain or suffering. Instead, motives of stimulus seeking, pleasure drive, or self-destructiveness are and have been invoked on the psychological side, or biogenetic or addictive mechanisms on the physiological side, to account for why individuals become so dependent on substances of abuse. Notwithstanding the scientific advances that have allowed the measurement of genetic and physiological factors, clinical work with and diagnostic studies of addicts, guided by a modern psychodynamic perspective, offer a basis to conclude that the need to control or reduce emotional suffering is an important motivating factor in addictive disorders. Pleasure- or stimulus-seeking and self-destructive motives are indeed apparent in addictions, but in my opinion they are more often by-products or secondary to problems in self-regulation in which the capacities for managing feelings, self-esteem, relationships, and self-care loom large.[1-3]

In this chapter I explore how self-medication factors play an important role in individuals becoming dependent on alcohol and drugs, with an emphasis on alcoholism. The self-medication hypothesis implies that individuals prefer or depend on different drugs because each class of drugs, much like the classes of drugs legitimately used in psychiatry, have a distinctive action and effect which interacts with specific painful feeling states and related psychiatric disorders. I use clinical examples to demonstrate that self-medication factors are as important with alcohol dependence as they are with other addictive drugs. I will compare and contrast the appeal of alcohol with other classes of drugs that are misused and abused (i.e., narcotics and stimulants).

2. The Challenge of Self-Regulation

Because humans are governed less by instincts and more by coping skills and capacities acquired from the caretaking environment, requirements for human survival and adaptation place a lifelong challenge on humans for self-regulation. Regulating emotions or feeling life is one of the most central of these challenges. I believe self-medication factors in addictive disorders are intimately related to human self-regulation problems, and, in particular, to the regulation of affects or feeling life. Accordingly, in this chapter I place and discuss self-medication factors and substance abuse in a broader context of the human need for self-regulation.

Clinical investigators working with alcoholics and addicts over the past three decades have accumulated observations and findings suggesting a self-medication hypothesis of addictive disorders.[4–9] Many of these reports stressed major developmental impairments and severe psychopathology and associated painful affect states that made reliance on drugs likely and compelling. Subsequent diagnostic and treatment studies provided supporting and empirical evidence that addicts suffer with coexisting psychiatric disorders and structural psychopathology.[10–20]

Despite the documented association between substance abuse and psychopathology, I have more recently become convinced that there is a wide range of emotional vulnerability or susceptibility to addictive and alcoholic disorders. Admittedly, the cases of severe psychopathology represent an extreme, but they and the less severely or minimally affected individuals with psychopathology are all more or less subject to human experiences and processes involving distress and suffering. It is distress and suffering that is at the heart of alcoholism and addiction, and cases of more extreme psychopathology are examples of where the emotional pain is greater for such individuals as a consequence of their psychopathology.

The self-medication hypothesis takes into consideration how the effects or actions of the different classes of drugs (i.e., stimulants, opiates, and sedative–hypnotics) interact with states of distress to make them appealing and to cause certain individuals to become dependent on them. The self-medication perspective of drug–alcohol dependence places heavy emphasis on painful affects, but other self-regulating factors involving self-esteem, self-other relationships, and self-care also interact with affect states in substance use and misuse. I will expand on these other factors subsequently.

As we have indicated, our emphasis in exploring self-medication factors in alcoholism and addictions is on suffering and its psychological determinants. There are clearly other determinants, however, in addition to the psychological factors that cause or contribute to the development of dependency on alcohol and drugs. These include genetic, environmental, and cultural factors which may either protect against or heighten a person's vulnerability to substance use disorders. Exploration of these factors goes beyond the scope of this chapter, and we limit ourselves to the psychological factors. However, a comprehensive explanation or theory of substance dependence must ultimately attempt to integrate and account for how all of these factors interact.

3. Old and New Theories of Human Distress

3.1. Drives and Conflict

Early psychoanalytic theory of the mind advanced by Sigmund Freud emphasized instinctual factors (i.e., pleasure and aggressive drives) and a topographic view of the mind in which much of mental life and psychic process was considered to be unconscious. Freud and his followers later placed greater emphasis on internal processes and states involving wishes and needs and a more detailed appreciation of structural factors and functions involved in regulating psychic life and adjustment to reality. In these earlier psychodynamic formulations, psychic suffering and human distress were viewed for the most part in terms of conflict psychology. Distress was felt to be the result of human drives or wishes pressing for discharge but opposed by inhibitions or repression.

Early psychoanalytic approaches to relieving conflict and distress emphasized making unconscious mental life (i.e., fantasies, wishes, and desires) conscious, and verbalizing and working through pent-up sexual and aggressive drives. Employing free association and cathartic techniques, the objective was to reduce or minimize tensions, conflict, and distress which resulted from excessive control or repression of drives and related impulses.

3.2. Affects and Structure

There has been a decided shift from these early psychodynamic theories, which stressed drives and conflict, and reducing or keeping drives at a minimum as a means to avoid distress and conflict. Contemporary psychodynamic theory has placed affects and feeling life center stage and more systematically considers the ways ego and self-structures develop and unfold to optimally regulate affects (i.e., feeling life), self-esteem, relationships, and adaptation to external reality.

Although modern psychodynamic clinicians still employ free association to access the nature and source of emotional distress, greater efforts are placed on actively building empathic connections and contact with patients to help them identify their feelings and needs, to derive a better sense of self and others, and to develop a sense of safety and comfort. Emphasis in contemporary clinical approaches focuses more on fostering improved capacities for containment of feelings and self-regulation. Rather than releasing or reducing drive tensions to minimal levels, modern approaches stress the maintenance of optimal (vs. maximum or minimal) affects and helping individuals grow in their capacity to control and transform distress.

3.3. Development and Adaptation

The degree to which individuals can tolerate distress and find relief from human suffering is proportional to the degree they have been able to develop and internalize capacities to regulate feelings, to establish and maintain a healthy regard for self and others, and to take care of themselves. These capacities are incorporated as mental structures and functions in our personality organization and reflect our ego capacities and sense of self.

The development of ego and sense of self begins in infancy and continues over a lifetime. The attitudes and functions that are internalized derive primarily from our parents and, subsequently, from association with other significant individuals and groups. If the growing-up environment is optimally constant, nurturing, and relatively free of major trauma or neglect, ego functions and the sense of self coalesce to give us a mature and adaptable character structure. In contrast, major developmental flaws, defects, and distortions occur in a person's character structure as a function of environmental inconstancy, trauma, and neglect.[21] Our focus on problems in self-regulation and the use of substances for the purpose of self-medication is based on this appreciation of these developmental processes and disabilities. These developmental flaws and deficits in the character structure of substance abusers are responsible for the difficulties they experience in adapting to their internal emotional life and external world of reality. It is on this basis that addicts and alcoholics attempt to correct these flaws through the use of substances, a "correction" they feel they cannot achieve on their own.

4. Common Factors in Alcoholism and the Addictions

The common factors in alcoholism and the addictions center around the use of substances as a means to achieve and maintain self-regulation. However, considering how disregulated, disorganized, and out of control addicts and alcoholics appear, it is hard to believe that they could be using these substances for purposes of regulating themselves. In fact, it is on the basis of this latter observation that many argue that substances cause distress and disregulation rather than the other way around.[22,23] Such accounts, in my estimation, focus excessively on the admitted regression in psychological function associated with long-term use of drugs, some drugs (e.g., stimulants and sedative–hypnotics) causing more regression than others.[11] They fail to take enough into account the more enduring and relatively immutable personality structures of such individuals which reveal long-standing difficulties in managing their inner psychological life and their external behaviors. Systematic study of such factors reveals that many of the protracted states of dysphoria (or "hypophoria") associated with drug withdrawal are some of the same states that coexisted with other determining personality traits and features predating the substance dependence.[24,25]

I would argue that the regular reliance on any drug causes a "dis-use" atrophy in a person's capacity to achieve a subjective or behavioral end in more ordinary ways. That is, the more individuals depend on a drug or alcohol to calm, activate, relate to others, play, and so forth, the less they develop capacities to achieve them normally, and more often and tragically they undermine any existing capacities they might have developed. But as we gain an appreciation of substance abusers' lifelong difficulties in coping with distress, their initial and subsequent reliance on drugs becomes more understandable. In this section I review how sectors of vulnerability in personality organization common to alcoholics and addicts, involving feeling life (affects), self-esteem, self-other relations, and self-care, can predispose individuals to use and become dependent on substances.

4.1. Affects

The nature of the distress or suffering associated with alcoholism and addiction, I feel, is closely linked with the complex ways in which individuals with these problems experience, tolerate, and express their feelings (i.e., affects). They seem to suffer in the extreme, either feeling too much or feeling too little. Some seem to be more chronically "disaffected"[26] or unable to name their feelings ("alexithymia")[27] and seem more pervasively devoid of feelings; others seem, more often than not, overwhelmed with intense affects, such as rage, shame, loneliness, and depression, and yet others "flipflop" between the extremes of emotional flooding and emptiness.[1-7]

Individuals who suffer in these ways use drugs and alcohol to help them cope with emotions. Depending on one's state and the doses of drugs used, drug–alcohol effects may, in some instances, attenuate or allow feelings. When individuals feel a need to repeatedly resort to drugs or alcohol to achieve such effects, it is usually a sign that they suffer with developmental deficits and handicaps and thus need drug–alcohol effects to achieve and maintain states of feeling that they cannot achieve on their own. That is, drugs and alcohol are used as a "prosthetic"[4] to compensate for deficits in regulating affect life.

We will elaborate subsequently on the differences in the effects of the various classes of drugs, including alcohol, and how they interact with specific affect states to make them compelling. However, there is one more general aspect of drug–alcohol use involved in controlling feelings that I believe is important to review. I am referring to a paradoxical aspect of drug–alcohol dependency, namely, that as much as substances may be used to relieve distress and painful affect states, such a reliance also perpetuates and often worsens such states. Although at first this result might seem to be a case of enduring some distress in exchange for even momentary relief, more recently I have realized that substance abusers employ this negative effect in the service of controlling their suffering. In this instance, at least part of the "tradeoff" in accepting the pain of drug use involves converting the passive experience of not knowing or being able to access feelings, to an experience where one actively controls feelings, even if the feelings they produce are painful. This seems to apply especially to those patients I described who more often do not seem to feel or are devoid of feelings. Rather than just relieving painful affects when they are overwhelming, drugs and alcohol, and the distress they entail, may also be adopted as a way of being in control, especially when they feel out of control because affects are vague, elusive, and nameless.[28,29]

4.2. Well-Being and Self-Esteem

Basic states of well-being and positive self-regard derive from earliest stages of development. Addicts and alcoholics suffer with developmental deficits involving a failure to internalize the comforting, soothing, validating, and mobilizing aspects of their parenting or caretaking environment.[1]

I have been repeatedly impressed that drug and alcohol-dependent individuals are vulnerable around problems in soothing and calming themselves, especially when they are stressed and overwrought, and conversely, that they may also suffer with initiative and activation problems when their safety or well-being depends on taking action. Deriving from these basic states, but related to subsequent developmental challenges and need for mastery, substance abusers also suffer because they have not developed a sufficient capacity for self-esteem or self-love where they enjoy a confidence in themselves and their potential, and a balanced valuation of their importance in relation to self and others.[21,30]

Drug and alcohol effects interact with affect states and characterological or characteristic defenses related to states of disharmony, immobilization, and self-esteem in ways that relieve or alter the suffering entailed with these states. I discuss these interactions more specifically below. When substance abusers speak of the "high" or euphoria that they experience with drugs or alcohol, they are probably referring to the self-soothing, comfort, repair, and sense of well-being and power they cannot obtain or sustain within themselves or from others unless they resort to drugs or alcohol.[31-34]

4.3. Relationships

The problems addicts and alcoholics have in relation to regulating their feelings and maintaining their self-esteem make relating to and depending on others a precarious, if not erratic, experience. As much as they need others to know how they feel, they often fear and distrust their dependency, disavow their need, and act in counterdependent ways. Their defenses of self-sufficiency and disavowal leave them isolated and cut off, and they disguise from self and others their need for nurturance and validation, which is often excessive, given their developmental deficits. Consequently, there is a tendency to be inconsistent in satisfying their own and others' needs in relationships. They alternate between being selfless and demanding, but more chronically dissatisfied and cut off, and thus more susceptible to using drugs and alcohol to process emotions around their needs and wants.[1,2]

4.4. Self-Care

Because of the obvious dangers associated with acute and chronic use of drugs and alcohol, substance abusers are often accused (and they also accuse themselves) of harboring self-destructive motives. Some have suggested that addictive behavior is a form of "suicide on the installment plan." This kind of cynical, negative, destructive motive attributed to addicts derives from early drive psychology[35] and detracts from an empathic understanding of addicts' vulnerabilities. Addictive behavior is governed less by self-destructive motives but is more the result of developmental failures and deficits that leave certain individuals ill equipped to protect and take care of themselves. Along these lines we have proposed that addicts and alcoholics suffer with deficits or deficiencies in a capacity for self-care.[1,21,36] Although we first identified and described self-care deficits in opiate addicts,[1] we have continued to observe this vulnerability to varying degrees, in all substance abusers, including alcoholics and cocaine addicts.

The capacity for self-care or self-protection involves certain ego functions which serve and ensure survival. These functions include signal anxiety, judgments, reality testing, control, and the ability to make cause–consequence connections. The capacity for self-care is acquired and internalized from early and subsequent phases of childhood development, and it derives from the nurturing and protective roles and function of the child's parents. If adequately developed, the capacity for self-care assures appropriate planning, action, and anticipation of events to avoid mishaps or danger. Healthy self-care is apparent in adults in appropriate degrees of anticipatory affects, including embarrassment, shame, fear, worry, and so forth, when facing hazardous or harmful situations.[1,3,21,36]

As I have indicated, deficits or vulnerabilities in the capacity for self-care cut across all substance abusers. However, the degree of deficiency or disability in self-care may be variable over time in any one individual, but it is more global and pervasive in some types of addictions than others, for example, in certain polydrug addicts and more-so in intravenous drug abusers. Self-care functions may be better established in some individuals, but they may lapse or deteriorate under conditions of major stress, depression, or as a consequence of prolonged drug–alcohol use. These functions may also be overridden because for certain individuals survival concerns become subordinate to needs for relief from painful affect states or a drivenness to achieve or perform, which drug effects may enhance.[3] Whether this involves a lapse or is the result of more severe impairment, self-care problems in substance abusers are apparent in addicts and alcoholics in their failure or inability to adequately worry about, fear, or consider the long- and short-term complications and dangers associated with drugs and alcohol.

5. Drugs and Self-Medication

Most individuals who become and remain dependent on drugs and alcohol have experimented or tried many drugs and even continue to use more than one drug. However, if asked, most addicts will indicate they prefer a particular drug. Exploring psychological characteristics of such individuals reveals that the drug they select or prefer is a function of characteristic defenses, organization in personality style (or structure), and related affect states which dominate their inner emotional life and their relationships with others. Addicts and alcoholics have a special "discovery" that specific painful feeling states may be relieved or that pleasant, special states of well-being may be achieved through a particular drug.

If an analogy for personality structure and affects can be made to a container and the contents, respectively, one could then say that drugs exercise their effects in the way they alter or modify the container and the contents, the two main factors with which drugs interact. For some individuals, the container is too porous and the contents (e.g., rage and anger) pour out too readily, causing self and others much distress and disharmony. For others, the container is overly restrictive and sealed and thus constricts the experiencing and communication of a range of contained emotions. And for yet others, certain emotions or energy are depleted and diminished. Drugs and alcohol can modify or act on either the container (structure) or the contents (affects). There may be some duplication and overlap in effects from drugs, and depending on dose and setting, two different drugs might produce similar effects but based on different mechanisms of action. For example, both alcohol, in low to moderate doses, and cocaine enhance socialization. Alcohol dissolves the container and lets feelings out, whereas cocaine mobilizes the content and produces increased energy and euphoric feeling. Both effects enhance social interaction. On the other hand, alcohol in heavy doses, like opiates, may have a containing or muting effect on intense, painful emotions. Notwithstanding some of these similarities, the self-medication hypothesis rests on the assumption that the three main classes of drugs of abuse (i.e., stimulants, opiate–analgesics, and sedative–hypnotics) have distinctly different actions and effects.

The process whereby substance abusers discover that the particular action of a drug suits them best has been variously described as the "drug-of-choice,"[4] "the preferential use of drugs,"[6] "the self-selection process,"[37] and most recently, "the drug of commitment,"[34] In this section I discuss the appeal of stimulants and opiates, and in the next section, the appeal of the sedative–hypnotics, in particular, alcohol.

5.1. Stimulants

Within one decade cocaine has gone from being a relatively low-profile, elite, exclusive drug of glamorous, fast-living, and famous people, to a drug that pervades all strata of our society. Because it is the most widespread and prevalent stimulant of abuse, I will consider it the representative drug of the stimulant class of drugs.

The main desired effects of cocaine derive from its activating and energizing properties. It probably has wide appeal because its stimulating effects allure both low-energy- and high-energy-type individuals. For the former, cocaine helps to overcome fatigue and depletion states associated with depression[9,37] or relieves feelings of boredom and emptiness[7]; for high-energy individuals, cocaine provides increased feelings of assertiveness, self-esteem, and frustration tolerance[4] or "augments a hyperactive, restless lifestyle and an exaggerated need for self sufficiency (p. 100)."[38]

The affect states that respond to the stimulating action of cocaine are more often than not related to an individual's personality organization and defensive style which probably predispose to characteristic-associated states of depression, boredom, emptiness, and hyperactivity and make drug-seeking behavior and involvement more likely. Although an extensive review of these personality factors is not possible, the following are examples of factors that can contribute to cocaine use: (1) states of boredom and emptiness with which certain cocaine addicts suffer could be the basis on which they are described as "sensation" or "stimulus-seeking" personalities; (2) individuals who are overcompensating, ambitious, and driven in their character style use stimulants to augment their drive to achieve, or to compensate for their not infrequent collapse in self-esteem and depression when their ambitions fail; and (3) cocaine may act paradoxically to calm certain restless, emotionally labile individuals with attention deficit disorder.[3,9]

> *Case Vignette.* Sam, a 39-year-old, successful businessman, 1 year into recovery, poignantly demonstrated many of these features of distress and lifelong character flaws that set him up to "love" cocaine. Despite being very personable, handsome, and successful in his businesses, he complained of always being afraid of people, "out of touch with his desires and needs and pleasing people." Despite many sexual liaisons, he said until recently he never felt close to anyone, and more recently when he did, he "lost" himself in the relationship. He described how minor or major external events could rapidly flip his self-esteem. At these times he would fuel an insatiable need for love and admiration with cocaine. Action and activity, he said, was his main mode of coping, and cocaine provided the means to get started and continue moving. The drug would help him to overcome his overbearing depression and to feel empowered and attractive enough to literally cruise around and find a woman to satisfy his needs.

5.2. Opiate–Analgesics

In contrast to the stimulants, opiates principally have a muting and containing action. Although opiates mute and relieve physical pain (and on this basis we might surmise that they generally alleviate emotional pain—and they do), I have been impressed that they have a much more specific effect and appeal. Working more exclusively with narcotic addicts in the early 1970s in a methadone treatment program, I became impressed with how many of the narcotic addicts conveyed and demonstrated the muting and containing action of opiates on aggression and violent feelings.[8,39] A subsequent series of reports[7,40,41] described how individuals who prefer and have become dependent on opiates have had long-standing histories as victims of physical abuse and violence and in many cases often turned into the perpetrators of violence. Such people, whether victims or perpetrators, suffer with acute and chronic states of associated aggressive and rageful feelings. Individuals predisposed to opiates discover that these intense, disorganizing affects are significantly contained or attenuated when they first use opiates, and on this basis they described this action as "calming—feeling mellow—safe—[or]—normal for the first time."

In my experience, the problem with aggression in such individuals is a function of an excess of this intense affect—partly constitutional and partly environmental in origin—which interacts with ego and self structures that are underdeveloped or deficient and thus fail to contain this affect. Opiates are compelling because their anti-aggression/rage action mutes uncontrolled aggression and reverses internal psychological disorganization and the external threat of counteraggression with which these intense emotions are associated.[9,40]

> *Case Vignette.* A 47-year-old psychologist described graphically how her preference for the containing and soothing effects of opiates compensated for her inability to process emotional distress. Although she was more subdued at the time she offered the following complaints and concerns, early in treatment she had powerfully displayed an intensely angry and intemperate self when frustrated.
>
> Anticipating a stressful, overseas flight that day, she complained, "There's no place in my brain for [dealing with] discomfort." She was expecting to experience a "cranky sleeplessness" on the flight and worried that she would target her husband with her feelings. She was anticipating that her only alternative would be to use drugs. She pointed to a print portraying a mother comfortably and comfortingly holding a child and lamented that she could not calm or sooth herself. Not insignificantly she contrasted her lot to that of two other patients in group therapy who used alcohol to overcome inhibitions and to socialize.

6. Alcohol and Self-Medication

The patient in the last vignette perceptively and intuitively grasped how alcohol affects individuals who prefer it differently from the way it affects those who prefer opiates. Whereas opiate addicts brim with intense and most often angry feeling, alcoholics suffer because they more often are restricted and overcontained in the ways they experience and express emotion. Sedative–hypnotics including alcohol have appeal because these drugs relieve tense, anxious states associated with rigid, overdrawn defenses. The psychoanalyst Fenichel[42] quotes an unknown source that "the superego is that part of the mind that is soluble in alcohol." This quote corresponds better to the dynamics that are emphasized in early psychoanalytic formulations. These early views stressed that an overdrawn conscience could leave individuals conflicted and tense about sexual and aggressive drives and impulses and that alcohol acted on releasing individuals from their restrictive superego defenses. More recent formulations focus on ego defenses and the subjective aspects of self and self–other experiences.

In this section I chiefly use alcohol as the main and representative drug for the sedative–hypnotic class of substances. Beyond alcohol, the main types of drugs abused in this class have been the barbiturates (e.g., secobarbital) and the barbiturate-like (e.g., glutethimide) drugs. More recently, these drugs have been replaced by benzodiazepines. The abuse potential of the benzodiazepines is variable and to some degree seems to be a function of pharmacokinetics. On the other hand, a recent report suggested that states of distress ("probably—discomfort with people and one's surroundings, discontentment and dysphoria," p. 336) are greater in alcoholics and are probably the main determinants as well in the abuse of benzodiazepines. In this report, Ciraulo and associates[43] provided empirical support for self-medication factors in alcoholism. They showed that alcoholics react with a more positive change to the benzodiazepine alprazolam than controls do and therefore are more likely to abuse this drug. Notwithstanding the differences in form (i.e., a pill versus a drink) and meaning, there are enough similarities to use alcohol as the representative drug of this class of drugs to explore their appeal as self-medication agents.

6.1. Affects and Alcohol

Whereas early psychodynamic formulations stressed the dissolving or disinhibiting effect of alcohol on rigid superego mechanisms of defense, more contemporary formulations have placed greater emphasis on alcohol's effect on constricted ego defenses and subjective feelings involving the sense of self and self in relationships with other people. A modern song by Jimmy Buffet captures how alcohol releases feelings and allows him (and most likely others) to enjoy a better sense of well-being within himself:

> I drink a lot of whiskey
> It gives me such a glow
> It makes me quite immobile
> But it let's my feelings show.
> "Brahma Fear"

As I have suggested, some substance abusers, like this artist and others, suffer because they cannot feel their feelings. Our current understanding of why it is that certain individuals cannot feel and need substances to do so is not entirely clear. Some argue that certain patients who are totally out of touch with feelings are "disaffected" and use drugs and activity to ameliorate feelingless, lifeless states related to primitive defenses against anxieties associated with rage and terror.[26] This formulation is reminiscent of conflict psychology, but on a more archaic level. Others[5] have proposed that feeling life is underdeveloped in alcoholics and that affects, when underdeveloped, tend to remain somatized, not differentiated (i.e., alcoholics cannot distinguish anxiety from depression) and not verbalized ("alexithymia"). Whether deriving from conflict or developmental deficits, sedative–hypnotic abusers' descriptions of their experience may better convey how their preferred drugs alter their feelings, as the following example demonstrates:

> *Case Vignette.* A 30-year-old divorcée, brought up by a restricted and restricting mother and an alcoholic father, withdrew from her family and engaged in much promiscuous activity while a teenager to avoid, in particular, her mother's harsh and critical attitudes. She married in her early twenties and almost totally reversed her behavior and attitudes, adopting strict measures of propriety. By her late twenties, dissatisfaction in her unsatisfactory marriage ultimately left her with a chronic sense of dysphoria and disabling migraine headaches. She dramatically discovered that the barbiturates in a commonly prescribed drug for headaches relieved more than her physical distress. Describing the drug effects, she said, "It's wonderful—[it] relieves the boredom and fills the void."

6.2. Well-Being, Self-Esteem, and Alcohol

For some, the principal reason for using alcohol or related drugs is to just feel, as the previous case example and Jimmy Buffet's song suggests. For others, it is to feel better inside oneself or to feel better about oneself. Much of this had to do with splits in personality organization which wall off comforting, soothing, and validating parts of self and do not allow a person to provide these functions for self. Krystal and Raskin[5] and Krystal[32] have proposed that this class of drugs has appeal because the drugs dissolve exaggerated defenses of denial and splitting. For some, alcohol allows the brief and therefore safe experience of loving and aggressive feelings which are otherwise "walled off" and leave such individuals feeling cut off and empty. Others discover that the soothing effect of alcohol calms internal clamor and emotional "noise," as the following example shows:

> *Case Vignette.* A 40-year-old psychiatrist described her nightly dependence on a bottle of wine as a means of achieving a sense of "bliss, harmony, and oneness." She emphasized that it was the only time she felt "all right," and that she drank "to maintain a blissful oneness with the

world." Although in her recovery she was discovering that Alcoholics Anonymous, jogging, and music could get her outside of the "inner [emotional] noise," she described how she still had to fight the other alternative that would immediately "quiet the nose," namely, the alcohol.

6.3. Relationships and Alcohol

The notion of alcohol as a superego solvent partly explains why certain tense, neurotically inhibited individuals "enjoy" alcohol as a social lubricant and why this effect is enjoyed by many more in Western cultures for purposes of socializing and partying. Its main attraction, however, is more likely related to more deeply seated defenses related to discomfort and fears about human closeness, dependency, and intimacy. Both superego and ego defenses may, nevertheless, rigidly coalesce in such individuals to leave them feeling chronically distant, cut off, and cold in relationships with significant others. It is often under these conditions that certain predisposed people have a powerful and often dramatic realization as to what alcohol and sedative–hypnotics can do. A popular author–lecturer describes how a child rigidly internalizes harsh parental controls, and subsequently, how the resultant strictures in personality yield to the discovery of drug-alcohol effects:

> So you couldn't be mad, you couldn't be sad, you couldn't be glad. You became a walking uptight. Then when you put the chemical in your body—pow! You could relax for the very first time. You were functional! You could feel your feelings, dance, talk to girls. I'm alive! Alive! (p. 89).[44]

7. Conclusion

Self-medication factors play an important role in the development of a reliance on drugs and alcohol. Each class of drugs-of-abuse interacts with painful affect states and related personality factors to make an individual's preferred drug appealing and compelling. Addicts and alcoholics share in common general problems in self-regulation involving difficulties with affect life, self-esteem, relationships, and self-care. These self-regulation problems combine to make people more desperate, driven, isolated, and impulsive and more likely to assume the risks of drug–alcohol seeking and drug and alcohol-using behavior. Addiction-prone individuals discover which drug suits them best through the unique qualities of their affect experience, and these choices are what distinguish addicts and alcoholics from each other.

Given that all humans more or less struggle with self-regulation issues, what probably distinguishes substance abusers in general from nonsubstance abusers is the way capacities to experience and regulate feeling interact with the capacity to manage and contain behavior or impulses. We need to study further how, for example, basic states of well-being, a healthy regard for self and others, and mature self-care protect against addictive and alcoholic dependence. Considerable clinical and empirical evidence has accumulated over the past two decades indicating that it is probably the malignant combination of defects in regulating affects and self-care, or problems in managing feelings and impulses, that are the necessary and sufficient deficiencies to produce addiction and alcoholism. Addictive and alcoholic solutions, then, are a way of compensating for self-regulation problems that individuals cannot otherwise correct on their own.[33,34,45,46] Unfortunately, such solutions are short-lived and the attempts at self-correction backfire and fail.

References

1. Khantzian EJ: The ego, the self and opiate addiction: Theoretical and treatment considerations. *Int Rev Psychoanal* 5:189–198, 1978.
2. Khantzian EJ: An ego-self theory of substance dependence, in Lettieri EJ, Sayers M, Wallenstein HW (eds): *Theories of Addiction*. NIDA Monograph #30. Rockville, MD, National Institute on Drug Abuse, 1980, pp 29–33. Also published in revised form. Psychopathological causes and consequences of drug dependence, in Gottheil E, Druley KA, Skoloda TE, Waxman H (eds): *Etiological Aspects of Alcohol and Drug Abuse*. Springfield, IL, Charles Thomas, 1983, pp 89–97.
3. Khantzian EJ: Self-regulation factors in cocaine dependence: A clinical perspective, in *The Epidemiology of Cocaine Use and Abuse*. NIDA Mongraph. Rockville, MD, National Institute on Drug Abuse, 1988, in press.
4. Weider H, Kaplan EH: Drug use in adolescents: Psychodynamic meaning and pharmacogenic effect. *Psychoanal Study Child* 24:399–431, 1969.
5. Krystal H, Raskin HA: *Drug Dependence: Aspects of Ego Functions*. Detroit, Wayne State University Press, 1970.
6. Milkman H, Frosch WA: On the preferential abuse of heroin and emphetamine. *J Nerv Ment Dis* 156:242–248, 1973.
7. Wurmser L: Psychoanalytic considerations of the etiology of compulsive drug use. *J Am Psychoanal Assoc* 22:820–843, 1974.
8. Khantzian EJ: Opiate addiction: A critique of theory and some implications for treatment. *Am J Psychother* 28:59–70, 1974.
9. Khantzian EJ: The self-medication hypothesis of addictive disorders: Focus on heroin and cocaine dependence. *Am J Psychiatry* 142(11):1259–1264, 1985.
10. Woody GE, O'Brien CP, Rickels K: Depression and anxiety in heroin addicts: A placebo-controlled study of doxepin in combination with methadone. *Am J Psychiatry* 132:447–450, 1975.
11. McLellan AT, Woody GE, O'Brien CP: Development of psychiatric illness in drug abusers. *N Engl J Med* 201:1310–1314, 1979.
12. Dorus W, Senay EC: Depression, demographic dimension, and drug abuse. *Am J Psychiatry* 137:699–704, 1980.
13. Weissman MM, Slobetz F, Prusoff B, Merritz M, Howard P: Clinical depression among narcotic addicts maintained on methadone in the community. *Am J Psychiatry* 133:1434–1438, 1976.
14. Rounsaville BJ, Weissman MM, Kleber H, Wilber, C: Heterogeneity of psychiatric diagnosis in treated opiate addicts. *Arch Gen Psychiatry* 39:161–166, 1982.
15. Rounsaville BJ, Weissman MM, Crits-Cristoph K, Wilber C, Kleber H: Diagnosis and symptoms of depression in opiate addicts: Course and relationship to treatment outcome. *Arch Gen Psychiatry* 39:151–156, 1982.
16. Treece C, Nicholson B: DSM-III personality type and dose levels in methadone maintenance patients. *J Nerv Ment Dis* 168:621–628, 1980.

17. Nicholson B, Treece C: Object relations and differential treatment response to methadone maintenance. *J Nerv Ment Dis* 169:424–429, 1981.
18. Khantzian EJ, Treece C: DSM-III psychiatric diagnosis of narcotic addicts: Recent findings. *Arch Gen Psychiatry* 42:1067–1071, 1985.
19. Blatt SJ, Berman W, Bloom-Feshback S, Sugarman A, Wilber C, Kelber H: Psychological assessment of psychopathology in opiate addicts. *J Nerv Ment Dis* 172:156–165, 1984.
20. Woody GE, Luborsky L, McLellen AT, O'Brien CP, Beck AT, Blaine J, Herman I, Hole A: Psychotherapy for opiate addicts. *Arch Gen Psychiatry* 40:639–645, 1983.
21. Khantzian EJ, Mack JE: A.A. and contemporary psychodynamic theory, in Galanter M (ed): *Recent Development in Alcoholism, Vol 7.* New York, Plenum Press, 1989, pp. 67–89.
22. Vaillant GE: National history of male psychological health. VIII: Antecedents of alcoholism and "orality." *Am J Psychiatry* 137:181–186, 1980.
23. Cummings CP, Prokop CK, Cosgrove R: Dysphoria: The cause of the result of addiction. *Psychiatric Hosp* 16:131–134, 1985.
24. Martin WR, Hewett BB, Baker AJ, Haertzen CA: Aspects of the psychopathology and pathophysiology of addiction. *Drug Alcohol Dependence* 2:185–202, 1977.
25. Martin WR, Haertzen CA, Hewett BB: Psychopathology and pathophysiology of narcotic addicts, alcoholics, and drug abusers, in Lipton VA, DiMascio A, Killam KF (eds): *Psychopharmacology: A Generation of Progress.* New York, Raven Press, 1978.
26. McDougall J: The "dis-affected" patient: Reflection on affect pathology. *Psychoanal Q* 53:386–409, 1984.
27. Krystal H: Alexithymia and the effectiveness of psychoanalytic treatment. *Int J Psychoanal Psychother* 9:353–388, 1982.
28. Khantzian EJ: A clinical perspective of the cause-consequence controversy in alcoholic and addictive suffering. *J Am Acad Psychoanal* 15(4):521–537, 1987.
29. Khantzian EJ: Substance dependence, repetition and the nature of addictive suffering. Unpublished manuscript.
30. Mack JE: Alcoholism, A.A. and the governance of the self, in Bean MH, Zinberg NE (eds): *Dynamic Approaches to the Understanding and Treatment of Alcoholism.* New York, Free Press, 1981, pp 125–162.
31. Khantzian EJ, Mack JE, Schatzberg AF: Heroin use as an attempt to cope: Clinical observations. *Am J Psychiatry* 131:160–164, 1974.
32. Krystal H: Self-representation and the capacity for self care. *Annu Psychoanal* 6:209–246, 1977.
33. Woolcott P: Addiction: Clinical and theoretical considerations. *Annu Psychoanal* 9:189–204, 1980.
34. Spotts JV, Shontz FC: Drug induced ego states: A trajectory theory of drug experience. *Soc Pharmacol* 1:19–51, 1987.
35. Khantzian EJ, Treece C: Psychodynamics of drug dependence: An overview, in Blaine JD, Julius DA (eds): *Psychodynamics of Drug Dependence.* NIDA Monograph #12. Rockville, MD, National Institute on Drug Abuse, 1977, pp 11–25.
36. Khantzian EJ, Mack JE: Self-preservation and the care of the self - ego instincts reconsidered. *Psychoanal Stud Child* 38:209–232, 1983.
37. Khantzian EJ: Self-selection and progression in drug dependence. *Psychiatry Digest* 10:19–22, 1975.
38. Khantzian EJ: Impulse problems in addiction: Cause and effect relationships, in Wishnie H (ed): *Working with the Impulsive Person.* New York, Plenum Press, 1979, pp 97–112.
39. Khantzian EJ: Preliminary dynamic formulation of the psychopharmacologic action of methadone, in *Proceedings of the Fourth National Methadone Conference, San Francisco, 1972.* New York, National Association for the Prevention of Addiction to Narcotics, 1972.
40. Khantzian EJ: Psychological (structural) vulnerabilities and the specific appeal of narcotics. *Ann NY Acad Sci* 398:24–32, 1982.
41. Vereby K (ed): Opiods in Mental Illness: Theories, clinical observations, and treatment possibilities. *Ann NY Acad Sci* 168:621–628, 1982.
42. Fenichel O: *The Psychoanalytic Theory of Neurosis.* New York, Norton, 1945.

43. Ciraulo DA, Barnhill JC, Greenblatt DJ: Abuse liability and clinical pharmacokinetics of al-prazolam in alcoholic men. *J Clin Psychiatry* 49:333–337, 1988.
44. Bradshaw J: Our families, ourselves. *Self Center*, September/October 1988.
45. Khantzian EJ: A contemporary psychodynamic approach to drug abuse treatment. *Am J Drug Alcohol Abuse* 12(3):213–222, 1986.
46. Donovan JM: An etiologic model of alcoholism. *Am J Psychiatry* 143:1–11, 1986.

Treating Combined Alcohol and Drug Abuse in Community-Based Programs

Robert L. Hubbard

Abstract. The key issues in effective treatment of combined alcohol and drug abuse are identified as comprehensive diagnosis, effective services, and long-term recovery. Empirical data from community-based alcohol and drug treatment studies are presented, illustrating the extent of combined abuse, the lack of treatment for combined abuse, and the negative effects of combined abuse on treatment outcomes. Reconsideration is given to issues such as the concentration of diagnosis on a primary pattern of abuse, the orientation toward concurrent treatment of combined abuse, the requirement of immediate abstinence vs. gradual reduction of combined abuse patterns, and the role of relapse in recovery from combined abuse.

1. Introduction

The diagnosis and treatment of combined alcohol and drug abuse was identified as a major concern for community-based programs[1,2] in the 1980s. Current epidemiological trends and data from programs indicate that treatment of combined abuse will continue to be a major concern through the 1990s.

The combined abuse of alcohol and such drugs as marijuana, cocaine, and heroin persists in creating significant problems across health, legal, psychological, and social domains. The use of multiple drugs of abuse, especially marijuana and cocaine in combination with alcohol, is common. Among persons entering treatment, patterns of use became more complex during the 1970s and 1980s.[2] Between 1985 and 1987, treatment admissions for cocaine abuse in state-funded programs doubled.[3] A rapid proliferation of private, short-term inpatient "substance abuse" programs has emerged from what was a system based on traditional 12-step program to treat alcoholism.[4] Anecdotal reports indicate these programs now attract large numbers of working and middle-class cocaine abusers covered by private health insurance.[5] There

Robert L. Hubbard • Alcohol and Drug Abuse Research, Research Triangle Institute, Research Triangle Park, North Carolina 27709.

is increasing recognition of the need for alcoholism treatment in traditional publicly funded drug abuse treatment programs, particularly methadone and therapeutic community modalities.

Despite the clear evidence of increases in the problem of combined alcohol and drug abuse, and initial recommendations and guidelines for treatment and diagnosis, the nature and treatment of combined alcohol and drug abuse are still often misunderstood, ignored, or accorded less priority than the "primary" drug of abuse. Major clinical and research questions remain to be answered about combined alcohol and drug use.

- How should combined alcohol and drug abuse be diagnosed?
- What is the most effective treatment regimen for combined abuse?
- How can recovery rates be sustained?

This chapter builds on previous discussion of these issues in the combined treatment of multiple substance abuse.[1] The major emphasis is on a practical approach to treating combined alcohol and drug abuse problems in community-based programs. These programs often have limited access to state-of-the-art clinical and research knowledge.

2. Estimations and Nature of Alcohol and Drugs and Extent of Combined Use

The rapid escalation of drug use through the 1970s, coupled with the persisting high rates of alcohol abuse, resulted in large numbers of individuals who have the combined problems of alcohol and drug abuse. Estimates are that 18–20 million U.S. residents used marijuana in 1985 and 4–6 million used cocaine.[6] A national survey in 1984 reported that one in five men and 1 in 20 women report consuming 45 or more drinks a month.[7] These data and other information indicate that about 18 million residents are estimated to have alcohol problems. Ongoing studies of high-school seniors[8] and reviews of epidemiological research indicate younger abusers are very likely to abuse both alcohol and drugs.[9]

One can only speculate on the potential impact of combined abuse for treatment in the future. Five million youths aged 12–17 have tried marijuana and one million have tried cocaine.[6] Between 20 and 30% of high-school students report being drunk six or more times in a year.[10] Most youths who abuse drugs also evidence problems with alcohol. The effects of this rapid escalation in combined use and its consequences have only begun to be seen in the treatment system.[11,12] In the next 10–20 years it is likely that these younger abusers of both alcohol and drugs will dominate the treatment population. Available data only indicate the potential scope of the task for clinicians in the future.

The role of alcohol abuse among drug abusers has been well documented, particularly for opioid abusers. Estimates of the extent of alcohol use among drug abuse treatment clients vary, depending on the study, the treatment population, and the definition of alcohol use employed. In reviews of prior research,[14] reported rates of alcoholism among opioid abusers entering methadone clinics vary between 5 and 45%; rates of alcohol abuse among those entering methadone treatment vary between 20 and 53%[15]; and between 20 and 30% of heroin addicts are estimated to have a past or current drinking problem.[16] Regardless of the nature of the definition or the precision of the estimates, it can be concluded that a large proportion of methadone treatment clients are alcohol abusers or alcoholics.

The extensive research on multiple substance abuse population has described the array of drugs abused by those who are not involved with opioids. The National Drug/Alcohol Collaboration Project documented abuse of two or more drugs by 80% of the population.[1] In a sample of 11 outpatient drug-free treatment programs, 15% of the admissions who had not used opioids abused multiple nonopioids, including alcohol, 25% abused one nonopioid and alcohol, and about half abused marijuana and alcohol. The increasing epidemic of cocaine abuse is often accompanied by alcohol abuse. Alcohol can be used as a depressant to "control or titrate cocaine's antagonistic stimulant-depressant effect."[17] The data on the extent of alcohol abuse among cocaine admissions are limited. One study reports 27% of cocaine abusers entering treatment are alcohol abusers.[18]

Evidence of drug abuse among alcoholics and problem drinkers has been documented over the past 60 years.[19] Estimates were that about one in five abused drugs. The emergence of multiple drug abuse by younger clients suggests that this proportion will increase substantially through the 1990s. In a younger population of Driving While Intoxicated (DWI) arrestees referred to outpatient treatment, half reported some marijuana use, and about one in five reported cocaine or other stimulant use.[20] The belief that many cocaine abusers seek treatment in traditional alcohol treatment modalities suggests that the issues of combined use will become an increasing problem for alcohol treatment.

3. Combined Alcohol and Drug Problems in Two Samples of Community Programs

Although the existence of combined alcohol and drug abuse has received considerable attention, the role of combined use in treatment and its effects on outcomes have received less attention. Alcohol abuse among drug abuse treatment clients may significantly detract from the treatment process. Alcohol users are more frequently discharged from drug abuse treatment programs and have poorer treatment outcomes than those who do not use alcohol.[21] Drug abuse clients who are dually addicted or who have histories of alcohol abuse have higher rates of psychopathology, medical complications, and criminal activity than those without drinking problems.[22] The effects of drug abuse on alcohol treatment outcomes have seldom been explored. Key questions that need to be addressed by careful research include the following:

Is combined alcohol and drug abuse diagnosed?
If diagnosed, how is combined abuse treated?
If treated, how effective is the treatment?
What is the effect of continued abuse of alcohol on drug use and the effect of continued drug use on alcohol abuse after treatment?

Data from two studies of publicly funded, community-based treatment programs provide some early data on these questions. The first study[23] involved a national sample of 11,000 drug abuse treatment clients in 12 methadone, 14 residential, and 11 outpatient drug-free programs which were publicly funded. These clients entered treatment between 1979 and 1981 and were followed up to 5 years after leaving treatment. The second study[24] involved a random sample of 400 clients in a statewide system who had terminated treatment in residential and outpatient alcohol treatment programs.

Alcohol was commonly and extensively used by clients entering drug abuse treatment programs and may interfere with rehabilitation. Data on use, heavier drinking, and problems were obtained by self-report. Outpatient drug-free programs had a higher percentage of clients who use any alcohol (84%) than other modalities. Methadone clients were least likely to drink any alcohol (66%) and least likely to drink heavily. The highest proportions of heavy drinkers were found in the residential programs. The proportion of heavy drinkers among drinkers ranged from a low of 38% in methadone programs to a high of 61% in residential programs.

The high rates of heavy use are strong evidence that alcohol abuse was common. About 4 of 10 clients reported that they got drunk during the 3 months before entering treatment. However, about one in four residential and outpatient drug-free program clients reported being drunk on 20 or more days during that 3-month period.

Upon entry into a drug abuse treatment program, about one in five clients expressed a need for alcohol abuse treatment. The proportion perceiving a need for alcohol treatment varied among modalities, from about 36% of residential clients to about 7% of methadone maintenance clients. Overall, about one client in seven felt that alcohol use was either a primary or a secondary reason for seeking treatment; about a third of the residential clients felt that way.

In the statewide alcohol treatment system, over half of the residential clients used drugs in addition to alcohol: 30% were users of marijuana only and another 20% used other drugs in addition to marijuana. About one-third of outpatient clients had a secondary drug of abuse; 21% used only marijuana and another 8% used marijuana and other drugs. Although many programs treated both alcohol and drug abuse, all clients in this study were diagnosed by the programs as entering treatment primarily for alcohol problems.

Despite the evidence that combined alcohol and drug abuse is common among clients, treatment was seldom provided for more than one substance. In drug abuse treatment only 25% of residential and 10% of outpatient drug-free clients who reported problematic drinking received treatment for alcohol problems. Virtually no methadone clients received treatment for alcohol abuse. The analyses of alcohol abuse during and after treatment revealed little change and no effect of treatment duration. More detailed bivariate and multivariate analyses conducted for this chapter for the small numbers of clients receiving treatment for alcohol abuse showed this treatment did not significantly reduce their alcohol use.

A similar pattern emerged in the study of the statewide alcohol treatment programs. Although most of the programs provided services for both alcohol and drug abuse, less than half the clients reporting drug abuse received treatment for drug abuse. Again, multivariate analyses did not indicate a significant effect of the treatment on reducing drug abuse among clients treated principally for alcohol abuse.

The need to treat combined alcohol and drug abuse is illustrated in the results of analysis of outcomes. Multivariate logistic regression analyses were employed to examine the effects of patterns of "secondary" alcohol and drug abuse on the "primary" treatment outcome of alcohol or drug use. These models statistically controlled for sex, race, age, source of referral, prior treatment, pretreatment pattern of alcohol or drug abuse, and time in treatment. The odds of regular use of the primary drug of abuse are 2–3 times greater for drug abuse treatment clients who report heavier alcohol use after treatment than for clients who use alcohol less extensively. Similarly, alcohol treatment clients who use drugs after treatment are 3–4 times more likely to relapse in the year after treatment than those who abstain from drugs. These results suggest reduction of use of alcohol or drugs may reduce the chance of relapse for the other substances. The causal relationships and ordering of alcohol and drug abuse after treatment, however, need to be examined in more detail.

4. Issues in Treating Combined Alcohol and Drug Abuse

Three key issues must be considered when attempting to deal with combined alcohol and drug abuse. First, there must be a careful diagnosis of the nature and extent of combined abuse. Second, therapeutic regimens and services must be developed that effectively treat the combined abuse. Finally, combined abuse must be considered in the evaluation of the recovery process and the need for subsequent aftercare and treatment readmission.

4.1. Diagnosis

The diagnosis of alcohol dependence or abuse is difficult and there are few agreed-upon approaches. Similarly, the extension of these dependence measures to drug abuse is even more difficult. Given the problematic nature of defining a particular type of abuse or dependence, it is even more difficult to develop a system to clearly diagnose alcohol and drug dependence. One of the problems is the difficulty in obtaining accurate reports. Inaccurate or incomplete information on the complex array of alcohol and drug abuse can confound an appropriate diagnosis. These difficulties have been outlined previously[1] and are not repeated here. The following discussion assumes that accurate and complete information can be obtained. If accurate information is available, the question becomes how to best organize it to develop a useful diagnosis.

A number of problems confound the diagnosis of combined alcohol and drug abuse. Individuals may abuse or be dependent on a particular substance and have problematic use of the other. The distinction of dependence on a particular drug, however, becomes blurred because of the concurrent or sequential use of both. Alcohol and drugs may serve different functions in the combined abuse pattern, making a clear definition of dependence difficult. A further problem involves the self-definition of the client because of social norms or the definition for administrative and fiscal purposes imposed by a bifurcated treatment system. Thus, problems and dependence symptoms may be attributed to one substance solely because of an attribution process rather than a careful self-diagnosis by the client or in-depth interviews by the clinician.

A final problem is the difficulty in separating the usage patterns causing various symptoms or indicators of dependence. A number of studies have demonstrated that substances are used together and their combined use, in fact, describes a dependence pattern.[25] For example, cocaine and alcohol,[6] alcohol and marijuana,[26] heroin and cocaine are all patterns of abuse that cannot be easily disentangled.

Because of the difficult problems in developing any meaningful separation, current efforts to describe and diagnose abuse dependence within current frameworks are outmoded. One of the major stumbling blocks to describing abuse and dependence for combined alcohol and drug abuse is the emphasis on the primary drug of abuse. In place of the focus on a primary drug, a more detailed typology needs to be developed considering the full array of drugs that are being abused. This is not to say an index pattern of alcohol or a particular drug (i.e., heroin, cocaine) should not be specified. An index pattern serves a useful purpose. An index pattern would be identified and various combinations of drugs and alcohol within that pattern could be identified. For example, alcohol can be the index drug and subtypes would include the use of various other types of drugs such as alcohol–cocaine patterns. Various cocaine patterns could be identified as the index pattern and amplified also by different levels and types of alcohol abuse. Ideally, both approaches should be considered.

Second, it is equally important in diagnosing combined alcohol and drug dependence to understand the functional significance of patterns of alcohol and drugs. Because of the synergistic and interactive effects of various drug and alcohol combinations,[2] consideration of the functional role of each may need to be incorporated into the diagnosis. Not only should the index drug be identified, but those important functional combinations should also be indicated, especially for combined use of alcohol and cocaine or alcohol and marijuana. Various functional combinations may suggest very different types and levels of clinical interventions. Our current knowledge of effective clinical approaches to combined abuse is limited.

A third approach to diagnosis is a consideration of the consequences of combined abuse. In most diagnostic frameworks, consequences are the primary behaviors used to identify dependence. Alcohol and drugs, however, each have different personal and social significance. One key distinction is the illegality of most drugs and the legal availability of alcohol. Types of consequences must be considered within the criminal and medical frameworks. Consequences may be due more to social norms or individual attitudes rather than to actual dependence.

In summary, it is critical to obtain accurate information for diagnosis. The basic diagnostic framework, however, must go beyond accurate descriptive information. Information must be organized in such a way that it can be used by the clinician and the client for maximum benefit in treatment. The use of a primary alcohol or drug categorization may, in fact, perpetuate stereotypes and the separation of alcohol and drug abuse treatment. A full description of the total array of drugs used with their functional significance is recommended in order to describe various types of dependence in place of a simple alcohol, drug, or multiple substance dependence model.

4.2. Treatment

The current thinking on the treatment of multiple substance abuse suggests that alcohol and drugs should be treated as a combined problem. Most programs are increasingly recognizing that both alcohol and drug abuse must be treated.[27,28] A critical question is how each or both should be treated and when.

Typically substance abuse treatment programs emphasize abstinence from all substances and treat both drugs and alcohol similarly.[4] The typical regime would be a 28-day inpatient program followed by longer-term aftercare and outpatient continuing care. On the other hand, most traditional publicly funded drug abuse treatment programs have focused on drugs that are perceived as more serious, such as opioids[28] and cocaine.[29] Alcohol in many ways was seen as unimportant or as a secondary problem to be treated at a later time or with an ancillary service. The wisdom of both approaches may need to be combined.

Clearly, there is a need for concurrent consideration of alcohol and drug abuse. On the other hand, in many ways both the pharmacological and social implications of alcohol and drug abuse are so different than they may require separate consideration.[30] The functions of combined abuse can suggest whether a concurrent or sequential approach is most appropriate. A sequential program that focuses on the more serious substance in terms of life functioning may need to occur first. There is substantial evidence that heroin addiction can be substantially reduced without concurrent reductions in alcohol abuse.[31] Within a long-term continuum of care approach, it may be more effective to reduce first the principal abuse pattern with follow-up services to reduce residual use.

Ideally, abstinence is a goal at each point in treatment. Realistically, in drug abuse treatment programs, this would be difficult if impossible to achieve with a single treatment episode. Furthermore, in alcohol treatment programs, relapse is often a fundamental part of the recovery process.[32] Anecdotal reports indicate that clients abusing alcohol may feel that, because they are alcoholics, marginal use of other drugs may not interfere with the recovery process from alcohol. The fact that many recovering abusers may test this hypothesis must be considered in the assessment of the recovery process.

In summary, the separate and sequential treatment of alcohol and drugs needs to be carefully examined. Alcohol and drugs are considered separately, both within the abuser's life-style and in society at large. Further, alcohol and drugs differ in their legal availability. Pharmacologically there is a major difference in readdiction liability for various substances. Given these differences, it is logical to have a clear separation of the major patterns of abuse. Whether to treat alcohol and drugs concurrently or sequentially is, in fact, a clinical decision for which little evidence is now available. Concurrent treatment is a fundamental aspect of an abstinence-oriented 12-step approach essential to the goals of alcoholism and substance abuse treatment programs. The sequential approach is a fundamental aspect of the social functioning model more prevalent in community-based drug abuse treatment programs. Regardless of the approach, it is critical that patterns of alcohol and drug abuse be treated with a carefully developed treatment plan and followed up with appropriate clinical intervention. Clearly the goal should be abstinence during and after treatment. The fundamental question is: What is the most effective, long-term treatment regimen for long-term recovery?

4.3. The Recovery Process

Fundamental to the recovery from alcohol and drug abuse is a clear understanding of the role alcohol and drugs play in relapse. Little research describes the temporal ordering of alcohol and drug abuse in relapse. In many cases they may cooccur. If so, it is more likely that this is a combined dependence symptom rather than an alcohol and drug problem. One of the fundamental aspects of the recovery process is to integrate the social support systems for individuals recovering from abuse of both alcohol and drugs. The simple differentiation of Alcoholics Anonymous (AA), Narcotics Anonymous (NA), or Cocaine Anonymous, however, implies a primary drug problem.

This may be counterproductive to successful social support for recovery from combined abuse of alcohol and drugs. The integration of alcohol issues into NA programs and of drug issues into AA programs needs to be encouraged. Because of the traditional values of both fellowships, this may require substantial reeducation and reorientation.

The second major question involves how to treat relapse to the "secondary" drug or alcohol abuse pattern. In an integrated program, this relapse would suggest the need for increased aftercare or treatment readmission in order to preclude subsequent relapse to the primary abuse pattern. A full understanding of this more complex recovery process from combined abuse is necessary. Unfortunately, the concentration on specific drugs of abuse has precluded the overall understanding of the nature of this more complex recovery process. Further clinical and research understanding of how the recovery process from combined alcohol and drug abuse compares and contrasts with the recovery from dependence primarily on alcohol and drugs is needed.

5. Summary

The task facing clinicians now treating alcohol and drug abuse is far more complex than in the past. In an era of increasing questions about the effectiveness of alcohol treatment and drug abuse treatment, another layer of complexity is not welcome. Given the complex patterns of alcohol and drug abuse, consideration of this complexity is essential. In the next decade combined alcohol and drug problems will be the normative problem which must be treated. Much of our knowledge and beliefs about treatment and recovery may, in fact, not apply to individuals with complex combined alcohol and drug abuse patterns. Clinicians and program directors must work to further integration of combined alcohol and drug abuse treatment. How this is best accomplished is a clinical decision which must be based on a sound, empirical understanding of processes and effectiveness. Much conventional wisdom and current approaches may need to be discarded or revised. In fact, the challenge of combined alcohol and drug abuse suggests that we step back and take a new look at many of the basic types of approaches that have heretofore been the mainstay of the treatment system. Specifically, these include the concentration on a primary drug of abuse, the orientation toward concurrent treatment of combined abuse, the requirement of immediate abstinence vs. gradual reduction of combined abuse patterns, and the role of relapse in recovery from combined abuse. If we consider each of these issues carefully and develop empirical knowledge, we can hope to develop more effective treatment for combined alcohol and drug abuse.

References

1. Carroll JFX: Treating multiple substance abuse clients, in Galanter M (ed): *Recent Developments in Alcoholism, Vol 4*. New York, Plenum Press, 1986, pp 85–103.

 2. Hubbard RL, Bray RM, Craddock SG, Cavanaugh ER, Schlenger WE, Rachal JV: Issues in the assessment of multiple drug use among drug treatment clients, in Braude MC, Ginzburg HM (eds): *Strategies for Research on the Interaction of Drugs of Abuse* Washington, DC, U.S. Department of Health and Human Services, NIDA Research Monograph 68, 1986 pp 15–40.
 3. NASADAD: State resources and services related to alcohol and drug abuse problems, fiscal year 1987: An analysis of state alcohol and drug abuse profile date. Washington, DC, NASADAD, 1988.
 4. Cook CCH: The Minnesota model in the management of drug and alcohol dependency: Miracle, method or myth? Part I. The philosophy and the program. *Br J Addict* 83:625–634, 1988.
 5. Blume SB: Alcohol problems in cocaine abusers, in Washton, AM, Gold MS (eds): *Cocaine: A Clinician's Handbook.* New York, Guilford Press, 1987, pp 202–207.
 6. NIDA: *National Household Survey on Drug Abuse: Main Findings 1985.* Rockville, MD, National Institute on Drug Abuse, 1988.
 7. Hilton ME, Clark WB: Changes in American drinking patterns and problems, 1967–1984. *J Stud Alcohol* 48:515–522, 1987.
 8. Johnston LD, O'Malley PM, Bachman JG: *Highlights from Drugs and American High School Students, 1975–1983.* DHHS Pub. No. (ADM) 84-1317. Washington, DC, Supt. of Documents, U.S. Government Printing Office, 1984.
 9. Clayton RR: Multiple drug use: Epidemiology, correlates and consequences in Galanter M (ed): *Combined Alcohol and Drug Use Problems.* New York, Plenum Press, 1986, pp 1–38.
10. Rachal JV, Guess LL, Hubbard RL, Maisto SA, Cavanaugh ER, Waddell R, Benrud CH: *Adolescent Drinking Behavior, Vol I; the Extent and Nature of Adolescent Alcohol and Drug Use: The 1974 and 1978 National Sample Studies.* Research Triangle Park, NC, Research Triangle Institute, 1980.
11. Kleinman PH, Wish ED, Deren S, Rainone GA: Multiple drug use: A symptomatic behavior. *J Psychoactive Drugs* 18:77–86, 1986.
12. Holland S, Griffin A: Adolescent and adult drug treatment clients: Patterns and consequences of use. *J Psychoactive Drugs* 16:79–89, 1984.
13. Barr HL, Cohen A: *The Problem Drinking Drug Addict.* NIDA Services Research Administrative Report. Rockville, MD, National Institute on Drug Abuse, 1979.
14. Stimmel B, Cohen M, Sturiano V, Hanbury R, Korts D, Jackson G: Is treatment for alcoholism effective in persons on methadone maintenance? *Am J Psychiatry* 140:862–866, 1983.
15. Hunt DE, Strug DL, Goldsmith DS, Lipton DS, Robert K, Truitt L. Alcohol use and abuse: Heavy drinking among methadone clients. *Am J Drug Alcohol Abuse* 11:37–53, 1985.
16. Belenko S: Alcohol use by heroin addicts: Review of research findings and issues. *Int J Addiction* 14:965–975, 1979.
17. Smith DE: Cocaine-alcohol abuse: Epidemiological, diagnostic and treatment considerations. *J Psychoactive Drugs* 18:117–129, 1986.
18. Kirstein LS: Inpatient cocaine abuse treatment, in Washton AM, Gold MS (eds): *Cocaine: A Clinician's Handbook.* New York, Guilford Press, 1987, pp 96–105.
19. Kaufman E: Alcoholism and the use of other drugs, in Pattison EM, Kaufman E (eds): *Encyclopedia Handbook of Alcoholism.* Garden Press, 1982, pp 696–705.
20. Hoffman NG, Ninonuevo F, Mozey J, Luxenberg MG: Comparison of court-referred DWI arrestees with other outpatients in substance abuse treatment. *J Stud Alcohol* 48:591–594, 1987.
21. Bihari B: Alcoholism and methadone maintenance. *Am J Drug Alcohol Abuse* 1:78–87, 1974.
22. Roszell DK, Calsyn DA, Chaney EF: Alcohol use and psychopathology in opioid addicts on methadone maintenance. *Am J Drug Alcohol Abuse* 12:269–278, 1986.
23. Hubbard RL, Bray RM, Cavanaugh ER, Rachal JV, Craddock SG, Collins JJ, Allison M: *Drug Abuse Treatment Client Characteristics and Pretreatment Behaviors.* Washington, DC, U.S. Department of Health and Human Services, Treatment Research Monograph Series, 1986.
24. Hubbard RL, Anderson J: *A Followup Study of Individuals Receiving Alcoholism Treatment.* Research Triangle Park, NC, Research Triangle Institute, 1988.

25. Miller NS, Dackis CA, Gold M: The relationship of addiction, tolerance, and dependence to alcohol and drugs: A neurochemical approach. *Substance Abuse Treatment* 4:197–207, 1987.
26. Zweben JE, O'Connell K: Strategies for breaking marijuana dependence. *J Psychoactive Drugs* 20:121–127, 1988.
27. Zweben JE, Smith DE: Changing attitude and policies toward alcohol use in the therapeutic community. *J Psychoactive Drugs* 18:253–260, 1986.
28. Gordis E: Methadone maintenance and patients in alcoholism treatment, in *Alcohol Alert.* Rockville, MD, NIAAA, August 1988.
29. Washton AM, Gold MS (eds): *Cocaine: A Clinician's Handbook.* New York, Guilford Press, 1987.
30. Hubbard RL, Marsden ME: Relapse to use of heroin, cocaine, and other drugs in the first year after treatment, in Tims FM, Leukefeld CG (eds): *Relapse and Recovery in Drug Abuse.* Washington, DC, U.S. Department of Health and Human Services, NIDA Research Monograph 72, 1986, pp 157–166.
31. Hubbard RL, Marsden ME, Cavanaugh ER, Rachal JV, Ginzburg HM: Role of drug-abuse treatment in limiting the spread of AIDS. *Rev Infect Dis* 10:377–383, 1988.
32. Marlatt GA, Gordon JR: *Relapse Prevention: Maintenance Strategies in Addictive Behavior Change.* New York, Guilford Press, 1984.

15

Structured Outpatient Treatment of Alcohol vs. Drug Dependencies

Arnold M. Washton

Abstract. This chapter describes the rationale, indications, design, and use of a structured outpatient treatment approach as an effective alternative to residential treatment for alcohol and drug dependencies. An increasing demand for outpatient treatment services is being created by a combination of clinical and economic factors, including the influx of employed drug abusers who do not need or desire residential care and mounting financial pressures to contain health care costs. To be effective as a primary treatment modality, outpatient programs must be highly structured and intensive and able to deal with the full spectrum of alcohol and drug addictions. Perpetuating the historical separation between alcoholism and drug abuse treatment programs is unnecessary and counterproductive, although certain modifications in treatment approaches are needed to accommodate the distinctive characteristics of particular classes of drugs and the people who use them. The "outpatient rehab," a treatment model that approximates the intensity of inpatient treatment on an outpatient basis, may help to maximize the clinical efficacy and cost-effectiveness of outpatient treatment as a viable alternative to residential care. Initial treatment results with this model are encouraging.

1. Introduction

Two of the most significant developments to emerge in the chemical dependency treatment field in recent years are the increasing utilization of structured outpatient treatment programs as an alternative to traditional residential care and the increasing integration of alcoholism and drug abuse treatment into generic programs capable of treating the full spectrum of chemical addictions and cross-addictions.

The major impetus for these developments can be attributed to significant changes in the population of patients appearing for treatment, caused mainly by the recent cocaine epidemic. Because cocaine does not produce a

Arnold M. Washton • The Washton Institute On Addictions, New York, New York 10016.

withdrawal syndrome that requires medical management in a hospital, and, a great many cocaine addicts are employed, there is an escalating demand for outpatient treatment modalities as an alternative to residential care. Furthermore, because cocaine is often used in combination with other drugs such as alcohol, heroin, or marijuana, an increasing number of chemically dependent patients are multiple drug/alcohol users. This is narrowing the traditional gap between the alcoholism and drug abuse treatment fields. More and more programs are treating the full spectrum of addictions rather than restricting their programs to one particular form of chemical dependency such as alcoholism, cocaine addiction, or heroin addiction.

This chapter focuses on several key issues concerning structured outpatient treatment of chemical addictions, including the relative effectiveness and indications for outpatient vs. inpatient treatment; similarities and differences between alcoholism vs. drug addiction treatment; the basic ingredients of an effective outpatient program; and the successive stages of outpatient treatment from initial evaluation and early abstinence through relapse prevention and advanced recovery. This chapter deals only with abstinence-oriented treatment techniques: neither detoxification methods nor pharmacological treatments for the various chemical addictions are addressed; these topics are covered elsewhere in this volume. Owing to space limitations, this chapter cannot cover all of the essential details in designing effective outpatient treatment programs, and the reader is referred to other recent publications[1-3] for more detailed information about program design, patient assessment, and outpatient treatment techniques.

A basic thesis of this chapter is that the most common chemical addictions among patients who seek treatment (e.g., alcoholism, heroin addiction, and cocaine addiction) share more similarities with one another than differences and, therefore, separate programs for each addiction are unnecessary and counterproductive. But there are still important differences that must not be overlooked in the treatment. Ideally, programs should be able to deal with the full spectrum of addictions and cross-addictions by incorporating drug-specific treatment components into a comprehensive, abstinence-oriented treatment approach.

The information in this chapter is based largely on my own clinical experience of the past 13 years, mainly in outpatient settings, involving patients from diverse racial, ethnic, and socioeconomic backgrounds with all types of chemical addictions. My patients have spanned the gamut from unemployed ghetto heroin addicts to professionals, business executives, and adolescents addicted to cocaine, alcohol, or marijuana. During the past 2 years, my efforts have focused on developing intensive outpatient programs—"outpatient rehabs"—a primary modality of treatment that seeks to maximize the clinical effectiveness, patient acceptability, and cost-effectiveness of chemical dependency treatment for employed adults and their families, irrespective of the patient's primary drug of choice.

2. Outpatient vs. Inpatient Treatment

Traditional 28-day residential treatment programs and longer-term thera-peutic community programs have dominated the alcoholism and drug abuse treatment fields for decades. Although there is still a raging controversy about the relative effectiveness and indications for inpatient vs outpatient treat-ment, increasing attention is being paid to outpatient treatment modalities owing to a complex interplay between clinical and economic factors, accentu-ated in part by the cocaine epidemic.

1. Acceptability to patients. As compared to traditional inpatient (resi-dential) care, outpatient programs are more acceptable, especially to patients who are employed, because it does not force them to be separated from job and family. The patient's participation in treatment can remain confidential, sparing unnecessary embarrassment and stigmatization that might result from a sudden, conspicuous, prolonged absence from the workplace. By eliminating these barriers, outpatient programs can increase the chances that an active drug/alcohol abuser will enter treatment and avoid the conse-quences of continued drug/alcohol use, such as job loss.

2. Clinical effectiveness. Outpatient treatment is more clinically effective and appropriate as a primary treatment modality for a wider segment of the addicted population than previously thought—it is fast becoming recognized as the modality of choice for most chemically dependent people seeking help, particularly those who are functional, employed adults. Moreover, treating addicts and alcoholics exclusively as inpatients may not prepare them ade-quately for reentry into the "real world" where drug cues and drug supplies are again ubiquitous. In cases where abstinence could have been initiated as an outpatient, residential treatment may merely postpone the inevitable task of learning how to cope successfully with daily life without using alcohol or drugs. Residential treatment insulates and protects the patient from stressors and triggers, thus creating a false sense of security that may act as setup for immediate relapse after discharge. The fact that relapse rates following com-pletion of residential treatment remain extraordinarily high[4,5] suggests that outpatient programs substantially more intensive than the usual once-a-week "aftercare" program are required to prevent relapse and foster a more lasting recovery, whether or not the patient receives prior residential treatment.

Outpatient treatment following a residential program is often viewed as an add-on, thus the term "aftercare," suggesting that the essential part of the treatment has already been completed and that further treatment is entirely optional, especially if the patient has done well in the inpatient program. When residential treatment is viewed more properly as the starting point or "launch-ing pad" for recovery, the critical role of outpatient treatment, whether or not preceded by residential treatment, becomes more apparent. According to this view, the major purpose of a residential program is to prepare the patient to make good use of an outpatient program. Despite continuing controversy about the relative efficacy and indications for inpatient versus outpatient treatment, major reviews of treatment outcome studies[4,5] indicate that success rates in outpatient programs are consistently equal to or better than those in residential programs, except for patients who are severely dysfunctional or require hospitalization for serious medical or psychiatric problems.

However, outpatient and inpatient programs should not be pitted against one another. The important question is not whether outpatient treatment should be used instead of inpatient treatment, but rather to define the appropriate clinical indications for each. Ideally, a continuum of care should be available which includes the options of a short-term residential program (14–30 days), a halfway house or partial hospitalization program, an intensive outpatient program, a relapse prevention program, and a longer-term follow-up program. The key to preventing relapse is in providing frequent weekly contacts, urine testing, support groups, and individual/family counseling throughout the first 6–12 months of recovery in order to combat the stressors and triggers that restimulate the desire for alcohol and drugs.

3. Cost. Outpatient treatment is much less expensive than residential care. More treatment can be provided with fewer dollars in an outpatient program. This is an important consideration for publicly funded treatment systems, which usually lack adequate funds to meet the ever-increasing demand for treatment. However, even in private treatment programs many patients do not benefit from the inherently lower cost of outpatient treatment because most health insurance policies and other sources of "third-party" payment still provide full coverage for inpatient treatment, but little or no coverage for outpatient treatment. Ironically, this means that only the most expensive form of treatment is accessible to patients who often do not need hospitalization in the first place. Because of mounting economic pressures to contain health care costs, greater emphasis is now being placed on developing more cost-effective alternatives to costly inpatient treatment, including intensive outpatient treatment programs.

3. When Is Outpatient Treatment Appropriate?

Because intensive outpatient treatment programs are still scarce in most areas, the choice of treatment modality for a given patient is often restricted by availability (or nonavailability) of certain options rather than clinical considerations alone. Although outpatient treatment would be utilized more extensively if it were more available, there are still many patients who do need residential treatment as a prerequisite to making use of an outpatient program. The following clinical indications for outpatient treatment can be applied in those cases where good outpatient programs are available (a description of what constitutes a good outpatient program is discussed later in this chapter in Section 5, "Ingredients of Effective Outpatient Treatment").

Outpatient treatment is indicated in the following circumstances:

1. When the patient is not physically dependent on alcohol, sedative–hypnotics, or other drugs associated with potentially dangerous withdrawal syndromes. Although opiate withdrawal is not itself physically damaging or life-threatening, and some patients can be safely and effectively detoxified as outpatients, the level of physical discomfort makes it impossible for many of them to achieve abstinence as outpatients.

2. When the patient is not experiencing medical or psychiatric problems of a serious nature that require inhospital diagnosis and/or treatment. Patients who are actively suicidal, homicidal, psychotic, or otherwise psychiatrically unstable should not be admitted to an outpatient program without prior hospitalization. Similarly, some patients have systemic infections and other medical conditions that require inpatient care.

3. When the patient is sufficiently motivated and functional so that he/she can continue to work productively and live at home during outpatient treatment. Except for patients who are extremely dysfunctional, unmotivated, or incapable of resisting drug hunger, the appropriateness of outpatient treatment in any given case is best evaluated during an initial "trial" period (usually the first week or two) in treatment. As in residential programs, many patients who at first seem poorly motivated respond favorably to positive peer pressure early in treatment. Moreover, there is no evidence that inpatient is more effective than outpatient treatment with individuals who are poorly motivated.

4. When the patient does not have a recent history of repeated failures in a structured outpatient treatment program. Those who have failed to achieve or maintain abstinence in nonspecific outpatient psychotherapy should not automatically be considered inappropriate for an outpatient program: many respond favorably to a more structured approach and do not require residential treatment.

5. When the patient has completed a residential program. As mentioned earlier, patients who complete residential treatment should immediately enter a structured outpatient program in order to prevent reentry problems that precipitate relapse and to foster continued recovery. Whenever possible, inpatients should attend outpatient group meetings during the last 2 weeks of residential treatment in order to facilitate a smooth transition from inpatient to outpatient care.

4. Alcoholism vs. Drug Addiction Treatment

4.1. Treatment Philosophy and Goals

The disease model of addiction and the requirement of total abstinence, traditionally used in alcoholism treatment programs, is finally gaining greater acceptance in drug abuse treatment programs, and this is helping to narrow the gap between these historically separate sectors of the chemical dependency treatment field. Alcohol is now regarded by most treatment professionals as simply one of many different types of mood-altering drugs.

Moreover, with the proliferation of illicit drug use over the past 3 decades, fewer patients who appear for treatment are using only one mood-altering substance: Multiple drug/alcohol use is now the norm and cross-addictions involving a variety of different substances are extremely common. "Pure" drug addicts and alcoholics are rapidly becoming extinct, especially since the cocaine outbreak. Very few cocaine addicts, for instance, are involved only with cocaine. Likewise, an increasing number of primary alcoholics are using cocaine and/or other drugs. Cocaine addicts typically drink alcohol (or take tranquilizers, sleeping pills, marijuana, or opiates) to "come down" from the unpleasant stimulant effects of high-dose cocaine. Alcoholics use cocaine in part to "wake up" from the depressant effects of alcohol. Cocaine enables them to prolong consciousness and drink more alcohol. Similarly, heroin addicts mix cocaine and heroin in the same syringe (a drug combination known as a "speedball") in order to enhance the euphoria and counteract the undesirable side effects of each drug.

This growing trend toward multiple drug/alcohol use has encouraged more widespread acceptance by treatment providers of total abstinence from all mood-altering chemicals, not just the patient's drug of choice, as the only effective treatment goal. In the 1960s and 1970s, many drug abuse treatment programs required patients to abstain completely from their drug of choice (usually heroin), but ignored or permitted the use of alcohol, marijuana, and even cocaine—since these drugs were not perceived as dangerous or as damaging to the patient's recovery. The fact that drinking or use of other drugs could set off craving for the patient's drug of choice, reduce his/her ability to resist temptation, or lead to substitute addictions was not adequately recognized. This lack of attention to the relapse dangers posed by use of any mood-altering chemical, coupled with the lack of application of the disease model as the fundamental basis for treatment, were probably significant contributors to the notoriously low success rates in drug treatment programs.

The disease model states that once a person has crossed the line from chemical use to chemical addiction, he/she can never return to controlled use without rekindling the addiction. Furthermore, this model holds not only for the person's drug of choice, but for all psychoactive or mood-altering substances, thus underscoring the need for total abstinence as the first and foremost treatment goal. Alcohol use must be seen as a major factor in promoting relapse to drugs just as drug use must be seen as a major factor in promoting relapse to alcohol. Furthermore, increasing emphasis on treating "the disease within" is one of the most pivotal developments to gain greater acceptance in recent years. There is now a discernible shift away from merely helping patients to get off drugs and an increasing emphasis on helping them stay off over the long term. Stopping drug use is easy enough in most cases, especially when there are no withdrawal symptoms, as with cocaine. The key to long-term recovery is not stopping, but staying stopped (i.e., preventing relapse). This requires special treatment efforts to counteract relapse tendencies. Relapse prevention is perhaps the most critical issue in addiction treatment today. Traditionally, programs have avoided even mentioning the topic of relapse for fear that it would communicate an expectation of failure. In recent years, however, much effort has been channeled into identifying factors that precipitate relapse and developing treatment strategies to avoid and/or cope with them.[6–8]

4.2. Treatment Techniques

The integration of treatment techniques for patients who have chosen different primary drugs is far from complete. For example, despite a long record of success in treating primary alcoholics, many traditional alcoholism treatment programs find cocaine addicts difficult to treat effectively. Treatment approaches that have historically worked well for alcoholics cannot be expected to work well for cocaine addicts without substantial modification. Cocaine addicts are not just alcoholics who have accidentally chosen a different drug. Asking them to merely substitute the word "cocaine" for "alcohol" in treatment lectures and group meetings is unfair and inadequate. Similarly, programs designed primarily to treat heroin addiction have experienced poor results with cocaine addicts, but for different reasons. Many of these programs are accustomed to utilizing pharmacological agents such as methadone or other substitute drugs, rather than abstinence-oriented treatment techniques, as the fundamental basis for treatment. In addition, many of the so-called "drug-free" treatment programs, designed originally to help the recently detoxified heroin addicts stay clean, have not modified or expanded their treatment approaches to accommodate the needs of cocaine addicts, alcoholics, and polydrug abusers. The treatment often remains overly focused on the patient's withdrawal complaints and puts too little emphasis on total abstinence, relapse prevention, and life-style change.

Are substantially different strategies required to treat alcoholism, cocaine addiction, heroin addiction, and other chemical dependencies effectively? The answer is—fundamentally, no. The basic ingredients of good treatment are pretty much the same for all addictions, irrespective of the patient's drug of choice, at least insofar as abstinence-oriented treatment is concerned. Although the patient's drug of choice is a significant factor, treatment based on the disease model and the requirement of total abstinence can be utilized effectively with all chemical addictions.

What modifications are required depending on the patient's primary drug of choice? Perhaps the most important one is for the clinician to know at least as much about the patient's drug of choice as the patient does. Users of illegal drugs, in particular, can readily sense when a clinician is naïve about drugs, including drug effects, medical consequences, methods of preparation and use, and the language of the illicit drug market. The clinician must have a sophisticated clinical knowledge of all addictive drugs, both legal and illegal, and be able to educate the patient about relevant clinical aspects of drug use, rather than vice versa.

A comparison of clinically relevant differences between alcoholism and cocaine addiction is outlined below to illustrate some of these points. These two addictions were chosen for comparison, in particular, because of the relevance of this issue to the many alcoholism treatment programs that are seeing an increasing number of patients whose primary addiction is to cocaine.

1. Cocaine and alcohol are pharmacological opposites. Cocaine is a potent CNS stimulant—alcohol is a potent CNS depressant. Cocaine is often taken to enhance performance—and may actually do so during the early "honeymoon" period of use. By contrast, alcohol disrupts brain function and almost always disrupts behavior and performance. Unlike alcohol, cocaine leaves no telltale odor on the user's breath and does not impair motor coordination in a way that would make it obvious to others that the user is intoxicated. Cocaine use can be very difficult to detect on the basis of visual observation alone, except perhaps when usage is extreme. People do not take alcohol in order to feel energetic and perform better at work. People do not take cocaine in order to feel relaxed and tranquilized. The particular pharmacological effects of a drug that the user seeks out are not insignificant, incidental, or accidental. An attempt must be made to understand the user's attraction to a drug in order to treat the problem effectively. That is, the clinician should seek to understand the particular "fit" between the person and the drug in terms of the role that the drug use plays in the individual's life and the ways in which the chosen substance may have been used in part to compensate for certain deficits in coping skills or may have satisfied unrealistic desires for a "magic solution" to real-life problems. Also, the basic pharmacological difference between cocaine and alcohol means that cocaine-specific education must be included in the treatment of all cocaine addicts. The education should focus on cocaine first and other drugs second, instead of vice versa.

2. Cocaine addiction develops and progresses much more rapidly than alcoholism. Alcoholism often develops and progresses over an extremely long period of time, which may span many years. Alcoholics entering treatment may report 10- to 15-year histories of heavy drinking, with an extensive list of personal losses and consequences associated with their gradual progression into addictive disease. By contrast, cocaine addiction develops rapidly—sometimes even with a few months after first use. This is especially true with the more intensive routes of administration such as freebase smoking and I.V. use. Unlike alcoholics, cocaine addicts sometimes report no long trail of drug-related dysfunction and no long, drawn-out progression from initial use into full-blown addiction. In recounting their history of use, many are hard-

pressed to identify exactly when the problem developed—it seems that all of a sudden they went from controlled use to out-of-control use with little or no transition period. When cocaine addiction develops very rapidly, it can some-times make it more difficult for both the user and the family to accept the fact that the problem truly exists (i.e., it can intensify denial), not only because the problem progresses so quickly, almost before anyone knows what's happen-ing, but also because many of the adverse psychosocial consequences of the compulsive cocaine use have not had time to catch up with them yet.

3. Cocaine addicts tend to identify best with other cocaine addicts, at least at the beginning of treatment. Just as alcoholics benefit greatly from the presence of role models who are themselves recovering alcoholics, cocaine addicts benefit similarly from having the same opportunity for role modeling and identification with peers who are successfully recovering from cocaine addiction. This means that, whenever possible, cocaine addicts should be placed into recovery groups that include at least several other cocaine addicts. In addition, whenever possible, programs treating cocaine addicts should include at least some members of the counseling staff who are themselves recovering cocaine addicts in solid recovery. However, cocaine addicts should not be segregated into separate treatment programs or separate treatment groups from alcoholics and other chemically dependent patients. In fact, this is distinctly contraindicated. Many cocaine addicts already suffer from an exaggerated sense of uniqueness and elitism—they consider themselves to be a "cut above" heroin addicts and alcoholics. It is usually helpful for cocaine addicts to see that their chemical dependency is a variation of addictive dis-ease and not a special problem in itself.

4. Cocaine addiction is associated with powerful urges and cravings that dominate the early abstinence period. The beginning phase of outpatient treatment with cocaine addicts often must deal exclusively with the patient's intense cravings and urges for cocaine. By contrast, the beginning phase of treatment with alcoholics often focuses on detoxification and on restoration of normal cognitive functions that were disrupted by chronic alcohol use. Unlike alcohol, there is no medically dangerous cocaine withdrawal syndrome to manage and there is no need for substitute drugs to gradually wean the patient from cocaine. But abrupt cessation of cocaine use typically brings on powerful cravings and urges which, if not handled effectively, lead to immediate relapse.

5. Cocaine is illegal, alcohol is not. As a result, cocaine addicts are often more guarded and suspicious toward treatment staff and extremely con-cerned about issues of confidentiality (especially patients who have both dealt and used illegal drugs). These concerns should not dismissed categorically as cocaine-induced paranoia. Involvement with illegal drugs often engenders deceptive, manipulative, and devious behavior which may not be seen as often in alcoholics. Clinicians must be prepared to deal with this type of behavior without being judgmental or personally offended.

Clinicians must be familiar with the terminology used in describing the sale, purchase, preparation, and use of street cocaine in its various forms. For example, it is important to know that cocaine hydrochloride powder is typically purchased in quantities of a gram (roughly equivalent to a couple of heaping tablespoons), an ounce (28 g), a "quarter" (7 g), or an "eighth" (3.5 g). Heavy users, especially those who intend to convert cocaine powder into smokable freebase, often buy the drug in quantities larger than a gram because they get a price break. Clinicians should also know the differences between cocaine powder, cocaine freebase, and crack, as well as the reagents and paraphernalia associated with the preparation and use of each, topics covered in greater depth elsewhere.[1]

5. Ingredients of Effective Outpatient Treatment

The basic ingredients of effective outpatient treatment include the following components:

1. A structured treatment program. In order to successfully recover from chemical dependency, most patients require a structured treatment program—preferably, one that is highly structured. The level of intensity, structure, accountability, and specific focus on recovery issues that most drug addicts and alcoholics require is usually offered only in specialized addiction treatment programs as compared to general psychiatric clinics or private practice. Most people who seek chemical dependency treatment recognize their need for external structure and are often relieved by the clear framework provided by a program that addresses the addiction problem directly. Ideally, the rules and expectations of the program regarding abstinence, attendance, and so forth should be concretized, in writing, at the very outset of treatment in the form of an agreement or treatment contract that the patient (and family) signs. More important, the basic rules and guidelines of the program must be implemented—fairly and consistently. Failure to set appropriate limits with addicts is a dangerous form of enabling which supports rather than discourages continued drug use. But rigid, irrational limit setting motivated by a clinician's frustration and annoyance can be even more harmful. Striking an appropriate balance between firmness and flexibility is essential.

Although most patients will require a structured program, some will accept only individual treatment from a private practitioner. It is certainly possible to treat addicts and alcoholics successfully in private practice, but it requires a therapist who is skilled and experienced in treating chemical dependency and able to offer the appropriate level of treatment structure and intensity, including individual, family, and group counseling as well as supervised urine testing. Treating chemical dependents with individual therapy alone, without the support of self-help meetings, group therapy, and family involvement, is often unsuccessful or only temporarily ameliorative. It is not uncommon for patients who enter a treatment program to report previous unsuccessful attempts in psychotherapy with practitioners who either ignored or postponed dealing with the drug problem—feeling that the "real" underlying psychological problems giving rise to drug use as a symptom had to be ameliorated first—or the therapist simply refused to deal with the chemical dependency problem at all. In all such cases, as one might expect, the patient's addiction only gets worse despite attempts at "treatment." Because addicts and alcoholics typically complain of depression, anxiety, and extreme difficulty in relationships, the general psychotherapist (especially one whose approach is psychodynamically oriented) is often a prime target for getting "hooked in" to the patient's enabling system by focusing on the multitude of interpersonal and self-esteem problems being generated (or exacerbated) by the chemical use rather than on the chemical use itself. Therapists who are not experienced and skilled in treating chemical addictions should be categorically avoided by patients suffering with these problems—unless the therapist refers the patient to an addiction treatment program and works cooperatively with the program in a joint treatment plan, temporarily putting aside all attempts at insight-oriented psychotherapy in favor of supportive counseling that reinforces the patient's attempts to achieve and maintain immediate abstinence from all mood-altering chemicals.

2. Treatment in stages. Recovery from chemical addiction does not occur all at once or instantaneously—no matter what the treatment approach. Treatment should proceed in a stepwise fashion, in stages where the patient and program focus sequentially on specific tasks and goals, as described later in this chapter.

3. Immediate abstinence without delay. It is imperative to insist on total abstinence from all mood-altering substances as the first and foremost step in treatment. Attempts to cut down, rather than stop, alcohol/drug use altogether are rarely successful. Any involvement whatsoever with psychoactive chemicals is likely to pull the patient back into compulsive use. Once the invisible line into addiction is crossed, the ability to return to occasional or "controlled" use is usually lost forever and cannot be condoned as a reasonable treatment goal. Many patients enter treatment harboring the hidden intention of resuming occasional use someday—when current pressures to stop all usage subside and the addiction problem is "cured" by the treatment program. It is essential to educate patients about this common error in thinking and to help them realize that chemical dependents never get a second "honeymoon" with their drug of choice. As long as drug/alcohol cravings are being reinforced, even occasionally, they will continue to exert an irresistible pull back to regular use.

4. Abstinence from all psychoactive drugs. Not only must patients give up their drug(s) of choice, but they must be told to abstain from all other mood-altering chemical as well. Requiring total abstinence ensures the widest margin of safety against potential relapse and prevents the development of substitute addictions. In addition, recovery from the addictive disease can occur only under conditions of total abstinence. The major goal of recovery is to develop and maintain a reasonably satisfying productive life-style without

the use of any mood-altering chemicals. Obviously, this process is stalled while the addict is continuing to use any drugs whatsoever.

Among cocaine addicts who enter treatment, for example, many vehemently object to the idea of giving up all other drugs, especially alcohol and marijuana. "After all," some argue, "I've never had a problem with alcohol or marijuana. I never used them daily, compulsively, or to the point where they interfered with my life. I don't understand why I can't continue to have a single glass of wine or beer with dinner and why I can't smoke a joint once in a while to relax after a hard day at work. I'm not an alcoholic or a 'garbagehead' like some of the other people in this program. My only problem is cocaine. The program's rule of total abstinence is unwarranted and irrational in my case. Why should I stay abstinent from everything?"

The major reasons for insisting on total abstinence as the safest course for recovery in these and other cases, are as follows:

a. Use of any psychoactive drug can trigger strong cravings for one's drug of choice. For example, most cocaine addicts have used other drugs (especially depressants such as alcohol, tranquilizers, sleeping pills, or opiates) to counteract the unpleasant stimulant aftereffects of cocaine or to alleviate the depression and irritability characteristic of the cocaine "crash." By being paired or associated with cocaine literally hundreds or thousands of times, these drugs acquire the ability (through the process of associative conditioning) to elicit powerful urges and cravings for cocaine. They become "reminders" or "triggers" for cocaine in the user's brain—setting off a chain reaction that usually starts with drug cravings and ends with drug use. Even patients who have no history of alcohol abuse prior to cocaine addiction may find that a single glass of beer or wine sets off irresistible cravings for cocaine.

b. Other drugs can reduce the patient's ability to resist temptation for their primary drug. Most mood-altering drugs have a "disinhibiting" effect on the user's attitude and behavior. That is, when high on any drug most people tend to feel "looser" and more likely to act on their impulses. Thus, the use of any mood-altering drug is likely to render the successfully abstaining patient more vulnerable to offers of their primary drug. Getting high on any drug inevitably puts the patient one step closer to full-blown relapse.

c. Other drugs provide substitute highs which can lead to substitute addictions. While abstaining from their drug of choice, many patients begin to regard other drugs increasingly appealing as a source of substitute highs. This is especially true for primary drug addicts who see alcohol as the only "legitimate," socially acceptable way left to get high. Alcohol is legal, readily available on most occasions, and its use is often socially encouraged even by family members and friends, who make the mistake of thinking that the drug addict's problem is limited only to their drug of choice. In patients who have a history of chemical dependencies that preceded their current drug of choice (e.g., alcoholism prior to cocaine addiction), use of any mood-altering substances is likely to rekindle these problems. Some patients are in denial about their previous addictions while others may purposely keep this information hidden from their therapist or peers in order to better rationalize the safety of continued use.

5. Education. All treatment for chemical addiction should include a strong educational component. The purpose of this education must be to provide the patient with a basic framework for understanding his/her addiction problem in a way that facilitates the treatment and recovery process. Education can be a powerful treatment tool for bringing about changes in attitude and behavior. It also helps to actively involve the patient as a participant in his/her own treatment. Family members should receive education as well. Topics covered in education sessions should include the basic pharmacology and effects of addictive drugs; basic principles of addictive disease and recovery; early warning signs of relapse and how to prevent relapses from occurring; an introduction to self-help programs; the family dynamics of addiction; enabling and codependency; and an overview of medical and psychosocial consequences of addiction.

6. Family involvement. Immediate involvement of the patient's family, whenever possible, is an essential feature of effective outpatient treatment. Lack of family involvement may lead to sabotage and undermining of the treatment by well-meaning family members who are actually supporting ("enabling") the patient's addiction while trying to help. Chemical dependency is almost always a family disease in terms of its etiology, maintenance, and negative impact. In many cases, successful recovery for the addict is extraordinarily difficult or impossible without the participation of key family members. In addition to supplying useful information that confirms, refutes, or elaborates upon the patient's report, family members are often themselves sorely in need of advice and guidance on how to deal with the addict's manipulative and exploitive behavior. They are sometimes contributing to the perpetuation of the addiction or otherwise enabling the patient's drug use by (a) giving the addict money that goes directly or indirectly to drugs; (b) making excuses to others for the addict's irresponsible behavior; (c) doing other things to shield the addict from the negative consequences of his/her drug use; and (d) acting out their own anger and feelings of helplessness on the addict in a way that allows the addict to conveniently blame family members rather than take personal responsibility for the problems in his life. Not only must family members learn how to help the addict more constructively, but they must also be helped to find more adaptive ways to deal with their justifiable feelings of anger, frustration, helplessness, and sadness which stem from their futile attempts to "fix" the addict's problem.

7. Urine testing. Outpatient treatment must include supervised urine testing at frequent intervals in order to reliably detect the use of any drugs or to verify abstinence. Urine testing in an outpatient program must be mandatory, not optional. It is an extremely valuable treatment tool that has significant clinical benefits for the patient. The purpose of urine testing is not to catch the addict in a lie, but rather to help him/her exert better control over impulses to use drugs by establishing accountability for any drug use that

may occur. This often helps to break through the denial and self-deceit that are characteristic of addictive disease and contributive to continuing drug use. Simply knowing that any drug use will be detected in the urine, the patient may be better able to resist temptation in an otherwise difficult situation. This is probably why most patients who enter an outpatient program are relieved rather than offended by the requirement of urine testing. When the program requires urine testing, without exception, patients know that they will not be able to relapse without being noticed—a comforting fact to most—despite their continuing ambivalence about giving up drugs. In addition to serving as a built-in safety mechanism, urine testing also prevents patients from devaluing a therapist or program whom they have been able to deceive and manipulate. Moreover, urine testing provides the patient with a concrete measure of treatment progress. Patients often ask to see the laboratory reports verifying that their urine is "clean." Also, family members often breathe a little easier knowing that the addict is on a schedule of urine surveillance. They can give up their attempts to guess "did he or didn't he" and to always feel obligated to stay on the lookout out for even the slightest behavioral signs that the addict may have used drugs again.

In order for urine testing to be of maximum clinical value, several procedural guidelines should be followed: (a) All samples should be witnessed (observed) in order to prevent falsification—samples "brought in" by patients should never be accepted. (b) A sample should be collected at least every 3–4 days so as not to exceed the sensitivity of laboratory detection methods for most drugs. (c) Testing should be done by enzyme immunoassay or radioimmunoassay procedures to ensure accuracy—less expensive tests, such as thin-layer chromatography are not accurate enough for short-acting drugs like cocaine.[9] (d) Urine testing should be continued throughout the entire course of treatment.

8. Group and individual therapy. A combination of group and individual therapy is optimal for most patients. Group therapy is virtually the core of most treatments for chemical dependency. A recovery group provides an opportunity for patients to identify with peers, receive group support and reassurance, learn about addiction and recovery, and confront maladaptive attitudes and behaviors. Individual therapy allows the treatment to be tailored to the specific individual needs and problems of each patient, such as psychological, sexual, and interpersonal problems that may have existed before the addiction or developed as a result of it.

9. Self-help groups. All outpatients should be strongly encouraged to become involved in the 12-step program of Cocaine Anonymous (CA), Narcotics Anonymous (NA), or Alcoholics Anonymous (AA). Exposure to these self-help programs should be routinely provided by all professional treatment programs. Self-help meetings offer an invaluable source of support and assistance at no cost to anyone who attends. Self-help is not a substitute for professional treatment, or vice versa.

10. Alternative activities. Physical exercise, sports, and other recrea-

tional activities are an important part of building a healthier life-style that supports a lasting recovery from chemical dependency. Physical activity can relieve stress, improve mood, and instill positive feelings of having greater control over one's life.

11. Nutritional, medical, and dental care. Neglect of one's physical health and general well-being is common during active addiction. Many patients have lost a significant amount of body weight, ignored chronic medical problems, and perpetuated or intensified poor eating habits. A comprehensive medical, dental, and nutritional evaluation is indicated in most cases, followed by proper treatment and counseling.

12. Pharmacological therapy. A "magic bullet" to cure chemical addictions will probably never be found. But patients who have coexisting psychiatric disorders that may be responsive to nonaddictive therapeutic medications should not be deprived of these medications, when clinically appropriate. The indications for using psychotropic medications to treat psychiatric disorders in recovering addicts are the same as for any other patient, but clinicians must be careful not to prescribe any medications with acute mood-altering effects since all such medications have the potential for being abused.

6. Stages of Outpatient Treatment

The following description of treatment stages is based on the "outpatient rehab" program offered at The Washton Institute, a highly structured and intensive program that lasts 6–12 months. Each stage of the program focuses on specific issues and goals most relevant to a particular stage of the recovery process.[1] There are no rigid dividing lines between the different stages of treatment, and patients may enter at different stages and progress through them at different rates. Dividing the program into phases is helpful not only in defining its basic framework, but also in allowing patients to experience a sense of accomplishment and reward by marking their progress with the completion of each phase. Supervised urine samples are taken regularly throughout the program. Patients are encouraged to attend self-help meetings and their participation is facilitated by making such meetings regularly available to them on the premises of the program.

6.1. Assessment and Crisis Intervention

This stage of treatment lasts from 1 to 2 weeks, depending on the patient's clinical status when he/she first applies for treatment. For example, patients who have already achieved several days of abstinence on their own before the initial interview are usually ready to enter the intensive treatment program immediately. On the other hand, those who are still very much in the throes of active drug/alcohol use may require daily individual contact for at least several days in order to see whether they are indeed able to make use of outpatient treatment.

A vital issue in the assessment is to find out exactly what brings the person to treatment at this particular point in time: why today rather than last week or last month? This information helps to pinpoint the source of greatest distress for the patient, including those factors most likely to be motivating his/her current attempt to seek help. It may also identify a source of leverage that is helpful in preventing the patient from dropping out of treatment prematurely. Other issues covered in the initial assessment include: (1) the current pattern of all drug/alcohol use, including the frequency, amount, chronicity, circumstances, and route of administration; (2) the presence and severity of all drug-related medical and psychosocial problems; (3) the history of previous drug/alcohol use and the progression from initial use to regular use and dependency; (4) a detailed description of previous periods of abstinence and/or treatment episodes, including the circumstances and precipitants of relapse; (5) the presence and severity of nonchemical addictions, including compulsive gambling, sexuality, eating, spending, and working, and any previous treatment for these problems; (6) a detailed psychiatric history and assessment of current psychiatric status; (7) a detailed family history with regard to psychiatric illness and substance abuse; (8) the nature of current relationships and contacts with friends and family; (9) educational and occupational history, including current indebtedness and involvement in drug dealing; (10) current and pending legal status; and (11) the patient's expectations of treatment, desire for change, and current beliefs about the nature and severity of his/her drug or alcohol problem. These and other assessment issues are discussed in detail elsewhere.[1,3]

It is essential for patients entering outpatient treatment to become abstinent without delay. No meaningful treatment can take place while patients remain preoccupied with obtaining, using, and recuperating from alcohol/drugs and no therapeutic progress can be made until an initial period of abstinence is achieved. Attempts to deal with personal problems other than alcohol/drug use must be temporarily postponed in the interest of focusing entirely on attaining abstinence. The initial crisis intervention plan for establishing abstinence usually consists of having daily or almost daily contact with the patient, daily urine monitoring, and, when possible, immediately enlisting the support of close family members and friends to set up temporary external controls (with the patient's consent) aimed at thwarting the patient's impulses to use drugs. This may include having someone accompany the patient at all times for a few days or at the very least requiring the patient to account for all time not spent at home or at work with "check-in" calls; taking control of the patient's finances and access to money; and a contingency written contract that requires the patient to enter a residential treatment program if he/she is unable to achieve abstinence during the early phase of outpatient treatment. Patients are instructed to avoid all people, places, and things associated with their drug/alcohol use; to avoid bars, parties, and hangouts since contact with any of these is likely to reinitiate drug/alcohol use; to discard all drug supplies, drug paraphernalia, liquor/wine bottles, and beer cans in their car, home, or office; to immediately break off contact with dealers and users, even those who are considered by them to be good friends.

The key ingredient in successful outpatient treatment is structure. The challenge is to provide the active drug/alcohol user with a specific framework for translating his/her stated intentions or desires to become abstinent into a specific action plan—one that can be followed through application of simple self-control, environmental control, and avoidance strategies on a day-to-day basis. Compliance with that structure or action plan is essential, but completely voluntary in the outpatient setting. The patient's compliance can be markedly enhanced through early contact with a friendly, engaging, knowledgeable clinician who is willing to "start where the patient is": someone who can recognize and deal with the patient's ambivalence about giving up drugs and not respond with aloofness, irritation, or frustration; someone who can offer specific information about the physical and psychological effects of the patient's drug(s) of choice and responds to the patient's eagerness to talk about these concrete issues in part as a vehicle for establishing a beginning therapeutic alliance. Education and supportive counseling (usually on a one-to-one basis) during the initial crisis phase of treatment play a crucial role in engaging the patient in the treatment program and preventing premature dropout.

It is essential that new patients make a commitment to abstain from the use of all mood-altering chemicals (including alcohol and marijuana) for at least the duration of the treatment program, even if they claim to have no history of problems with certain chemicals. Strong resistance or unwillingness to make even a short-term commitment to total abstinence or adopt a "wait and see" attitude is often indicative of strong reservations about giving up drugs/alcohol at all. Patients who are ambivalent, but at least minimally motivated for treatment, usually accept the requirement of total abstinence, even if they intend to comply with it only temporarily, since they usually view this requirement as a sensible practice. Total abstinence offers the widest margin of safety, but its value is often not fully appreciated by patients until later stages of recovery.

6.2. Early Abstinence

After a few days of abstinence have been achieved, patients are usually ready to enter the 8-week Intensive Program consisting of an early abstinence group that meets four times a week. The primary function of this group is to foster initial changes in the patient's attitude, life-style, and behavior in order to break the vicious cycle of addiction and establish stable abstinence. A substantial part of the group's activities is psychoeducational. Patients are helped to understand the how and why of total abstinence; deal with immediate and delayed withdrawal effects; identify both external (environmental) and internal (emotional) cues that elicit drug hunger; utilize techniques to combat and "short-circuit" cravings and urges; utilize self-help and other social supports; and accept the identity of a recovering person.

Group sessions are supplemented at least once weekly with individual counseling sessions that offer a more concentrated, personalized focus on the needs, problems, and life circumstances of each patient. Family members attend an 8-week Family Counseling Program whose purpose is to educate family members about addiction, recovery, relapse, and enabling; to teach family members how to help the primary patient without destructive enabling; and to help family members cope with the negative impact of the patient's addiction on their own mental and physical well-being.

6.3. Relapse Prevention

This stage of treatment overlaps with the previous one, but focuses more specifically on the task of preventing relapse as the foundation for longer-term recovery.[6] Patients attend a twice-weekly relapse prevention groups for 16 weeks (i.e., until at least 6 months of recovery have been achieved) in conjunction with individual and/or family counseling once a week.

Topics addressed in the group include (1) techniques for dealing with urges, cravings, and self-sabotaging setups for drug/alcohol use; (2) early identification of relapse warning signals and useful strategies for coping with them; (3) debunking relapse myths; e.g., relapse means failure, relapse is inevitable, relapse erases all progress up to that point, relapse is a sign of poor motivation; (4) the desire to "test control" or use "occasionally" again; (5) selective memory for the "good highs"—known as "euphoric recall"; (6) the tendency to feel "cured" and to withdraw energy and commitment from the treatment process prematurely; (7) the tendency to downplay the importance of maintaining total abstinence from secondary drugs of choice and to construct rationalizations for renewed or continued use; (8) resistance to making major life-style and attitude changes, including the creation of a social support network of nonusers; (9) resistance to reaching out for help including involvement in the 12-step programs of AA, NA, or CA; (10) dealing with negative mood states, interpersonal stress, job stress, and social pressures to use alcohol/drugs; and (11) learning how to have fun without alcohol/drugs. Recovery groups are an ideal place for these topics to be addressed because group members not only supply peer identification, role modeling, and positive social pressure for one another, but they are adept at confronting one another's resistances and "blindspots"—including subtle forms of self-sabotage—and at offering each other acceptable ways to overcome these difficulties.

6.4. Advanced Recovery

After attaining solid abstinence and an increased ability to cope with the ups and downs of daily life, patients often need and want to tackle some of the more highly charged psychological issues that may keep their relapse potential unnecessarily high if not addressed. Many clinicians feel that no attempts at psychotherapy should be made with addicts or alcoholics until at least 6–12 months of abstinence have been achieved. Although it is advisable to avoid focusing on highly charged topics in early recovery, any clinician who is skilled in treating chemical dependency will have been using psychotherapeutic skills during every step of the process, but with a finely tuned sense of timing and an ability to decide when certain issues need to be addressed.

Following completion of the relapse prevention program, patients enter an advanced recovery program, which consists of a once-weekly, recovery-oriented psychotherapy group in combination with once-weekly, individual psychotherapy sessions (sometimes interspersed with couples or family therapy sessions, according to the patient's needs). The length of participation in this phase of treatment is open-ended, but requires a commitment of at least 3 months for each new participant. The spectrum of issues addressed in this part of the program is, of course, highly individualized, often including emotion-laden topics such as dependency, depression, anger, sexuality, self-esteem, separation–individuation, traumatic events (e.g., incest and other forms of emotional or physical abuse), parental addictions, relationship problems, and critical career/job decisions.

The therapist must be mindful of the increased danger of relapse when such issues are addressed. A good sense of timing is especially critical here: for example, knowing when to press harder on certain issues vs. backing off; knowing when to be confrontational vs. supportive; and so forth. It is unlikely that all of the patient's personal problems will be solved by the end of his/her participation in this program. A reasonable set of goals include solidifying changes in attitude, life-style, and behavior that are consistent with long-term recovery; achieving a level of personal stability and understanding that leads to effective problem solving; and, deepening the patient's commitment to the recovery process, including reaching out for help when needed.

7. Final Comment

The basic principles and techniques of effective outpatient treatment for chemical dependency are virtually the same whether the patient's drug of choice is alcohol, cocaine, heroin, or other mood-altering substance. Patients should not be segregated from one another into separate treatment programs based on their primary drug of choice. However, in creating treatment programs that can deal effectively with the full range of chemical addictions, adequate consideration must be given to important differences between classes of drugs and the populations that use them. This is especially important in the early phase of treatment, when drug-specific education and counseling components must be incorporated into the overall program in order to prevent premature dropout and improve retention.

An intensive outpatient program is the treatment of choice for functional alcohol/drug abusers who can continue to work and live at home while receiving treatment. Contrary to traditional beliefs, primary outpatient treatment programs that are sufficiently structured and intensive can be effective alternative to costly residential care. According to this view, residential treatment is reserved primarily for those patients who are severely dysfunctional or otherwise require hospitalization because of serious medical or psychiatric problems. Moreover, the major role of a residential program is as that of a "launching pad" for recovery which prepares the patient to make use of an outpatient program rather than the place where the major portion of the recovery process has already been completed.

A new model of treatment, the "outpatient rehab," incorporates the high level of structure and intensity needed to maximize the effectiveness of outpatient treatment. Clinical and economic considerations are creating a growing trend toward greater utilization of outpatient treatment models. The efficacy of outpatient rehabs has not yet been evaluated systematically, but initial experience at this facility is yielding encouraging results: thus far, among 100 consecutive applicants for treatment, over 80% have successfully completed the 6-month program and the number of patients who require residential treatment has been cut by more than half.

Inpatient and outpatient treatment should not be viewed as competitive or as substitutes for one another. When a full spectrum of care is available, treatment decisions can be made based on an optimal match between the patient's clinical needs and the particular modality of treatment best suited to meet those needs.

References

1. Washton AM: *Cocaine Addiction: Treatment, Recovery, and Relapse Prevention.* New York, Norton, 1989.
2. Washton AM: Outpatient treatment techniques, in Washton AM, Gold MS (eds): *Cocaine: A Clinician's Handbook.* New York, Guilford Press, 1987, pp 106–117.
3. Washton AM, Stone N, Hendrickson EC: Cocaine abuse, in Donovan D Marlatt GA (eds): *Assessment of Addictive Behavior.* New York, Guilford Press, 1988, pp 364–389.
4. Miller WR, Hester RK: Inpatient alcoholism treatment: Who benefits? *Am Psychologist* 41:794–805, 1986.
5. Annis HM: Is inpatient rehabilitation of the alcoholic cost effective? *Adv Alcohol Substance Abuse* 5:175–190, 1986.
6. Washton AM: Preventing relapse to cocaine. *J Clin Psychiatry* 49:34–38, 1988.
7. Marlatt GA, Gordon J: *Relapse Prevention.* New York, Guilford Press, 1985.
8. Gorski T, Miller M: *Staying Sober: A Guide for Relapse Prevention.* Independence , MO, Independence Press, 1986.
9. Verebey K: Drug detection by laboratory methods, in Washton AM, Gold MS (eds): *Cocaine: A Clinician's Handbook.* New York, Guilford Press, 1987, pp 214–228.

Behavioral Treatment of Alcohol and Drug Abuse
What Do We Know and Where Shall We Go?

Reid K. Hester, Ted D. Nirenberg, and Ann M. Begin

Abstract. Over the last 20 years there has been a substantial increase in the use of alcohol and drugs in industrialized nations and a concomitant shift in the emphasis of treatment for alcohol and drugs. Rather than seeking treatment for alcohol alone or a single class of drug, many individuals are seeking treatment for alcohol and/or a number of drugs. While theoreticians have been exploring the similarities in the addictive behaviors, clinical researchers are only just beginning to do so. Unfortunately, most treatment research has focused almost exclusively on alcohol abusers or drug abusers, with little research conducted to date with alcohol and drug abusers. Behavioral interventions developed for alcohol abuse are now being tested with drug abusers, and vice versa.

The purpose of this chapter is fourfold: (1) to briefly discuss the similarities in the assessment of alcohol and drug abuse; (2) to describe behavioral interventions that have been supported by research and briefly review this treatment outcome research; (3) to discuss the theoretical similarities in behavioral interventions for alcohol and drug abuse; and (4) to make recommendations for future advancements in treatment and research.

1. Introduction

The past two decades have witnessed a dramatic increase in the use of psychoactive substances in industrialized nations and a concomitant need for services directed toward substance abuse treatment. Consistent with this increase in multiple drug use by the population has been a shift in the emphasis of treatment. For many years the treatment of alcohol and drug abuse was

Reid K. Hester • Behavior Therapy Associates, Albuquerque, New Mexico 87110.   Ted D. Nirenberg • Department of Psychiatry and Human Behavior, Brown University, Providence, Rhode Island 02906; and Substance Abuse Treatment Center, Roger Williams General Hospital, Providence, Rhode Island 02908.   Ann M. Begin • Butler Hospital, and Department of Psychiatry and Human Behavior, Brown University, Providence, Rhode Island 02906.

considered separately. Most abusers in treatment were abusing alcohol or drugs, and the combined alcohol and drug abuser or polydrug user was relatively rare. More recently, however, this pattern has changed dramatically. Today many individuals who seek treatment are abusing alcohol and a variety of other drugs, including cocaine, marijuana, stimulants, sedative/hypnotics, and hallucinogens.[1–4]

Theoreticians and clinicians have begun to explore the similarities between the addictive behaviors. Indeed, the notion of chemical dependence as encompassing alcohol and drugs seems to have become commonplace in many treatment centers in the United States. In the last 10 years there also has been an attempt to integrate diverse theoretical perspectives about addictive behaviors. Rather than emphasizing the differences, theoreticians are exploring the similarities between the addictive behaviors.[5,6]

Despite these changes, there appears to have been relatively little dialogue between those clinical researchers whose focus was on alcoholism and those whose focus was on drug abuse. Given the considerable amount of literature in the two fields (e.g., an alcoholism treatment literature review by Miller and Hester[7] contained over 600 references), keeping informed of advances in knowledge even in subsections of each of these fields is extremely difficult. This chapter attempts to bridge this gap by reviewing issues in the assessment of alcohol and drug abuse; providing a brief description of those behavioral treatments that have received consistent support in controlled studies in the area of alcoholism; briefly reviewing the treatment outcome research; identifying similarities and differences in the interventions for alcohol and drug abuse; and, finally, making recommendations for future advancements in the treatment and research of substance abuse.

2. Assessment of Alcohol and Drug Abuse

While substance abusers as a group share many commonalities, individual differences between these individuals are significant. Alcohol and drug problems are multidimensional and frequently vary in intensity and etiology. A comprehensive assessment of a client's problem, therefore, is essential in order for a clinician to formulate the most effective treatment plan for a particular client.

While the direct consequences of alcohol and drug abuse are frequently responsible for a client's malaise, it generally is not the only problem. Whether another problem is the etiological source of the substance abuse or vice versa, concurrent problems must be addressed. It is therefore essential to provide a comprehensive assessment of the client's general life functioning (e.g., marital, employment, social, affective functioning) and to incorporate this information in treatment planning.

Behavioral clinicians utilize assessment before and during treatment in a continuous and interactive manner. Initial assessment provides information helpful in matching clients to (1) the goals of treatment, (2) the treatment setting, and (3) specific interventions. Subsequent assessment is used to evaluate the accuracy of the initial assessment and ongoing treatment strategies. Continuous assessment can provide feedback to the client and clinician about the impact of their efforts. Successful strategies can be reinforced and unsuccessful strategies can be reformulated.

Understanding alcohol and drug abuse requires assessment of the antecedents and consequences of substance use as well as the actual alcohol or drug use behavior itself. In regard to alcohol and drug use, Sobell et al.[8] recommend that a minimum of 13 variables should be addressed. These include the following:

1. The specific quantities of alcohol and other drugs used and the frequency of use.
2. Usual and unusual substance use circumstances and patterns.
3. Predominant mood states and situations antecedent and consequent to substance use.
4. History of alcohol and drug withdrawal symptoms.
5. Medical problems associated with or exacerbated by substance use.
6. Identification of possible difficulties the client might encounter in initially refraining from substance use.
7. Extent and severity of previous substance abuse.
8. Multiple drug use.
9. Reports of frequent thoughts or urges to drink or take drugs.
10. History of previous responses to substance abuse treatment and self-initiated periods of abstinence.
11. Review of the positive consequences of substance abuse.
12. Other life problems.
13. Indicants of tolerance.

Specific techniques that have been used to assess these variables include (1) retrospective methods, such as self-reports, collateral reports, and official records; (2) assessment instruments, such as quantity–frequency,[9] time-line follow-back,[10] Michigan Alcoholism Screening Test (MAST),[11] Comprehensive Drinker Profile,[12] Drug Abuse Screening Test (DAST),[13] Addiction Severity Index (ASI),[14] Inventory of Drinking Situations,[15] Situational Confidence Questionnaire,[16] and Alcohol Expectancies;[17] (3) self-monitoring[18]; and (4) physiological assessments, such as breath alcohol, urine, and liver function tests. For a comprehensive review of alcohol and/or drug assessment instruments, refer to Jacobson[19,20] and Sobell et al.[8]

3. Behavioral Treatments for Alcohol and Drug Abuse

Alcoholism treatment methods currently supported by controlled outcome research include (1) aversion therapies; (2) behavioral self-control training; (3) behavioral marital and family therapy; (4) community reinforcement approach; (5) social skills training; and (6) stress management training. Cue exposure methods are also included since they have received positive support in drug abuse research.

3.1. Aversion Therapies

3.1.1. Alcohol Abuse.
The aversion therapies include chemical aversion, electrical aversion, and covert sensitization. In chemical aversion, the most common form of aversive conditioning, the client is usually given emetine, which produces nausea and emesis, and pilocarpine, which closes the sphincter from the stomach to the intestinal tract. As the client starts to become nauseous, he or she is given alcohol to sniff, sip, and swallow. As nausea continues and emesis begins to occur, the client continues to smell and drink the alcohol. This pairing of drinking and nausea and vomiting continues for about 30–60 min. Five conditioning sessions are usually held within 10 days, but the number of sessions is adjusted according to the client's responses. If a conditioned response develops, the client begins to experience nausea and/or revulsion to the smell, taste, and sometimes even the sight of alcoholic drinks. In electrical aversive conditioning, the client has electrodes attached to his or her arm and is given electrical shocks during the process of smelling and sipping the drink, although the drink is not consumed. In covert sensitization, the client is seated in a comfortable chair in a quiet room and instructed to relax and vividly imagine a variety of scenes that have been tailor-made to match his or her own drinking behaviors and sensations. In these scenes, the client's subjective experiences of drinking are associated with intense feelings of nausea. Behavioral ratings of nauseous responses are taken, along with self-report and physiological measures of reactivity. As with chemical aversion, the desired goal is to develop a conditioned response to the sight, smell, and taste of alcohol. The overall purpose of all three conditioning paradigms is to reduce or eliminate an individual's desire for alcohol.

Evaluations of chemical aversion therapy have been reported for over 50 years and have documented consistently high abstinence rates.[7] Two controlled studies[21,22] also have documented higher rates of abstinence relative to comparison groups but not as high as those in the uncontrolled studies.

The uncontrolled and controlled studies of electrical aversion present a much more confusing picture. An early study[23] reported a better outcome for subjects given electrical aversion therapy in addition to hospital treatment compared to those given only hospital treatment, but noted that they fared no better than a control group given noncontingent shock treatment (which theoretically should not work). Other investigators have found no significant differences in outcome for subjects given electrical aversion therapy compared to other treatments (e.g., Refs. 22, 24,25). Finally, an unpublished, but important study by Marlatt[26] found substantial reductions in drinking at follow-up in subjects receiving electrical aversion relative to those receiving noncontingent shock treatment and a hospital ward control group.

Outcome studies in covert sensitization also present something of a confused picture perhaps due, at least in part, to differences in the treatment procedures defined as "covert sensitization." When procedures have been carefully defined along the lines of classical conditioning, the picture has been much more consistent and positive. The development and strength of a conditioned response during the conditioning process has been found to be associated with a more favorable outcome at follow-up.[27–29]

3.1.2. Drug Abuse. Aversion procedures have also been used frequently in the treatment of drug abuse. This extensive use has been linked to such theoretical assumptions as conditioned withdrawal reactions to drug cues and the strong reinforcing effects of some drugs, as well as being linked to such pragmatic issues as court-mandated treatment for drug abusers.[30]

Two chemically aversive stimuli, apomorphine (an emetic) and Scoline (which produces respiratory paralysis), have produced positive outcomes at least in case studies.[31–33] For example, Thompson and Rathod[33] gave heroin addicts Scoline to produce brief respiratory paralysis immediately following a cookup ritual. Eight of ten heroin addicts were reportedly drug-free (by frequent urinalysis) at follow-up intervals ranging from 3 to 30 weeks, while the six control subjects all relapsed. Unfortunately, the control subjects were not randomly assigned, so the positive results are equivocal. Morakinyo[34] has also used chemical aversion therapy in the treatment of cannabis dependence with positive results.

Electrical aversive stimuli have been used in the treatment of drug addiction, but these studies also have been uncontrolled case studies. Wolpe[35] reported that a Demerol abuser, who shocked himself on nine different occasions when a drug craving was experienced, relapsed after 12 weeks, though craving apparently decreased. Spevak and colleagues[36] reported that two of three male adolescent amphetamine abusers who were treated with electric shock relapsed during the 7 months following treatment. O'Brien et al.[37] reported two case studies in which heroin addicts, following relaxation training, received electrical shock which was paired with stories about the act of injecting heroin. One subject was reported drug free at 14 months, although she was treated by systematic desensitization for a drug-related fear and received a booster treatment. The other subject was drug free at 6 months but refused booster treatment. Since studies have utilized electric shock in conjunction with other therapeutic components, such as behaviorally oriented group therapy and relaxation training,[38] the impact of the aversive conditioning technique cannot be determined.

In covert sensitization, the drug abuser is instructed to imagine aversive stimuli such as vomiting while also imagining drug-related scenes or behavior. Such covert conditioning methods have been reported in several single case studies.[39–41] In studies with more than one subject, Steinfeld[42] reported a decrease in self-reported drug use in two polydrug users, and Deuhn[43] reported 18 months of abstinence in six of seven LSD users. In another study,[44] intravenous amphetamine addicts were asked to imagine a typical injection situation and then to imagine that they felt no drug effects. Three of the four subjects were drug free at a 9-month follow-up.

Maletzky[45] has noted that imaginal scenes may not be sufficiently vivid to induce a conditioned aversive reaction. To address this concern, the sensitization procedure has been enhanced by having the subjects sniff valeric acid, a harmless procedure that elicits vivid, noxious olfactory cues. In another variant of the technique, covert sensitization was conducted under hypnosis.[46]

Other aversive methods used to treat drug abusers have included implosive therapy[47] and confrontational feedback.[48,49] Unfortunately, while there have been several encouraging studies using aversive methods in the treatment of drug problems, studies typically have been single case reports. Controlled experimental evaluations have been rare. Moreover, none of the studies using chemical or electrical stimuli with drug abusers have demonstrated physiological evidence of a conditioned aversion.

3.2. Behavioral Self-Control Training

3.2.1. Alcohol Abuse. Behavioral self-control training (BSCT)[50–53] can be used to pursue either a drinking goal of moderation or a goal of abstinence. It consists of behavioral strategies which include self-monitoring, goal setting, specific changes in drinking behavior, rewards for goal attainment, functional analysis of drinking situations, and the learning of alternative coping skills.

For example, clients initially are shown how to monitor their own drinking. They are given self-monitoring cards on which they write down the date and time of each drink, the amount of alcohol in each drink, where they are, and with whom they are drinking. They set limits on their drinking, which include the number of drinks per occasion and estimated peak blood alcohol concentrations. Following this, clients are instructed in a variety of behavioral strategies to control their rate of drinking. Examples include drinking weaker drinks, spacing them out across time, sipping rather than gulping drinks, alternating nonalcoholic drinks with alcoholic drinks, limiting the total time they spend drinking, and refusing social pressures to drink. Clients are next encouraged to set up a system of rewards for achieving the goals they set for themselves. Once this is done, clients are about 6 weeks into the program and have a large amount of self-monitoring data. This information provides the basis for a functional analysis of drinking. Using their self-monitoring cards, they are asked to identify antecedent events to heavy drinking as well as both the short- and long-term consequences of their drinking. By becoming aware of environmental, interpersonal, and intrapersonal factors that have been associated with excessive drinking, they can begin to plan ahead with alternative coping strategies rather than to merely react to them with heavy drinking. Finally, clients are encouraged to learn new coping strategies to deal more effectively with high-risk situations for relapse into heavy drinking.

There have been more controlled studies of the effectiveness of BSCT procedures than of any other treatment for alcoholism. Caddy and Lovibond[54] reported superior outcome for subjects participating in a BSCT program relative to untreated controls. Brown[55] and Coghlan[56] documented a superior outcome for Driving While Intoxicated (DWI) offenders given BSCT relative to those given an alcohol education program. In a series of studies, Vogler and his colleagues[57,58] reported rates of moderate drinking ranging from 21 to 68% at 12-month follow-up for subjects in a BSCT program. Sanchez-Craig and her colleagues[52,59] found substantial improvements in subjects given BSCT procedures (with goals of either abstinence or moderation) at up to 2-year follow-up. Miller and Hester[60] have conducted a series of studies comparing different modes of delivery of BSCT, again with positive results.

Perhaps the most controversial study of BSCT procedures has been that of Sobell and Sobell.[61] Using inpatient gamma alcoholics, they randomly assigned them either to individualized behavior therapy with a goal of controlled drinking or to one of three comparison groups who received treatment with a goal of abstinence. They documented greater improvement in the experimental group relative to the control groups, although the findings were questioned by Pendery and her colleagues.[62] Pendery et al.'s conclusion that the experimental group fared poorly after treatment appears accurate, but they failed to note that the control groups who received abstinence-oriented treatment did worse than the experimental group. In view of this and other studies of BSCT procedures that have utilized moderation goals with gamma alcoholics, using BSCT procedures with a moderation goal does not appear to be the most appropriate treatment for such subjects. On the other hand, the consistently positive outcome studies of BSCT have documented the best outcome in subjects who have lower levels of problem severity.

3.2.2. Drug Abuse. Wilkinson and LeBreton[4] have used a behavioral self-control training model in the treatment of 49 multiple drug abusers who were randomly assigned to the treatment, as part of a larger study. Self-monitoring cards were adapted to permit recording of several drug classes, for the identification of cravings and refusals of drugs, and for consumptions. Subjects were asked to record the time of events, dose, and context. Treatment components consisted of the self-monitoring of drug use, setting specific goals for reduced use, and identifying cognitive and behavioral strategies for avoiding drug use in situations of high risk. Although subjects were classified as successful ($N = 11$ at Session 1 and 10 at Session 2), improved ($N = 20$ and 15, respectively), and unimproved ($N = 18$ and 13, respectively), and attempts to discern the variables that were predictive of outcome were described, no outcome data were reported on comparison or control groups.

To the authors' knowledge, no other studies have been reported investigating the efficacy of self-management techniques as a unimodal treatment with drug abusers. The efficacy of such interventions remains to be tested.

3.3. Behavioral Marital and Family Therapy

3.3.1. Alcohol Abuse.   O'Farrell and Cowles[63] have described behavioral marital and family therapy as a series of strategies that can be implemented during three broadly defined stages of recovery: (1) recognizing that a problem exists and that something needs to be done about it, (2) stopping the abusive drinking, and (3) long-term maintenance of change. During the first stage, the spouse or significant other is seen individually if the alcohol-abusing spouse is unwilling to come to treatment or even discuss the possibility of treatment. The nonabusing spouse is instructed in strategies to reduce physical abuse to himself or herself and in how to increase the alcohol abuser's motivation to change. During the second stage of recovery, the first goal of therapy is to reduce or eliminate the abusive drinking and to change alcohol-related patterns of interactions. A subsequent goal is to change general patterns of interaction to reduce conflict and provide an environment supportive of sobriety. The final goal during the second stage of recovery is to teach the couple and/or family how to deal with conflicts without drinking. The focus of treatment during the long-term maintenance stage is on relapse prevention and marital or family issues commonly encountered during long-term recovery.

Other behavioral approaches to marital and family therapy[64-66] may place greater emphasis on various aspects of the change process, but all have a goal of changing the environmental contingencies for drinking and sobriety and of training behaviors that reduce conflict and improve communications between the alcohol abuser and his or her spouse or family.

Controlled studies of behavioral marital and family therapy consistently have documented positive results in the experimental groups relative to control groups. The most recent well-designed studies have been conducted by McCrady and her colleagues[65,67] and O'Farrell and his colleagues.[68,69] Both groups have documented an improved outcome for subjects either receiving marital therapy or having the spouse involved in treatment relative to either individual therapy or no spouse involvement. While these improvements are significant during the early course of follow-up (i.e., within the first 6 months), at 18-month to 4-year follow-ups, the differences between the two groups disappear. One explanation is that gains in the marital therapy groups diminish although there is continued improvement in the control groups. Also, the impact of behavioral marital and family therapy may not be sufficient to maintain gains without either additional booster sessions or additional treatment specifically designed to prevent relapse. This need for some form of ongoing treatment contact, even if only on a monthly or quarterly basis, has been recognized and presently is being studied.

3.3.2. Drug Abuse.   Despite frequently reported use of family therapy in drug abuse treatment agencies, few controlled outcome studies have been reported. Recently, Todd[70] presented a 10-session family treatment approach based on behavioral principles for drug abuse.[71,72] However, while behavioral components to the family therapy intervention were underscored, structural family therapy also was utilized in this intervention. In one controlled treatment outcome study, family therapy was found to have a significant impact on heroin abuse.[71,72] For the best treatment condition (paid family therapy), 67% of the cases showed a successful outcome in abstinence from use of illegal opiates for at least 80% of one time interval. This contrasted with 33% in the non–family treatment condition and 39% in the control condition. Results for legal opiates (including detoxification from methadone) were similar: paid family therapy, 62% success; non–family treatment, 27% success; control, 28% success. Finally, a dramatic finding was related to the difference in death rates between clients in the family and non–family treatment groups. For non–family treatment clients, there was a 10% death rate, compared to 2% for clients whose families were involved in treatment. Szapocznik et al.,[73] also utilizing structural family therapy, compared the relative effectiveness of one-person family therapy and conjoint family therapy with adolescents who abused drug(s) (e.g., marijuana, barbiturates, alcohol). While the two approaches were found to be equally effective, the specific effects on drug abuse were not delineated.

While preliminary work appears promising, the research on the efficacy of behavioral marital or family therapy with drug abusers has been very limited.

3.4. The Community Reinforcement Approach/Contingency Management

3.4.1. Alcohol Abuse.
The community reinforcement approach (CRA) to the treatment of alcohol abuse[74] is a group of behaviorally based procedures designed to alter the contingencies for drinking in such a way that sobriety is rewarded and drinking results in a "time out" from positive reinforcers. CRA may include a behavioral compliance program to ensure that the abuser takes disulfiram, reciprocity marriage counseling, a job club for unemployed clients, social skills training, advice on social and recreational activities, a nonalcoholic social club, and training in controlling urges to drink. Specific components of the CRA are chosen based on the client's needs.

Four controlled studies have evaluated the effectiveness of the CRA for alcohol abusers.[75–78] The first study compared the CRA when added to an inpatient alcohol treatment program to the inpatient program without the CRA.[79] Patients receiving the CRA had significantly better outcome during follow-up. It was later tested on an outpatient basis with similar success.[76] In one of the studies the procedures were dismantled in an attempt to determine their relative effectiveness, and it was found that for married clients, the disulfiram compliance program alone was as effective as the comprehensive CRA. Single clients, however, did not do as well with just the disulfiram compliance program, but had outcomes equal to those of the married clients when given the entire battery of CRA procedures.

3.4.2. Drug Abuse.   While the CRA has been shown to be successful to date, such efforts have been directed toward alcohol rather than other drug abuse. A considerable literature in the drug abuse field does exist, however, on the usefulness of contingency contracting, an operant intervention technique that seeks to reinforce desired behavior by controlling behavioral consequences. Thus, when treatment providers or other significant others have control over meaningful reinforcers or punishers, response contingencies may be established to control drug use and abuse.

In general, contingency contracts used in drug treatment settings have included several target behaviors, such as informing the therapist of the subject's whereabouts and contacting the therapist if exposed to a situation that might precipitate drug use or if drugs are actually used.[80–83] In an exemplary, multifaceted contingency-management program known as the Drug Project, Boudin[84] incorporated sequential levels of contracting including managerial, transitional, and personal contracts.

Crowley[85] has reported on extensive experience in treating drug-abusing physicians. In the case of a physician–addict, he or she might be asked to provide the therapist with a signed letter which indicates that if the letter is mailed by the therapist to the medical board, he or she has relapsed and should be suspended from medical practice. The client agrees to attend specific treatment sessions and to provide urine specimens at specific intervals. The therapist agrees to certify that the client is drug-free and capable of continuing medical practice unless there is evidence of relapse or a failure to provide drug-free urine specimens, in which case the therapist mails the previously written letter to the appropriate medical board. Obviously, such contracts work best in treating clients who have something to lose, and may be unnecessarily punitive, thereby reducing the clients' willingness to become involved in treatment.[86]

Previous research also has indicated that contingency contracting is useful in improving the effectiveness of methadone maintenance treatment.[87] Several small experimental studies have shown that methadone take-home doses, sometimes combined with other clinic privileges, can reduce or eliminate illicit drug use,[88–90] though the change is sometimes small[91,92] and usually confined to the period during which the contingency is being used.[93] Magura and colleagues[94] recently reported that contracting had a favorable, though transient, effect primarily on non-cocaine-abusing methadone patients.

Other studies, such as that of Dolan et al.,[95] have utilized contingency contracts that specified aversive consequences (e.g., detoxification and removal from methadone treatment) in attempting to decrease illicit drug use among methadone patients. In this study of 21 subjects selected on the basis of having a positive urinalysis during a 60-day baseline, illicit drug use was significantly reduced during the 30-day intervention and remained below baseline levels during a 60-day follow-up. Finally, the reader is referred to a review by Bickel and colleagues[96] on the combined use of behavioral and pharmacological treatment to reduce alcohol consumption in alcoholic methadone patients.

In general, contingency management methods have achieved modest success with drug abusers, attaining some value in terms of behavior management during treatment. However, their efficacy in contributing to successful treatment outcomes once the abusers are discharged into the community is generally unknown.

3.5. Social Skills Training

3.5.1. Alcohol Abuse.   Social skills training refers to behavioral training in a variety of coping skills designed to achieve personal goals and solve interpersonal problems. In general, it is considered an adjunct treatment. Chaney[97] conceptualizes skillful behavior as an interaction between a person's thoughts, feelings, and actions in an environment and with other people. Because of the heterogeneity of the general population of alcohol abusers, it is not possible to specify one set of social skills that is appropriate to teach all clients. There may, however, be sufficient similarity between individuals in particular treatment programs that a group of skills can be specified. This can be done through a situational analysis of relapse determinants.[98,99] Coping skills and situational problems are graded from simple and easy to complex and difficult, and training progresses from easier tasks to more difficult tasks. Clients' behavioral skills are measured prior to and following training. The training is conducted in groups, with each member taking an active part in role playing or behavioral rehearsal of a variety of different social situations. After a client role-plays a situation, he or she receives feedback from the group and therapist(s) which reinforces appropriate behaviors and provides constructive criticism. In addition to therapist-generated problem situations, clients are asked to present their own problem situations as sessions progress. As clients demonstrate appropriate coping skills in the group, they are given homework assignments to cope with similar situations outside of the group. This increases the probability that the skills that are trained generalize to the client's real world.

Controlled evaluations in alcoholism have consistently supported the effectiveness of social skills training as an adjunctive treatment for alcoholics.[100–102] Optimal elements include behavioral group practice, attention to cognitions about assertiveness, and assertiveness skills.

3.5.2. Drug Abuse.   Relapses to drug use often involve inadequate coping with interpersonal stress, social pressure, or negative emotional states.[103] Since drug abusers in residential drug treatment centers have shown deficits in social and coping skills and interpersonal cognitive problem solving, skill training has been advocated as an effective component of treatment for preventing relapse.[104–107] Drug abusers have been reported to find frustrating situations more difficult to handle effectively than do nonaddicts, suggesting the importance of being able to cope with interpersonal stressors.[108] Behavioral skill training programs for substance abusers that focus on problem solving and/or social skills training have the explicit goal of enhancing clients' ability to handle stressful events. Recent reviews[30] of treatment outcome research have noted that such programs have shown promising results.

In one uncontrolled study, Callner[109] found improvements in role-play assessments with assertiveness training. In a later experimental study, Callner and Ross[110] found increased assertiveness in drug abusers who were assessed in a role-playing test after undergoing assertion training. Lin and colleagues[111] found self-reported improvements in assertiveness after receiving social skills training in a residential facility. Smith[112] found improvement in problem-solving related to marijuana, decreased use and abuse of marijuana, and improved role-playing performance in marijuana-related situations among teenage marijuana abusers exposed to behavioral skills training. Hawkins et al.[105] reported that after receiving supplemental skills training and social-network-development aftercare, the role-play performance of drug abusers improved in situations involving avoidance of drug use, coping with drug relapse, social interaction, interpersonal problem solving, and coping with stress.

Reeder and Kunce[113] used a "vicarious behavior induction" method with heroin addicts in which subjects were exposed either to a videolecture, a taped lecture on coping behavior, or to a videomodel, a taped model successfully solving problems related to abstinence. Six-month outcome data showed that the videomodel subjects had significantly better employment and/or school attendance (46% vs. 18%). Finally, Platt and Metzer[114] reported that providing addicts with interpersonal cognitive problem solving skills may have a beneficial effect on their ability to cope with problems of daily living. They report that addicts can be taught interpersonal problem-solving skills and that such skills have been retained for at least 1 year.[115] Greatest skill acquisition was found to take place among those subjects who had entered the program with the lowest levels of interpersonal problem-solving skills. Unfortunately, the effects of interpersonal cognitive problem-solving training on drug use were not reported.

Few studies have focused on skills training as a treatment intervention for drug abusers. Of particular importance is the fact that few studies investigated the effects of skills training on quantity or frequency of drug use after the end of treatment.

3.6. Stress Management Training

3.6.1. Alcohol Abuse. Stress is a commonly used, loosely defined term in everyday language. For clinical purposes, stress has been broadly defined as the "entire process of interaction between external 'stressors' (e.g., work commitments, criticism, unrealistic demands) and an individual's reactions to these, or 'stress responses' "[116] Stress management training can be broadly described as training that teaches clients (1) active coping strategies to replace maladaptive stress responses; (2) life-style changes to reduce the severity and frequency of external stressors; and (3) how to alter the perceived degree of threat posed by the stressor. Specific strategies include training in relaxation skills, cognitive restructuring of self-statements, and assertive resistance to workloads and responsibilities that are unrealistic or excessive.

Outcome evaluations of stress management procedures have been inconsistent, largely as a result of investigating different procedures on different populations. For example, studies of the effectiveness of relaxation training have been mixed,[117,118] but subject populations have been diverse. Rosenberg[119] found that anxious subjects benefited significantly from relaxation training, while subjects with low levels of anxiety did not benefit relative to a control group. Overall, however, there is evidence to support the effectiveness of stress management training as an adjunct treatment for alcohol abusers.

3.6.2. Drug Abuse. Although various anxiety-management procedures have been evaluated with drug abusers, few studies have used relaxation training in the treatment of drug abusers except as part of a systematic desensitization treatment. For example, O'Brien et al.,[37] in the use of aversive conditioning, taught heroin addicts relaxation skills. Deep muscle relaxation also has been used effectively to lessen the effects of a bad LSD trip.[120] Systematic desensitization has been used to treat psychological side effects of a drug paranoia in a Drinamyl abuser[121] and LSD flashbacks,[36] as well as presumed correlates of drug use, such as fears of being independent[121] and social anxieties.[121,122] Biofeedback methods also have been used to induce relaxation,[123,124] but findings either have been unimpressive or have been reported through uncontrolled studies.

In one of the few controlled studies, Brautigam[125] evaluated the efficacy of meditation as a treatment for drug addiction using random assignment to meditation and control (group counseling) conditions. The meditators decreased their use of both "soft" and "hard" drugs in the 3 months following the initiation of meditation, while the controls' drug use remained at a high level. However, the short length of the follow-up period and discontinuation of meditation by 4 of the 10 experimental subjects weakens the positive results, especially since the author reported that in the 2-year period after the study, periodic relapse to drug use occurred for 80% of the meditators.

On the basis of the aforementioned studies, it is presently impossible to formulate any definitive conclusions regarding the efficacy of relaxation training as a treatment for drug abuse (see Klajner et al.[126] for a review of relaxation training in the treatment of substance abuse).

3.7. Cue Exposure

Drug Abuse. Former drug abusers often report symptoms of withdrawal and/or intense craving when exposed to stimuli previously associated with the act of drug injection.[127] This phenomenon of learned or "conditioned" withdrawal/craving has been widely reported and has been considered to be important in explaining relapse to drug use.[128-131] Such conditioning models posit that aspects of craving, tolerance, and withdrawal are learned responses that can be extinguished through proper procedures.

In support of this model, Sideroff and Jarvik,[132] in replicating a study done by Teasedale,[133] examined the effects of drug-related slides on the physiological and psychological states of abstinent opiate addicts. They reported increases in physiological correlates of distress (heart rate and galvanic skin response), as well as higher subjective ratings of anxiety, depression, and craving, in their opiate addicts when exposed to drug- vs. non-drug-related slides.

Childress et al.[131] is one of the few research groups that have investigated the potential effectiveness of extinction procedures with opioid and cocaine abusers. For opioid abusers, the graduated hierarchy of extinction stimuli included self-produced verbal imagery ("drug stories"), audiotapes of drug talk, color slides of cookup–injection rituals, videotapes of drug purchases, cookup and injection, and handling of drug objects in a cookup/tieoff procedure. Saline self-injection was optional. Cocaine stimuli were developed in a similar manner, using language, scenes, and paraphernalia directly from the client's street experience. Although data collection in their treatment-outcome study of abstinent, formerly opioid-dependent clients is still in progress and the cocaine study is in an early stage, Childress et al.[134] report that the extinction procedures "were effective in virtually eliminating both craving and withdrawal symptoms in response to the stimuli within 20 treatment sessions [a 3-week inpatient stay]."

Data from this series of studies are encouraging, particularly since the stimuli and procedures may easily be adapted to a clinic setting. However, extinction procedures have not been widely used. How long those reductions in conditioned craving and withdrawal to the drug-related stimuli last and how well those reductions in response will generalize to other drug-related stimuli in the client's postdischarge environment will need to be evaluated in well-controlled treatment outcome studies.

4. Similarities in Behavioral Alcohol and Drug Abuse Treatment

The previous two sections indicate that, by and large, the interventions for alcohol abuse that have been supported by controlled research are being adapted and tested for their effectiveness in drug abuse. The notable exception is cue exposure methods, which were first developed and tested with drug abusers. Cue exposure application with alcohol abusers is just now being considered.[135]

The interventions for alcohol and drug abuse can be conceptually divided into three categories: (1) those which focus directly on the drinking and drug use behaviors (antidipsotropic medications and methadone, aversion therapies, cue exposure, and behavioral self-control training); (2) those which focus on changing the environmental contingencies to encourage sobriety and discourage alcohol and drug use and reduce conflict within the client's home environment (behavioral marital and family therapies and the community reinforcement approach/contingency management); and (3) those which focus on increasing the coping skills of the client so that he or she can more effectively deal with situations that place him or her at high risk for relapse (social skills training and stress management training). Viewed from this conceptual perspective, these various approaches attempt to change (1) the client's ability to deal more effectively with antecedent events that in the past have been associated with alcohol and/or drug abuse; (2) the client's behaviors, thoughts, and feelings that are associated with the actual use of the alcohol and/or drugs; and (3) the consequences for sobriety vs. alcohol and/or drug use.

5. Future Directions in Treatment and Research

Treatment outcome research in alcoholism has become substantially more methodologically rigorous and sophisticated in the last decade. Unfortunately, the same cannot be said for the treatment outcome research in drug abuse. While alcoholism researchers frequently employ random assignment, adequate sample sizes, and minimum follow-ups of 1 year, this is usually not the case with the drug abuse research.

Both fields can be faulted, however, for not providing more detailed descriptions of their subject populations. In this regard, subjects need to undergo comprehensive pretreatment assessment which is multidimensional rather than unidimensional. Alcoholism researchers, in particular, often do not adequately assess polydrug abuse in their alcoholic subjects. Pretreatment client characteristics can and do interact differently with different treatments.[136] Without knowledge of potentially critical client characteristics, however, substantial error variance is likely to mask true treatment effects and client–treatment interactions.

There is also a need for long-term follow-ups. The current "gold standard" in alcoholism treatment research is a minimum of 12 months, a standard that should be adopted by drug abuse researchers. Two- to four-year follow-ups are also appropriate to determine the longer-range effects of treatment and to better understand how posttreatment life events interact with treatment effects in particular client populations. Claims of treatment effectiveness can no longer be based on changes in behavior during or immediately after completion of treatment.

Another variable that needs to be more adequately addressed in both fields is the use of additional treatment or booster sessions. Just as the optimal length and intensity of initial treatments need to be determined, so do the number, frequency, and duration of booster sessions. Appropriate use of booster sessions may optimize, maintain, or even increase initial treatment gains.

6. Summary

Three major conclusions can be drawn from the treatment outcome research in alcohol and drug abuse which are applicable to the future development of substance abuse treatment and research. First, it is clearly evident now that no single treatment is effective for everyone. Instead, there appear to be a number of promising alternatives. These alternatives need to be investigated with experimental rigor to determine their effectiveness with different populations of alcohol and/or drug abusers.

Second, a recent review[137] of the parameters of alcohol treatment (e.g., intensity, length, and setting) found that most alcohol abusers, when randomly assigned, do as well with shorter, less intensive, and outpatient treatments as they do with longer, more intensive, and inpatient treatments. The matching data suggest that alcohol abusers with more severe deterioration and/or social instability (e.g., homeless or unemployed) benefit more from longer, more intensive treatment while those clients with good social stability and less problem severity benefit at least as much, if not more, from briefer, less intensive interventions. If this also is the case with drug abuse treatment, then the limited resources for substance abuse treatment potentially can be used in more cost-efficient and cost-effective ways. Restructuring the delivery of treatment also would free up some of the limited resources for those clients who truly need more extensive treatment.

Third, there are compelling data from alcoholism treatment research to support the notion of matching clients to treatments.[138] When a client is appropriately matched to a specific treatment(s), the probability of a favorable outcome is significantly increased. Although still in its infancy, client–treatment matching research is one of the fastest-growing areas of research in alcoholism. It is highly likely that client–treatment matching issues also have the potential to improve the overall effectiveness of substance abuse treatments.

References

1. Farley EC, Santo Y, Speck DW: Multiple drug-abuse patterns of youths in treatment, in Bescher GM, Friedman AS (eds): *Youth Drug Abuse: Problems, Issues and Treatment.* Lexington, MA, Lexington Books, 1979, pp. 149–168.
2. Sadava SW: Concurrent multiple drug use: Review and implications. *J Drug Issues* 14:623–636, 1984.

3. Wilkinson DA, Martin G: Concordant findings with multiple outcome measures in evaluation of behavioral treatment of multiple drug abuse. Paper presented at the Third International Conference on the Treatment of Addictive Behaviors, North Berwick, Scotland, 1984.
4. Wilkinson DA, LeBreton S: Early indications of treatment outcome in multiple drug users, in Miller WE, Heather N (eds): *Treating Addictive Behaviors: Processes of Change*. New York, Plenum Press, 1986, pp 239–261.
5. Miller PM: Commonalities of addictive behaviors, in Nirenberg TD, Maisto SA (eds): *Developments in the Assessment and Treatment of Addictive Behaviors*. Norwood NJ, Ablex, 1988.
6. Miller WE, Heather N (eds): *Treating Addictive Behaviors: Processes of Change*. New York, Plenum Press, 1986.
7. Miller WR, Hester RK: Treating the problem drinker: Modern approaches, in Miller WR (ed): *The Addictive Behaviors: Treatment of Alcoholism, Drug Abuse, Smoking, and Obesity*, London, Pergamon Press, 1980. pp 11–141.
8. Sobell LC, Sobell MB, Nirenberg TD: Behavioral assessment and treatment planning with alcohol and drug abusers: A review with an emphasis on clinical application. *Clin Psychol Rev* 8:19–54, 1988.
9. Polich JM, Armor DJ, Braiker HB: *The Course of Alcoholism: Four Years after Treatment*. New York, Wiley, 1981.
10. Sobell LC, Maisto SA, Sobell MB, Cooper AM: Reliability of alcohol abusers' self-reports of drinking behavior. *Behav Res Ther* 17:157–160, 1979.
11. Selzer ML: Michigan Alcoholism Screening Test: The quest for a new diagnostic instrument. *Am J Psychiatry* 127:1653–1658, 1971.
12. Marlatt GA, Miller WR: Comprehensive drinker profile, in Lettieri DJ, Nelson JE, Sayers MA (eds): *NIAAA Treatment Handbook Series 2: Alcoholism Treatment Assessment Research Instruments* Washington, DC, U.S. Government Printing Office, 1987, pp. 167–188.
13. Skinner HA: The drug abuse screening test. *Addict Behav* 7:363–371, 1982.
14. McLellan AT, Luborsky L, Woody GE, O'Brien CP: An improved diagnostic evaluation instrument for substance abuse patients. *J Nerv Ment Dis* 168:26–33, 1980.
15. Annis HM: A relapse prevention model for the treatment of alcoholics, in Miller WR, Heather N (eds): *Treating Addictive Behaviors: Processes of Change*. New York, Plenum Press, 1986, pp 401–434.
16. Annis HM, Kelly P: Two scales for assessing the determinants of alcohol relapse episodes. Paper presented at the meeting of the American Psychological Association, Toronto, Canada, 1984.
17. Southwick L, Steele C, Marlatt A, Lindell M: Alcohol-related expectancies: Defined by phase of intoxication and drinking experience. *J Consult Clin Psychol* 49:713–721, 1981.
18. Nirenberg TD, Sobell L, Ersner-Herschfield S: Self-monitoring of alcohol consumption: Reactivity and reliability. Paper presented at the meeting of the World Congress on Behavior Therapy, New York, 1983.
19. Jacobson GR: A comprehensive approach to pretreatment evaluation: I. Detection, assessment and diagnosis of alcoholism, in Hester RK, Miller WR (eds): *Handbook of Alcoholism Treatment: Effective Alternatives*. Elmsford, NY, Pergamon Press, 1989, pp. 17–53.
20. Jacobson GR: A comprehensive approach to pretreatment evaluation: II. Other clinical considerations, in Hester RK, Miller WR (eds): *Handbook of Alcoholism Treatment: Effective Alternatives*. Elmsford, NY, Pergamon Press, 1989, pp 54–66.
21. Boland FJ, Mellor CS, Revusky S: Chemical aversion treatment of alcoholism: Lithium as the aversive agent. *Behav Res Ther* 16:401–409, 1978.
22. Cannon DS, Baker TB, Wehl CK: Emetic and electric shock alcohol aversion therapy: Six- and twelve-month follow-up. *J Consult Clin Psychol* 49:360–368, 1981.
23. Vogler RE, Lunde SE, Martin PL: Electrical aversion conditioning with chronic alcoholics: Follow-up and suggestions for research. *J Consult Clin Psychol* 45:467–479, 1977.
24. Hedberg AG, Campbell LM: A comparison of four behavioral treatment approaches to alcoholism. *J Behav Ther Exp Psychiatry* 5:251–256, 1974.

25. McCance C, McCance PF: Alcoholism in North-East Scotland: Its treatment and outcome. *Br J Psychiatry* 115:189–198, 1969.
26. Marlatt GA: A comparison of aversive conditioning procedures in the treatment of alcoholism. Paper presented at the annual meeting of the Western Psychological Association, Anaheim, CA, 1973.
27. Elkins RL: Covert sensitization treatment of alcoholism: Contributions of successful conditioning to subsequent abstinence maintenance. *Addict Behav* 5:67–89, 1980.
28. Elkins RL, Murdock RP: The contribution of successful conditioning to abstinence maintenance following covert sensitization (verbal aversion) treatment of alcoholism. *IRCS Med Sci Psychol Psychiatry Soc Occup Med* 5:167, 1974.
29. Miller WR, Dougher MJ: Covert sensitization: Alternative treatment approaches for alcoholics. Paper presented at the Second Congress of the International Society for Biomedical Research on Alcoholism, Santa Fe, NM, 1984.
30. Sobell MB, Sobell LC, Ersner-Hirshfield S, Nirenberg TD: Alcohol and drug problems, in Bellack AS, Hersen M, Kazdin AE (eds): *International Handbook of Behavior Modification and Therapy.* New York, Plenum Press, 1982, pp 501–533.
31. Liberman R: Aversive conditioning of drug addicts: A pilot study. *Behav Res Ther* 14:381, 1968.
32. Raymond M: The treatment of addiction by aversion conditioning with apomorphine. *Behav Res Ther* 1:287–291, 1964.
33. Thompson IG, Rathod NH: Aversion therapy for heroin dependence. *Lancet* 31:382–384, 1968.
34. Morakinyo O: Aversion therapy of cannabis dependence in Nigeria. *Drug Alcohol Dependence* 12:287–293, 1983.
35. Wolpe J: Conditioned inhibition of craving in drug addiction: A pilot experiment. *Behav Res Ther* 2:285–288, 1965.
36. Spevak M, Pihl R, Rowan T: Behavior therapies in the treatment of drug abuse: Some case studies. *Psychol Rec* 23:179–184, 1973.
37. O'Brien JS, Raynes AE, Patch VD: Treatment of heroin addiction with aversion therapy, relaxation training and systematic desensitization. *Behav Res Ther* 10:77–80, 1972.
38. Copemann CD: Drug addiction: II. An aversive counterconditioning technique for treatment. *Psychol Rep* 38:1271–1281, 1976.
39. Cautela JR, Rosensteil AK: The use of covert conditioning in the treatment of drug abuse. *Int J Addict* 10:277–303, 1975.
40. Kolvin T: "Aversive imagery" treatment in adolescents. *Behav Res Ther* 5:245–248, 1967.
41. Anant SS: Treatment of alcoholics and drug addicts by verbal conditioning techniques. *Int J Addict* 3;381–388, 1968.
42. Steinfeld GJ: The use of covert sensitization with institutionalized narcotic addicts. *Int J Addict* 5:225–232, 1970.
43. Deuhn WD: Covert sensitization in group treatment of adolescent drug abusers. *Int J Addict* 13:485–491, 1978.
44. Gotestam KG, Melin L: Covert extinction of amphetamine addiction. *Behav Ther* 5:90–92, 1974.
45. Maletzky BM: Assisted covert sensitization for drug abuse. *Int J Addict* 9:411–429, 1974.
46. Copemann CD: Treatment of polydrug abuse by covert sensitization: Some contraindications. *Int J Addict* 12:17–23, 1977.
47. Hirt M, Greenfield H: Implosive therapy treatment of heroin addicts during methadone detoxification. *J Consult Clin Psychol* 47:982–983, 1979.
48. MacDonaugh TS: Evaluation of the effectiveness of intensive confrontation in changing the behavior of drug and alcohol abusers. *Behav Ther* 7:408–409, 1976a.
49. MacDonaugh TS: The relative effectiveness of a medical hospitalization program vs a feedback-behavior modification program in treating alcohol and drug abusers. *Int J Addict* 11:269–282, 1976b.

50. Miller WR, Munoz RF: *How to Control Your Drinking*, rev. ed. Albuquerque, University of New Mexico Press, 1982.

51. Robertson I, Heather N: *So You Want to Cut down Your Drinking?* rev. ed. Edinburgh, Scottish Health Education Group, 1985.

52. Sanchez-Craig M: *Therapist's Manual for Secondary Prevention of Alcohol Problems: Procedures for Teaching Moderate Drinking and Abstinence.* Toronto, Canada, Addiction Research Foundation, 1984.

53. Vogler RE, Bartz WR: *The Better Way to Drink.* Oakland, CA, New Harbinger Publications, 1982.

54. Caddy GR, Lovibond SH: Self-regulation and discriminated aversive conditioning in the modification of alcoholics' drinking behavior. *Behav Ther* 7:223–230, 1976.

55. Brown RA: Conventional education and controlled drinking education courses with convicted drunk drivers. *Behav Ther* 11:632–642, 1980.

56. Coghlan GR: The investigation of behavioral self-control theory and techniques in a short-term treatment of male alcohol abusers. Unpublished doctoral dissertation, State University of New York at Albany (University Microfilms No. 7918818), 1979.

57. Vogler RE, Compton JV, Weissbach TA: Integrated behavior change techniques for alcoholism. *J Consult Clin Psychol* 43:233–243, 1975.

58. Vogler RE, Weissbach JA, Compton LV, Martin GT: Integrated behavior change techniques for problem drinkers in the community. *J Consult Clin Psychol* 45:467–479, 1977.

59. Sanchez-Craig M, Annis HM, Bornet AR, MacDonald KR: Random assignment to abstinence and controlled drinking: Evaluation of a cognitive–behavioural program for problem drinkers. *J Consult Clini Psychol* 52:390–403, 1984.

60. Miller WR, Hester RK: The effectiveness of alcoholism treatment: What the research reveals, in Miller WR, Heather N (eds): *Treating Addictive Behaviors: Processes of Change.* New York, Plenum Press, 1986, pp 121–174.

61. Sobell MB, Sobell LC: Individualized behavior therapy for alcoholics. *Behav Ther* 4:49–72, 1973.

62. Pendery ML, Maltzman IM, West LJ: Controlled drinking by alcoholics? New findings and a reevaluation of a major affirmative study. *Science* 217:169–175, 1982.

63. O'Farrell TJ, Cowles KS: Marital and family therapy, in Hester RK, Miller WR (eds): *Handbook of Alcoholism Treatment Approaches: Effective Alternatives.* Elmsford, NY, Pergamon Press, 1989, pp 183–198.

64. Sisson RW, Azrin NH: Family-member involvement to initiate and promote treatment of problem drinkers. *J Behav Ther Exp Psychiatry* 17:15–21, 1986.

65. McCrady BS, Moreau J, Paolino TJ Jr., Longabaugh R: Joint hospitalization and couples therapy for alcoholism: A four-year follow-up. *J Stud Alcohol* 43:1244–1250, 1982.

66. Thomas, EJ, Santa CA: Unilateral family therapy for alcohol abuse: A working conception. *Am J Fam Ther* 10:49–60, 1982.

67. McCrady BS, Paolino TJ Jr., Longabaugh R, Rossi J: Effects of joint hospital admission and couples treatment for hospitalized alcoholics: A pilot study. *Addict Behav* 4:155–165, 1979.

68. O'Farrell TJ, Cutter HS: Effect of adding a behavioral or an interactional couples group to individual outpatient alcoholism counseling, in O'Farrell TJ (ed): Spouse-involved treatment for alcohol abuse. Symposium conducted at the Sixteenth Annual Convention of the Association for the Advancement of Behavior Therapy, Los Angeles, 1982.

69. O'Farrell TJ, Cutter HS, Floyd FJ: Evaluating behavioral marital therapy for male alcoholics: Effects on marital adjustment and communication before to after treatment. *Behav Ther* 15:147–168, 1984.

70. Todd TC: A contingency analysis of family treatment and drug abuse, in Grabowski J, Stitzer ML, Henningfield JE (eds): *Behavioral Intervention Techniques in Drug Abuse Treatment.* NIDA Research Monograph 46 (pp. 104–114). DHHS Pub No. (ADM) 84-1282. Washington, DC Supt. of Docs., U.S. Government Printing Office, 1984.

71. Stanton MD, Todd TC: Structural family therapy with drug addicts, in Kaufman E, Kaufman P (eds): *Family Therapy of Drug and Alcohol Abuse.* New York, Gardner Press, 1979.

72. Stanton MD, Todd TC, et al: *The Family Therapy of Drug Abuse and Addiction*. New York, Guilford Press, 1982.

73. Szapocznik J, Kurtines WM, Foote F, Perez-Vidal A, Hervis O: Conjoint versus one-person family therapy: Further evidence for the effectiveness of conducting family therapy through one person with drug-abusing adolescents. *J Consult Clin Psychol* 54:395–397, 1986.

74. Sisson RW, Azrin NH: The community reinforcement approach, in Hester RK, Miller WR (eds): *Handbook of Alcoholism Treatment: Effective Alternatives*. Elmsford, NY, Pergamon Press, 1989, pp 242–258.

75. Azrin NH: Improvements in the community-reinforcement approach to alcoholism. *Behav Res Ther* 14:339–348, 1976.

76. Azrin NH, Sisson RW, Meyers R, Godley M: Alcoholism treatment by disulfiram and community reinforcement therapy. *J Behav Ther Exp Psychiatry* 13:105–112, 1982.

77. Hunt GM, Azrin NH: A community-reinforcement approach to alcoholism. *Behav Res Ther* 11:91–104, 1973.

78. Mallams JH, Godley MD, Hall GM, Meyers RJ: A social-systems approach to resocializing alcoholics in the community. *J Stud Alcohol* 43:1115–1123, 1982.

79. Hunt GM, Azrin NH: A community-reinforcement approach to alcoholism. *Behav Res Ther* 11:91–104, 1973.

80. Anker AL, Crowley TJ: Use of contingency in speciality clinics for cocaine abuse, in Harris LS (ed): *Problems of Drug Dependence*. National Institute for Drug Abuse. Research Monograph 41. Rockville, MD, Committee on Problems of Drug Dependence, Inc., 1982, pp. 452–459.

81. Pickens RW, Thompson T: Behavioral treatment of drug dependence, in Grabowski J, Stitzer M, Henningfield JE (eds): *Behavioral Intervention Techniques in Drug Abuse Treatment*. NIDA Research Monograph 46. (pp.53–67). DHHS Pub. No. (ADM) 84-1282. Washington, DC, Supt. of Docs., U.S. Government Printing Office, 1984.

82. Polakow RL, Doctor RM: Treatment of marijuana and barbiturate dependency by contingency contracting. *J Behav Ther Exp Psychiatry* 4:375–377, 1973.

83. Hall SM: Cooper JL, Burmaster S, Polk A: Contingency contracting as a therapeutic tool with methadone maintenance clients: Six single subject studies. *Behav Res Ther* 15:438–441, 1977.

84. Boudin HM: Contingency contracting with drug abusers in the natural environment: Treatment evaluation, in Sobell LC, Sobell MB, Ward E (eds): *Evaluating Alcohol and Drug Abuse Treatment Effectiveness: Recent Advances*. New York: Pergamon Press, 1980.

85. Crowley T: Contingency contracting treatment of drug-abusing physicians, nurses and dentists, in Grabowski J, Stitzer M, Henningfield JE (eds): *Behavioral Intervention Techniques in Drug Abuse Treatment*. NIDA Research Monograph 46. (pp.68–83). DHHS Pub. No. (ADM) 84-1284. Washington, DC, Supt. of Docs., U.S. Government Printing Office, 1984.

86. Kleber HD, Gawin FH: Cocaine abuse: A review of current and experimental treatments, in Grabowski J (ed): *Cocaine: Pharmacology, Effects, and Treatment of Abuse*. NIDA Research Monograph 50. (pp. 111–129). DHHS Pub. No. (ADM) 87-1326. Washington, DC, Supt. of Docs., U.S. Government Printing Office, 1987.

87. Stitzer ML, Bigelow GE, McCaul ME: Behavioral approaches to drug abuse, in Hersen M (ed): *Progress in Behavior Modification, Vol 14*. New York, Academic Press, 1983.

88. Bigelow G, Lawrence C, Stitzer M, Wells D: Behavioral treatments during outpatient methadone maintenance: A controlled evaluation. Paper presented at the annual meeting of the American Psychological Association, Washington, DC, 1976.

89. McCaul ME, Stitzer ML, Bigelow GE, Liebson IA: Contingency management interventions: Effects on treatment outcome during methadone detoxification. *J Appl Behav Anal* 17:35–43, 1984.

90. Stitzer ML, Bigelow GE, Liebson IA, Hawthorne JW: Contingent reinforcement of benzodiazepine-free urines: Evaluation of a drug abuse treatment intervention. *J Appl Behav Anal* 15:493–503, 1982.

91. Hall SM, Bass A, Hargreaves WA, Loeb P: Contingency management and information feedback in outpatient heroin detoxification. *Behav Ther* 10:445–451, 1979.

92. Milby JB, Garrett C, English C, Fritschi O, Clarke C: Take-home methadone: Contingency effects on drug-seeking and productivity of narcotic addicts. *Addict Behav* 3:315–320, 1978.
93. Stitzer ML, Bigelow GE, Liebson IA: Reducing drug use among methadone maintenance clients. Contingent reinforcement for morphine-free urines. *Addict Behav* 5:333–340, 1980.
94. Magura S, Casriel C, Goldsmith DS, Strug DL, Lipton DS: Contingency contracting with polydrug-abusing methadone patients. *Addict Behav* 13:113–118, 1988.
95. Dolan MP, Black JL, Penk WE, Robinowitz R, DeFord HA: Contracting for treatment termination to reduce illicit drug use among methadone maintenance treatment failures. *J Consult Clin Psychol* 53:549–551, 1985.
96. Bickel WK, Marion I, Lowinson JH: The treatment of alcoholic methadone patients: A review. *J Substance Abuse Treatment* 4:15–19, 1987.
97. Chaney EF: Social skills training, in Hester RK, Miller WR (eds): *Handbook of Alcoholism Treatment: Effective alternatives.* Elmsford, NY, Pergamon Press, 1989, pp 206–215.
98. Annis H: *Inventory of Drinking Situations (IDS-100).* Toronto, Canada, Addiction Research Foundation, 1982.
99. Annis HM: *Situational Confidence Questionnaire "FCQ-39."* Toronto, Canada, Addiction Research Foundation, 1987.
100. Chaney ER, O'Leary MR, Marlatt GA: Skill training with alcoholics. *J Consult Clin Psychol* 46:1092–1104, 1978.
101. Jackson P, Oei TPS: Social skills training and cognitive restructuring with alcoholics. *Drug Alcohol Dependence* 3:369–374, 1978.
102. Monti PM, Abrams DB, Binkoff JA, Zwick WR, Liepman MR, Nirenberg TD, Rohsenow DJ: Communication skills training with family and cognitive behavioral mood management training for alcoholics. *J Stud Alcohol,* in press.
103. Marlatt GA, Gordon JR: Determinants of relapse: Implications for the maintenance of behavior change. In Davidson PO, Davidson SM (eds): *Behavioral Medicine: Changing Health Lifestyles.* New York, Brunner/Mazel, 1980, pp 410–452.
104. Catalano RF, Hawkins JD, Hall J: Preventing relapse among former substance abusers. Paper presented at the annual meeting of the International Network of Social Network Analysts, Phoenix, AZ, 1984.
105. Hawkins JD, Catalano RF, Wells EA: Measuring effects of a skills training intervention for drug abusers. *J Consult Clin Psychol* 54:661–664, 1986.
106. Marlatt GA, Gordon JR: *Relapse Prevention: A Self-Control Strategy for the Maintenance of Behavior Change.* New York, Guilford Press, 1985.
107. Platt JJ, Metzger DS: Cognitive interpersonal problem-solving skills and the maintenance of treatment success in heroin addicts. *J Addict Behav* 1:5–13, 1987.
108. Kolko DJ, Sirota AD, Monti PM, Paolino RM: Peer identification and empirical validation of problematic interpersonal situations of male drug addicts. *J Psychopath Behav Assess* 7:135–144, 1985.
109. Callner DA: The assessment and training of assertive behavior in a drug addict population, in Cannon D (chair): Social skills training in a drug rehabilitation program. Symposium presented at the meeting of the American Psychological Association, Montreal, Quebec, Canada, 1973.
110. Callner DA, Ross SM: The assessment and training of assertive skills with drug addicts: A preliminary study. *Int J Addict* 13:227–229, 1978.
111. Lin T, Bon S, Dickinson J, Blume C: Systematic development and evaluation of a social skills training program for chemical abusers. *Int J Addict* 17:585–596, 1982.
112. Smith TE: Drug education with adolescent marihuana abusers. Doctoral dissertation, University of Washington, 1981. Seattle, Dissertation Abstracts International 42, 5251A, 1982.
113. Reeder CW, Kunce JT: Modeling techniques, drug-abstinence behavior, and heroin addicts: A pilot study. *J Counsel Psychol* 23:560–562, 1976.
114. Platt JJ, Metzer D: Cognitive interpersonal problem-solving skills and the maintenance of treatment success in heroin addicts. *Psychol Addict Behav* 1:5–13, 1987.

115. Platt JJ, Morell J. Flaherty E, Metzger D: Controlled sutdy of methadone rehabilitation process. Final report No. R01-DA01929, Washington, DC, NIDA, 1982.
116. Stockwell T, Towne C: Anxiety and stress management, in Hester RK, Miller WR (eds): *Handbook of Alcoholism Treatment Approaches: Effective Alternatives.* Elmsford, NY, Pergamon Press, 1989, pp. 222–230.
117. Blake BG: A follow-up of alcoholics treated by behaviour therapy. *Behav Res Ther* 5:89–94, 1967.
118. Miller WR, Taylor CA: Relative effectiveness of bibliotherapy, individual and group self-control training in the treament of problem drinkers. *Addict Behav* 5:13–24, 1980.
119. Rosenberg SD: Relaxation training and a differential assessment of alcoholism. Unpublished dissertation, California School of Professional Psychology, San Diego (University Microfilms No. 8004362), 1979.
120. Dreilinger C, Thayer LC: Relaxation techniques in drug related crises: A case report. *Drug Forum* 4:73–78, 1974.
121. Kraft T: Successful treatment of a case of drinamyl addiction. *Br J Psychiatry* 114:1363–1364, 1968.
122. Paynard C, Wolf K: The use of systematic desensitization in an outpatient drug treatment center. *Psychother Theory Res Pract* 11:329–330, 1974.
123. Khatami M, Mintz J, O'Brien CP: Biofeedback-mediated relaxation in narcotic addicts. *Behav Ther* 8:968–969, 1977.
124. Goldberg RJ, Greenwood JC, Taintor Z: Alpha conditioning as an adjunct treatment for drug dependence II. *Int J Addict* 12:195–204, 1977.
125. Brautigam E: Effects of the transcendental meditation program on drug abusers: A prospective study, in Orme-Johnson DW, Farrow JT (eds): *Scientific Research on the Transcendental Meditation Program: Collected Papers, Vol. 1.* Livingston Manor, NY, MIU Press, 1977.
126. Klajner R, Hartman LM, Sobell MB: Treatment of substance abuse by relaxation training: A review of its rationale, efficacy and mechanisms. *Addict Behav* 9:41–55, 1984.
127. O'Brien CP: Experimental analysis of conditioning factors in human narcotic addiction. *Pharmacol Rev* 27:535–543, 1975.
128. O'Brien CP, Childress AR, McLellan AT, Ehrman R, Ternes JW: Types of conditioning found in drug-dependent humans, in Ray B (ed): *Learning Factors in Substance Abuse.* NIDA Research Monograph 84. (pp. 44–61). DHHS Pub. No. (ADM) 88-1576. Washington DC, Supt. of Docs., U.S. Government Printing Office, 1988.
129. Meyer RE, Mirin SM: *The Heroin Stimulus: Implications for a Theory of Addiction.* New York, Plenum Press, 1979, pp 231–247.
130. Meyer RE: Conditioning phenomena and the problem of relapse in opioid addicts and alcoholics, in Ray B (ed): *Learning Factors in Substance Abuse.* NIDA Research Monograph 84. (pp. 161–179) DHHS Pub. No. (ADM) 88-1576. Washington, DC, Supt. of Docs., U.S. Government Printing Office, 1988.
131. Childress AR, McLellan AT, Ehrman R, O'Brien CP: Classically conditioned responses in opioid and cocaine dependence: A role in relapse? in Ray B (ed): *Learning Factors in Substance Abuse.* NIDA Research Monograph 84. DHHS Pub. No. (ADM) 88-1576. Washington, DC, Supt. of Docs., U.S. Government Printing Office, 1988, pp 25–43.
132. Sideroff S, Jarvik M: Conditioned response to a videotape showing heroin-related stimuli. *Int J Addict* 15:529–536, 1980.
133. Teasedale J: Conditioned abstinence in narcotic addicts. *Int J Addict* 8:273–292, 1973.
134. Childress AR, McLellan AT, Ehrman R, O'Brien CP: Extinction of conditioned responses in abstinent cocaine or opioid users, in Harris LS (ed): *Problems of Drug Dependence 1986.* NIDA Research Monograph 76. DHHS Pub. No. (ADM) 87-1508. Washington, DC, Supt. of Docs., U.S. Government Printing Office, 1987.
135. Monti PM, Binkoff JA, Abrams DB, Zwick WR, Nirenberg TD, Liepman MR: Reactions of alcoholics and non-alcoholics to drinking cues. *J Abnormal Psychol* 96:122–126, 1987.
136. McLachlan JFC: Benefit from group therapy as a function of patient-therapist match on conceptual level. *Psychother Theory Res Pract* 9:317–323, 1972.

137. Miller WR, Hester RK: Inpatient alcoholism treatment: Who benefits? *American Psychologist* 41(7):794–805, 1986.
138. Miller WR, Hester RK: Matching problem drinkers with optimal treatments. In Miller WR, Heather N (eds): *Treating Addictive Behaviors: Processes of Change*, New York, Plenum Press, pp 175–204.

Contents of Previous Volumes

Volume 1

I. The Role of Genetics in the Expression of Alcoholism   *Henri Begleiter, Section Editor*

Overview   *Donald Goodwin*

Twin Adoption Studies: How Good Is the Evidence for a Genetic Role?   *Robin M. Murray, Christine A. Clifford, and Hugh M. D. Gurling*

Pharmacogenetic Approaches to the Neuropharmacology of Ethanol   *Dennis R. Peterson*

II. The Behavioral Treatment of Alcoholism   *Edward Gottheil, Section Editor*

Overview   *Edward Gottheil*

How Environments and Persons Combine to Influence Problem Drinking: Current Research Issues   *G.N. Barucht*

Alcoholism: The Evolution of a Behavioral Perspective   *William H. George and G. Alan Marlatt*

Behavioral Treatment Methods for Alcoholism   *Glenn R. Caddy and Trudy Block*

Outcome Studies on Techniques in Alcoholism Treatment   *Gloria K. Litman and Anne Topham*

Contributions to Behavioral Treatment from Studies on Programmed Access to Alcohol   *Glenn R. Caddy and Edward Gottheil*

Current Status of the Field: Contrasting Perspectives   A. The Behavioral Therapist's View   *Mark B. Sobell and Linda C. Sobell*   B. The Future of Behavioral Interventions   *S.H. Lovibond*   C. A Medical Clinician's Perspective   *Robert A. Moore*   D. An Anthropological Perspective on the Behavior Modification Treatment of Alcoholism   *David Levinson*

III. Social Mediators of Alcohol Problems: Movement toward Prevention Strategies   *Alfonso Paredes, Section Editor*

Overview   *Alfonso Paredes*

Estimating Alcoholic Prevalence   *Charles J. Furst*

The Role of Alcohol Availability in Alcohol Consumption and Alcohol Problems   *Jerome Rabow and Ronald K. Watts*

Price and Income Elasticities and the Demand for Alcoholic Beverages   *Stanley I. Ornstein and David Levy*

Youth, Alcohol, and Traffic Accidents: Current Status   *Richard L. Douglass*

IV. Current Concepts in the Diagnosis of Alcoholism   *James A. Halikas, Section Editor*

Overview   *James A. Halikas*

Detection, Assessment, and Diagnosis of Alcoholism: Current Techniques   *George R. Jacobson*

Types and Phases of Alcohol Dependence Illness   *Wallace Mandell*

Neuropsychology of Alcoholism: Etiology, Phenomenology, Process, and Outcome   *Ralph E. Tarter and Christopher M. Ryan*

Volume 2

I. Experimental Social and Learning Models of Drinking   *Alfonso Paredes, Section Editor*

Overview   *Alfonso Paredes*

A Conditioning Model of Alcohol Tolerance   *Christine L. Melchior and Boris Tabakoff*

Social Models of Drinking Behavior in Animals: The Importance of Individual Differences   *Gaylord D. Ellison and Allen D. Potthoff*

Social Correlates of Drinking in Contrived Situations   *Alfonso Paredes and Carolyn Jenuine Hopper*

Alcohol-Ingestive Habits: The Role of Flavor and Effect   *Jack E. Sherman, Kenneth W. Rusiniak, and John Garcia*

Commentary on the Utility of Experimental Social and Learning Models of Alcoholism   *Frank A. Holloway, O.H. Rundell, Pamela S. Kegg, Dick Gregory, and Thomas Stanitis*

II. Alcohol and the Liver: Recent Developments in Preclinical and Clinical Research   *Richard A. Deitrich, Section Editor*

Overview   *Charles S. Lieber*

Alcohol-Induced Liver Injury: The Role of Oxygen   *Ronald G. Thurman, Sungchul Ji, and John J. Lemasters*

Hypermetabolic State and Hypoxic Liver Damage   *Yedy Israel and Hector Orrego*

Commentary on the Hypermetabolic State and the Role of Oxygen in Alcohol-Induced Liver Injury   *Esteban Mezey*

Alcohol-Induced Mitochondrial Changes in the Liver   *Ellen R. Gordon*

Effect of Ethanol on Hepatic Secretory Proteins   *Dean J. Tuma and Michael F. Sorrell*

Use of Colchicine and Steroids in the Treatment of Alcoholic Liver Disease   *John T. Galambos and Stan P. Riepe*

III. Aging and Alcoholism   *Edward Gottheil, Section Editor*

Overview   *Edward Gottheil*

Neurobiological Relationships between Aging and Alcohol Abuse   *Gerhard Freund*

Alcohol Consumption and Premature Aging: A Critical Review   *Christopher Ryan and Nelson Butters*

Aging and Alcohol Problems: Opportunities for Socioepidemiological Research   *Richard L. Douglass*

Life Stressors and Problem Drinking among Older Adults   *John W. Finney and Rudolf H. Moos*

Cross-Cultural Aspects of Alcoholism in the Elderly   *Joseph Westermeyer*

IV. Contributions from Anthropology to the Study of Alcoholism   *Linda A. Bennett, Section Editor*

Overview   *Linda A. Bennett*

Ethnohistory and Alcohol Studies   *Thomas W. Hill*

Social-Network Considerations in the Alcohol Field   *Carl A. Maida*

Alcohol Use in the Perspective of Cultural Ecology   *Andrew J. Gordon*

Selected Contexts of Anthropological Studies in the Alcohol Field: Introduction   *Dwight B. Heath*

Family Research and Alcoholism   *Joan Ablon*

Alcoholism-Treatment-Center-Based Projects   *Jack O. Waddell*

Cross-Cultural Studies of Alcoholism   *Dwight B. Heath*

Volume 3

I. High-Risk Studies of Alcoholism   *Donald W. Goodwin, Section Editor*

Overview   *Donald W. Goodwin*

Behavioral Effects of Alcohol in Sons of Alcoholics   *Marc A. Schuckit*

The EEG in Persons at Risk for Alcoholism   *Jan Volavka, Vicki Pollock, William F. Gabrielli, Jr., and Sarnoff A. Mednick*

Psychopathology in Adopted-Out Children of Alcoholics: The Stockholm Adoption Study   *C. Robert Cloninger, Michael Bohman, Soren Sigvardsson, and Anne-Liis von Knorring*

Premorbid Assessment of Young Men at High Risk for Alcoholism   *Joachim Knop*

Minimal Brain Dysfunction and Neuropsychological Test Performance in Offspring
   of Alcoholics   *Victor M. Hellelbrock, James R. Stabenau, and Michie N. Hesselbrock*

II. Prostaglandins, Leukotrienes, and Alcohol   *Richard A. Deitrich, Section Editor*

Overview   *Erik Anggard*

Synthesis of Prostaglandins and Leukotrienes: Effects of Ethanol   *Robert C.
   Murphy and Jay Y. Westcott*

Biochemical Interactions of Ethanol with the Arachidonic Acid Cascade   *Sam N.
   Pennington*

Brain Arachidonic Acid Metabolites: Functions and Interactions with Ethanol   *Jay
   Y. Westcott and Alan C. Collins*

III. Cardiovascular Effects of Alcohol Abuse   *David H. Van Thiel, Section Editor*

Overview   *David H. Van Thiel*

Alcohol, Coronary Heart Disease, and Total Mortality   *Ronald E. LaPorte, Jane A.
   Cauley, Lewis H. Kuller, Katherine Flegal, and David Van Thiel*

Alcohol Consumption and Cardiovascular Risk Factors   *Katherine M. Flegal and
   Jane A. Cauley*

Myocardial Effects of Alcohol Abuse: Clinical and Physiologic
   Consequences   *David H. Van Thiel and Judith S. Gavaler*

Biochemical Mechanisms Responsible for Alcohol-Associated
   Myocardiopathy   *David H. Van Thiel, J.S. Gavaler, and D. Lehotay*

IV. Cerebral Functioning in Social Drinkers   *Elizabeth Parker, Section Editor*

Overview   *Elizabeth Parker*

The Continuity Hypothesis: The Relationship of Long-Term Alcoholism to the
   Wernicke-Korsakoff Syndrome   *Nelson Butters and Jason Brandt*

The Impact of Fathers' Drinking on Cognitive Loss among Social
   Drinkers   *Elizabeth S. Parker, Douglas A. Parker, and Jacob A. Brody*

Alcohol Use and Cognitive Functioning in Men and Women College
   Students   *Roseann Hannon, Charles P. Butler, Carol Lynn Day, Steven A. Khan,
   Lupo A. Quitoriana, Annette M. Butler, and Lawrence A. Meredith*

CT Demonstration of the Early Effects of Alcohol on the Brain   *Lesley Ann Cala*

Cognitive Deficits and Morphological Cerebral Changes in a Random Sample of
   Social Drinkers   *Hans Bergman*

Brain Damage in Social Drinkers? Reasons for Caution   *Shirley Y. Hill and
   Christopher Ryan*

Statistical Issues for Research on Social Drinkers   *Ronald Schoenberg*

Functional Brain Imaging   *Robert M. Kessler*

Volume 4

I. Combined Alcohol and Drug Abuse Problems   *Edward Gottheil, Section Editor*

Overview   *Edward Gottheil*

Multiple Drug Use: Epidemiology, Correlates, and Consequences   *Richard R. Clayton*

Mechanisms of Depressant Drug Action/Interaction   *Eugene P. Schoener*

Sedative Drug Interactions of Clinical Importance   *Paul Cushman, Jr.*

Treating Multiple Substance Abuse Clients   *Jerome F.X. Carroll*

II. Typologies of Alcoholics   *Thomas F. Babor and Roger E. Meyer, Section Editors*

Overview   *Thomas F. Babor and Roger E. Meyer*

Classification and Forms of Inebriety: Historical Antecedents of Alcoholic Typologies   *Thomas F. Babor and Richard J. Lauerman*

Empirically Derived Classifications of Alcohol-Related Problems   *Leslie C. Morey and Harvey A. Skinner*

An Examination of Selected Typologies: Hyperactivity, Familial, and Antisocial Alcoholism   *Arthur I. Alterman and Ralph E. Tarter*

Alcoholic Typologies: A Review of Empirical Evaluations of Common Classification Schemes   *Michie N. Hesselbrock*

Alcoholic Subtypes Based on Multiple Assessment Domains: Validation against Treatment Outcome   *Dennis M. Donovan, Daniel R. Kivlahan, and R. Dale Walker*

III. The Alcohol Withdrawal Syndrome   *Alfonso Paredes, Section Editor*

Overview   *Alfonso Paredes*

The Alcohol Withdrawal Syndrome: A View from the Laboratory   *Dora B. Goldstein*

Clinical Neuroendocrinology and Neuropharmacology of Alcohol Withdrawal   *Jeffrey N. Wilkins and David A. Gorelick*

Clinical Assessment and Pharmacotherapy of the Alcohol Withdrawal Syndrome   *Claudio A. Naranjo and Edward M. Sellers*

Special Aspects of Human Alcohol Withdrawal   *David A. Gorelick and Jeffrey N. Wilkins*

IV. Renal and Electrolyte Consequences of Alcohol Abuse   *David H. Van Thiel, Section Editor*

Overview   *David H. Van Thiel*

Disorders of the Serum Electrolytes, Acid-Base Balance, and Renal Function in Alcoholism   *Thomas O. Pitts and David H. Van Thiel*

Urinary Tract Infections and Renal Papillary Necrosis in Alcoholism   *Thomas O. Pitts and David H. Van Thiel*

Disorders of Divalent Ions and Vitamin D. Metabolism in Chronic Alcoholism   *Thomas O. Pitts and David H. Van Thiel*

The Pathogenesis of Renal Sodium Retention and Ascites Formation in Laennec's Cirrhosis   *Thomas O. Pitts*

Volume 5

I. Alcohol and Memory   *Henri Begleiter, Section Editor*

Overview   *Henri Begleiter*

The Chronic Effects of Alcohol on Memory: A Contrast between a Unitary and Dual System Approach   *D. Adrian Wilkinson and Constantine X. Poulos*

The Etiology and Neuropathology of Alcoholic Korsakoff's Syndrome: Some Evidence for the Role of the Basal Forebrain   *David P. Salmon and Nelson Butters*

Cognitive Deficits Related to Memory Impairments in Alcoholism   *Marlene Oscar-Berman and Ronald J. Ellis*

Specificity of Memory Deficits in Alcoholism   *Walter H. Riege*

Ethanol Intoxication and Memory: Recent Developments and New Directions   *Richard G. Lister, Michael J. Eckardt, and Herbert Weingartner*

II. Alcohol Treatment and Society   *Robin Room, Section Editor*

Overview   *Robin Room*

Inebriety, Doctors, and the State: Alcoholism Treatment Institutions before 1940   *Jim Baumohl and Robin Room*

Sociological Perspectives on the Alcoholism Treatment Literature since 1940   *Norman Giesbrecht and Kai Pernanen*

The Social Ecology of Alcohol Treatment in the United States   *Connie Weisner*

The Great Controlled-Drinking Controversy   *Ron Roizen*

III. The Effects of Ethanol on Ion Channels   *Richard A. Deitrich, Section Editor*

Overview   *Richard A. Deitrich*

Calcium Channels: Interactions with Ethanol and Other Sedative-Hypnotic Drugs   *Steven W. Leslie*

Effects of Ethanol on the Functional Properties of Sodium Channels in Brain Synaptosomes   *Michael J. Mullin and Walter A. Hunt*

Involvement of Neuronal Chloride Channels in Ethanol Intoxication, Tolerance, and Dependence   *Andrea M. Allan and R. Adron Harris*

The Effects of Ethanol on the Electrophysiology of Calcium Channels   *R.S. Pozos and S.G. Oakes*

The Electrophysiology of Potassium Channels   *Peter L. Carlen*

IV. Hazardous and Early Problem Drinking   *Alfonso Paredes, Section Editor*

Overview   *Alfonso Paredes*

Studying Drinking Problems Rather than Alcoholism   *Dan Cahalan*

Social Drinking as a Health and Psychosocial Risk Factor: Anstie's Limit Revisited   *Thomas F. Babor, Henry R. Kranzler, and Richard J. Lauerman*

Methods of Intervention to Modify Drinking Patterns in Heavy Drinkers   *Hans Kristenson*

Techniques to Modify Hazardous Drinking Patterns   *William R. Miller*

Alcohol-Related Hazardous Behavior among College Students   *Jerome Rabow, Carole A. Neuman, Ronald K. Watts, and Anthony C.R. Hernandez*

Volume 6

I. Substance Abuse and Posttraumatic Stress Disorder   *Edward Gottheil, Section Editor*

Overview   *Edward Gottheil*

Posttraumatic Stress Disorder and Substance Abuse: Clinical Issues   *Edgar P. Nace*

The Interrelationship of Substance Abuse and Posttraumatic Stress Disorder: Epidemiological and Clinical Complications   *Terence M. Keane, Robert J. Gerardi, Judith A. Lyons, and Jessica Wolfe*

Biological Mechanisms in Posttraumatic Stress Disorder: Relevance for Substance Abuse   *Thomas R. Kosten and John Krystal*

Coping and Defending Styles among Vietnam Combat Veterans Seeking Treatment for Posttraumatic Stress Disorder and Substance Use Disorder   *Walter E. Penk, Robert F. Peck, Ralph Robinowitz, William Bell, and Dolores Little*

Posttraumatic Stress Disorder in World War II and Korean Combat Veterans with Alcohol Dependency   *Keith A. Druley and Steven Pashko*

II. Alcohol and Its Management in the Workplace   *Paul M. Roman, Section Editor*

Overview   *Paul M. Roman*

The Epidemiology of Alcohol Abuse among Employed Men and Women   *Douglas A. Parker and Gail C. Farmer*

Growth and Transformation in Workplace Alcoholism Programming   *Paul M. Roman*

Constructive Confrontation and Other Referral Processes   *Harrison M. Trice and Willim J. Sonnenstuhl*

Identification of Alcoholics in the Workplace   *Walter Reichman, Douglas W. Young, and Lynn Gracin*

Monitoring the Process of Recovery: Using Electronic Pagers as a Treatment Intervention   *William J. Filstead*

Posttreatment Follow-up, Aftercare, and Worksite Reentry of the Recovering Alcoholic Employee   *Andrea Foote and John C. Erfurt*

New Occupations and the Division of Labor in Workplace Alcoholism Programs   *Terry C. Blum*

III. Consequences of Alcohol Abuse Unique to Women   *David H. Van Thiel, Section Editor*

Overview   *David H. Van Thiel*

Effects of Moderate Consumption of Alcoholic Beverages on Endocrine Function in Postmenopausal Women: Bases for Hypotheses   *Judith S. Gavaler*

Effects of Alcohol Abuse on Reproductive Function in Women   *Nancy K. Mello*

Maternal Ethanol Use and Selective Fetal Malnutrition   *Stanley E. Fisher and Peter I. Karl*

Ethanol Metabolism and Hepatotoxicity: Does Sex Make a Difference?   *David H. Van Thiel and Judith S. Gavaler*

IV. Markers for Risk of Alcoholism and Alcohol Intake   *Richard A. Deitrich, Section Editor*

Overview   *Richard A. Deitrich*

Physiological and Psychological Factors as Predictors of Alcoholism Risk   *Marc A. Schuckit*

Brain Evoked Potentials as Predictors of Risk   *Robert Freedman and Herbert Nagamoto*

Molecular Markers for Linkage of Genetic Loci Contributing to Alcoholism   *David Goldman*

Blood Markers of Alcoholic Liver Disease   *Charles S. Lieber*

Discriminant Function Analysis of Clinical Laboratory Data: Use in Alcohol Research   *Zelig S. Dolinsky and Jerome M. Schnitt*

Acetaldehyde and Its Condensation Products as Markers in Alcoholism   *Michael A. Collins*

Volume 7

I. Alcoholics Anonymous: Emerging Concepts   *Chad D. Emrick, Section Editor*

Overview   *Chad D. Emrick*

A Sociocultural History of Alcoholics Anonymous   *Harrison M. Trice and William J. Staudenmeier, Jr.*

Alcoholics Anonymous: Membership Characteristics and Effectiveness as
    Treatment   *Chad D. Emrick*
Some Limitations of Alcoholics Anonymous   *Alan C. Ogborne*
Alcoholics Anonymous and Contemporary Psychodynamic Theory   *Edward J.
    Khantzian and John E. Mack*
Al-Anon and Recovery   *Timmen L. Cermak*

II. Family Systems and Family Therapy in Alcoholism   *Edward Gottheil, Section
    Editor*

Overview   *Edward Gottheil*
Family, Alcohol, and Culture   *Linda A. Bennett*
Alcoholism and Family Interaction   *Theodore Jacob and Ruth Ann Seilhamer*
Alcoholism and Family Factors: A Critical Review   *Jane Jacobs and Steven J. Wolin*
Outcomes of Family-Involved Alcoholism Treatment   *Barbara S. McCrady*

III. Serotonin and Alcohol Preference   *Richard A. Deitrich, Section Editor*

Overview   *Richard A. Deitrich*
Serotonin and Ethanol Preference   *William J. McBride, James M. Murphy, Lawrence
    Lumeng, and Ting-Kai Li*
Use of Serotonin-Active Drugs in Alcohol Preference Studies   *Joseph E. Zabik*
Serotonin Uptake Blockers and Voluntary Alcohol Consumption: A Review of
    Recent Studies   *Kathryn Gill and Z. Amit*

**IV. Clinical Pharmacology in the Treatment of Alcohol Dependence: Manipulation
    of Neurobehavioral Mechanisms of Drinking**   *Alfonso Paredes, Section Editor*

Overview   *Alfonso Paredes*
Serotonin Uptake Inhibitors Attentuate Ethanol Intake in Problem
    Drinkers   *Claudio A. Naranjo and Edward M. Sellers*
Serotonin Uptake Blockers and the Treatment of Alcoholism   *David A. Gorelick*
Benzodiazepines in the Treatment of Alcoholism   *David Nutt, Bryon Adinoff, and
    Marku Linnoila*
Does Lithium Carbonate Therapy for Alcoholism Deter Relapse Drinking?   *David
    C. Clark and Jan Fawcett*
Treatment of Chronic Organic Mental Disorders Associated with
    Alcoholism   *Peter R. Martin, Michael J. Eckardt, and Markku Linnoila*
Methodological and Ethical Issues in Alcohol Research   *Alfonso Paredes.*

Index

Abortion, 107
Abstinence as treatment, 279–280, 289–291
Acetylcholine, 227
Addiction, *see also separate substances*
  factors, common, 259–262
    affects, 260–261
    relationships, 261
    self-care, 262
    self-esteem, 261
    well-being, 261
  as psychiatric disorder, 257
  psychpathology, structural, 257
  is suicide on the installment plan, 262
Adolescence: *see* Adolescent
Adolescent, *see also* Polydrug abuse
  alcohol problems, 111–123, 177–179, 184
  behavior problems, 184–185
  correlates, psychiatric, 111–123
  covariates, social, 125–143
  DOMAIN model, 186
  drug use, 125–143
    age, 126–131
      onset, 127–129
      period, 129–131
    and family, 131–135
    and life events, 139–140
    peers, 131
    work roles, 131–135
  family background, 190
  mother's role, 191
  problem drinking: *see* alcohol problems
Adulthood, young: *see* Adolescent
Affect, 53, 258, 260–261
  disturbance: *see* Depression
Age
  and alcoholism, 113
  and drug use, 126–131
    onset, 127–129
    period, 129–131
Alcohol abuse, 47–68, 173–201
  acquisition techniques for animals, 7
  in adolescence, 111–123, 177–179, 182–184
  affects, 266–268
  assessment, 306–307

Alcohol abuse (*cont.*)
  aversion therapy, 308–309; *see also* treatment
  behavior, reinforced, 7–19
  benzodiazepine interaction, 233–239; *see also* Benzodiazepine and cigarette smoking, 26; *see also* nicotine interaction *vs. cocaine*, 292
  consequences, 149–150, 174–179
    listed, 175
    model, two-dimensional, 176–177
  correlates, psychiatric, 111–123
  and death, 164–166
  dependence, 28–33, 57, 277–281, 285–304
    criteria for, 69–83
    diagnosis difficult, 277–279
    overview, 105–109
    syndrome concept introduced in 1976, 71
  drinking
    behavior, 71–72, 195
      180 questionnaires exist, 71
    criteria, idiosyncratic, 174
    and disruption at work, 182
    models, 176–181
    pattern, 8, 156–157
    and polydrug use, 183
    postprandial, 8
    problems, 173–201
      and ego, 189
    variables, 195
  and drug abuse, concurrent, 145–171, 182–184, 273–283; *see also* Polydrug abuse
  and ethnicity, 146–147
  factors
    biochemical, 24–28
    social, 24
  and family history of alcoholism, 180–181
  and food, 8, 20–22
  and gender, 15–16, 113, 146–147, 189–190
  and genetics, 16–19
  and hallucination, 28, 30
  and heroin, 148–149, 153–154, 159–163; *see also* Heroin
  impairment, 180
  by Iroquois Indians, 248

Alcohol abuse (*cont'd*)
  and marijuana, 26
  and menstruation, 26
  and methadone maintenance, 148–149
  models (minitheories), 179–181
  and narcotics addicts, 145–171; *see also*
      Polydrug abuse
  and nicotine interaction
    behavioral, 222–223
    cross-tolerance, 223
    mechanism of, 224–228
    physiological, 222–223
    at receptor level, 221–231
    and receptor structure, 224
    self-administration, 222
  and occupation, 250
  patterns, 8, 148, 156–157
  and peer pressure, 180–181
  and pharmacology, behavioral, 5–46
  and phencyclidine (PCP), 27
  and polydipsia, schedule-induced, in ani-
      mal, 7–8
  problems
    in adolescence, 111–123
    listed, 175
  as prosthetic, 262
  recovery, 280–281
  reinforcement strategies, 7–19
  relapse, 281
  and relationships, 268
  and religion, 250
  as sedative, 266
  self-administration, 13–14
  self-esteem, 119, 267–268
  self-medication, 265–266
  and substitution, intravenous, 9–12
    oral, 8–9
  as superego solvent, 268
  and support systems, social, 280–281
  tension reduction theory, 179–181
  tobacco interaction, 205–219; *see also* ciga-
      rette smoking; nicotine interaction
    behavior, 211–219
    diseases, 216
    dose-related, 206
    studies, 206–209
    tolerance, 210
  treatment, 279–280, 285–327
    aversion therapy, 308–309
      chemical, 308
      electrical, 308
      emetine, 308
      pilocarpine, 308
      sensitization, covert, 308
    behavioral, 305–327

Alcohol abuse (*cont.*)
  treatment (*cont.*)
    community-based, 273–283
    methods, six, 307–318
    in the United States, 274–275
    vulnerability, 177
    and well-being, 267–268
Alcoholics Anonymous, 99
Alcoholism
  case histories, 92–97
  common factors, 259–262
    affects, 260–261
    relationships, 261
    self-care, 262
    self-esteem, 261
    well-being, 261
  correlates, psychiatric, 113–120
    age, 113
    behavior
      depressive, 120
      deviant, 119–120
    demographic, 113–115
    ethnicity, 113–114
    gender, 113
    parents, 115–116
    peers, 116–118
    personality, 118–119
    psychiatric, 119–120
    religion, 114
    socioeconomic status, 114–115
    values, personal, 118–119
  as disorder, behavioral, 146
  eradication efforts, 99
  family of origin, 147
  psychopathology, 188
    religion, 114
    religiosity, 118–119
  secondary, 92–94
  self-medication hypothesis, 255–271
  self-regulation hypothesis, 255–271
  tension reduction hypothesis, 179
  time factor, 194
Alexithymia, 260, 267
Alprazolam, 266
γ-Aminobutyric acid (GABA), 237
Amphetamine, 12, 13, 25, 32, 309, 310
Analgesic, 264–265; *see also* Opiate
Angel dust: *see also* Phencyclidine
Apomorphine, 309
Arousal, 53
  affective, 53
Aversion therapy, 307–310
  chemical, 308
  electrical, 308
  sensitization, covert, 309

Baboon, 15
Barbital, 16
Barbiturate, 266, 267
Beck Depression Inventory Score, 120
  and alcoholism, 120
Beer, 249, 250
  origin of, 246
Behavior
  vs. biology, 58, 61, 62
  deviant and alcoholism, 119–120
  drug-reinforced, 5–6
  reinforced, 7–9
  and treatment, 305–327
Belushi, John (comedian), 87–89
Benzodiazepine, 266
  and alcohol interaction, 233–239
  clinical consideration, 234–236
  cross-tolerance, 234–235
  driving ability, 235
  overdose, 235–236
  pharmacodynamics, 237–238
  pharmacokinetics, 236–237
Biology *vs.* behavior, 58, 61, 62
Bungarotoxin, 224–225

Caffeine, 16
Cannabis: *see* Marijuana
3-Carbo-*t*-butoxy-*b*-carboline, 238
Case histories
  Belushi, John, 87–89
  drug dependence, 87–89
  multiaxial system, 97–101
  polysubstance use, 89–91
  post-traumatic stress disorder, 91–94
  primary–secondary distinction, 91–94
  psychopathology, 94–97
Causality and alcoholism, 187, 190
Chlordiazepoxide, 27, 32, 234
Cholesterol, 226
CIDI: *see* Composite International Diagnostic
    Interview
Cigarette smoking, 20, 249
  and alcohol consumption, 205–219
  topography, 208
Citalopram, 25
Civil Addict Program of Southern California,
    151–157
  interview
    first, 152–155
    second, 155–157
  sample characteristic, 151–152
Classification of Diseases, 10th ed., 70
Coca, 246
  leaf chewing, 20
Cocaine, 9, 12, 14, 20, 22, 23, 25, 27, 28, 47,

Cocaine (*cont.*)
    48, 61–64, 73, 246, 249, 263–264,
    292–294, 318
  vs. alcohol, 292
  crack, 246
  "crash," 296
  dependence, 57
  form used by addict, 294
  outpatient treatment, 286
  as stimulant, 264
  treatment, 291
    for outpatient, 286
  use in United States in 1985, 274
  withdrawal syndrome absent, 285–286
Cohabitation and drug abuse, 133
Common factor model of drug use initiation,
    183
Community-based program for treatment,
    273–283
Community reinforcement approach, 308
  and contingency contract as treatment, 314
Comorbidity in patient, 95–97
Composite International Diagnostic Interview
    (CIDI), 51
  reliability, statistical, 73
  substance abuse module (CIDI-SAM), 72
Construct
  of dependence: *see* Dependence
  of hunger: *see* Hunger
  hypothetical, measures for, 48
Consumption of alcohol: *see* Alcohol abuse
Contingency contract as treatment, 314
Conventionality, measures of
  and alcoholism, 118–119
Coping, 192–193; *see also* Stress
  and drinking, 192–193
Correlates, psychiatric, in alcoholism: *see*
    Alcoholism
Covariates, social, in adolescence: *see*
    Adolescent
Crack: *see* Cocaine
Craving, 49
Cronbach's alpha value, 60–61
Cue exposure, 318
  and conditioned withdrawal/craving, 318
Culture
  and chastity, premarital, 251
  lag, 252
  and lying, 251
  as metaphor, 251–252
  is what people do, 251
Curiosity, 56

Delirium tremens, 28
Demerol abuser, 309

Dependence, 1–4
  across substances, 62
  on alcohol, 47–48
  aspect, motivational, 56
  assessment, 56–58
  concept, 47–68, 87–89
  constructs, 48–49, 64–65
  criteria, 51, 79–80
    for alcohol, 69–83
    for drugs, 69–83
    operationalization, 69–83
  data collection, 50–51
    theory-bound, 51–52
  definition, 51
  diagnosis, 49–51
    guidelines for, 49–50
    issues unresolved, 85–104
    multiaxial system, 97–101
    primary-secondary distinction, 91–94
    psychopathology, 94–97
    withdrawal, 56–58
      assessment, 56
  drug
    frequency unrelated to dependence, 59
    quantity unrelated to dependence, 58
  factors, social, 106
  on hunger, 51–54
  interview, problems with, 69–70
  methodology, 56–59
  motivation theory, 52–56; 65–66; see also
      Motivation
  new look at syndrome, 47–49
  observation of, 51
  results, 59–64
  scales, consistency, internal, 60–61
  on substances, 47–48; see also Polydrug
      abuse
  syndrome is unidimensional, 60
  theory, 51–52
    motivation, 52–56, 65–66
  unidimensional, 60
  variables
    behavioral, 50, 58–59, 62–64
    biological, 50, 58–59, 62–64
  and withdrawal, 28–33
Depression, mental, 94–95
  and alcoholism, 120, 188–189
  and substance abuser, 53
Deviance, social, 108–109
Diagnosis, axial, 101
  of dependence: see Dependence
Diagnostic interview schedule of NIMH, 72
Diagnostic and Statistical Manual, 3rd ed., Re-
      vised (DSM-III-R), 70, 86
Diazepam, 27, 32, 235–236

Differential reinforcement, 31–32
Dihydrocodeine, 33
Dis-ease as disease, 102
Distress theories and Freud, 258–259
  and alcoholism, 119
Drinamyl abuser, 317
Drinking: see Alcohol abuse
Drive
  motivation, 56
  reduction, 54
Drug abuse, illicit
  and abortion, 133
  age of first use, 152
  and alcoholism, concurrent, 182–184
  of antidepressant, 255
  assessment, 306–307
  aversion therapy, 308–309
    with apomorphine, 309
    chemical, 309
    electrical, 309
    with scoline, 309
  as behavior disorder, 146
  of choice for user, 245–254, 263
    and culture, 250–254
    factors of, 245–254
    as phenomenon, 247–248
    psychoactive, 246–247
  and cohabitation, 133, 138
  conditioning, classical, 48–49
  container analogy, 263
  and curiosity, 56
  and delinquency, 185
  dependence, 28–33; see also Dependence
  disruptive, 176
  drive motivation, 56
  effects, pattern of, 137–138
  by high-school students, 131, 135
  and homophily, 139
  incentive motivation, 56
  initiation model
    common factor, 183
    simplex, 183
  and job, 138
  and life events, 139–140
  and marriage, 132–135
    time of, 135, 138
  and peers, 139
  pharmacology, behavioral, 5–46
  and polydrug use, 187; see also Polydrug
      abuse
  and pregnancy, 133
  progression with age, 128
    from alcohol to marijuana to hard drugs,
      182
  as prosthetic, 262

Drug abuse (*cont.*)
  psychopharmacological
    antidepressant, 255
    mood-altering, 256
    tranquilizer, 255
  as reinforcer, 7–19
    maintenance of, 19–28
  response
    behavioral, 49
    biological, 48
  role transition of user, 136–138
  treatment, 273–327
    community-based program, 273–283,
      285–304
    methods, six, 307–318
    trend, historical, 130
  and unemployment, 134
  use, changing pattern of, 248–249
  variation, intracultural, 249–250

Education
  and control model, 253
  and model, sociocultural, 253
  as prevention, 252–254
Ego structure, 258–259
Emetine, 308
Emotion
  coping with, 260
  lack of, 261
Epidemiologic Catchment Area Survey,
  72
Estrogen, 25, 26
Ethanol, *see also* Alcohol abuse; Alcoholism
  –nicotine interaction at nicotine receptor
    level, 221–231
Ethnicity and alcoholism, 113–114, 145–171
Ethylketazocine, 15
Etonitazene, 22
Euphoria, 66

Family
  and adolescent, 190
  and drug use, 131–135
  therapy
    behavioral, 308, 312–313
    marital, 308, 312–313
  and vulnerability, 190–191
Feeding conditions, altered, 20–22
Feelings, 258–259
  lack of, 267
Feighner criteria, 72
Fluoxetine, 25
Fluvoxamine, 25
Food deprivation with animal models, 8, 20

Gender, 15–16, 146–147, 189–190
  and alcohol abuse, 15–16, 113, 146–147,
    164
  and drinking pattern, 189
  and drug abuse, 15–16
  men alcoholics, 189–190
  and vulnerability, 189–190
  women alcoholics, 189–190
Global assessment of functioning scale, 101
Glutethimide, 266
Guttman scale, 60, 182

Hallucination, alcoholic, 28, 30
Heroin abuse, 148–149, 166, 250, 275, 309,
  313
  and alcohol abuse, 149, 153, 154, 159–163
  consequences, 149–150
  decline of use, 130
  treatment, 291
Homophily and drug use, 139
Human animal and drug, psychoactive, 246–
  247
  beer, 246
  chocolate, 246
  coffee, 246
  tea, 246
  tobacco, 246
Hunger, 51–54
  and dependence on, 51–52, 54
  disorders of, 52
  and motivation, 48, 52
  as substance dependence, 52
Hyperexcitability, 29

Imidazobenzodiazepine RO 15-4513, 27
Incentive motivation, 56
International Classification of Diseases, 86
Interview, essentials of a good, 74–77
  operationalization of dependence
    criteria listed, 79–80
  questions
    evaluation, 77–78
    length, 75–76

Job and drug abuse, 138

Ketamine, 13
Khat, 247

Laudanum, 246
Learning theory, 53, 54, 65
Life events and drug abuse, 139–140
Lorprazolam, 237
LSD, 28, 247, 250, 310, 317

Macaca nemestrina, 24
Marijuana, 26, 73, 106–108, 127–132, 182,
　　185, 249, 250
　effects, 137–138
　and marriage, 132
　　time of, 135
　and parenthood, 132
　and pregnancy, 133
　tea, 248
　trend, historical, 130
　use in United States in *1985*, 274, 276
Marriage and drug use, 132, 133
Membrane fluidity, 226
Men alcoholics, 189–190
Mescaline, 28, 247, 249
Methadone, 208, 275, 276, 313, 314
　maintenance, 148–166
　　and alcohol abuse, 148–149
Methaqualone, 16
Methohexital, 9
Methylxanthine, 28
Midazolam, 238
Monkey, 22, 23
Morphine, 16, 24, 31, 33, 246
Mother's role and adolescent drinking, 191
Motivation
　acquired, 54–56
　　two-stage process, 55
　and affect, 53
　and arousal, 53
　behavior *vs.* biology, 53
　biology *vs.* behavior, 53
　construct, 52–53
　curiosity, 56
　definition of, 53–54
　and dependence, 56
　drive -, 56
　and hunger, 48
　incentive, 56
　theory, 52–56, 65–66
　　and related constructs, 52–53
Mouse, 15
　food deprivation, 20
　inbreeding, 18–19
Mushroom, 249
　hallucinogenic, 246
　　in Mazatec region of Mexico, 248
　"magic," 249
Nalorphine, 15
Naloxone
　challenge test, 57, 59
　hydrochloride injection, 57
Naltexone, 28
　Narcotics addict and alcohol abuse, 145–
　　171

Neuroadaptation, 54
Nicotine, 14; *see also* Cigarette smoking;
　　Tobacco
　receptor structure, 224–225
　　and alcohol, 226–228
　　and function, 225–226
　　and lipids, 225–226
NIMH Diagnostic Interview Schedule, 72
Nonconformity and alcoholism, 188
Nosology, 85

Operationalization, 50
　and borderline cases, 50
　limit of, 136–137
Opiate, 47, 48, 61–66
　addict, 318
　and alcohol abuse, 147
　as analgesic, 264–265
　dependence, 57
　　naloxone challenge test, 57
Opioid: *see* Opiate
Opium, 246–249
　wars, 246
Opponent-process theory, 54–55
Outpatient treatment, 285–304
　abstinence
　　early, 301–302
　　immediate, 295
　　total is essential, 295–296, 300
　activities, other, 299
　assessment, 299
　care, total, 299
　for chemical addicts, 285–304
　crisis intervention, 299
　effectiveness, 294–299
　　avoidance, total, of drugs, 296
　　education, 297
　　family support, 297
　　guidelines, 298
　　in stages, 295
　　structured program, 285–304
　　urine testing, 297–298
　indications for, 289
　vs. inpatient treatment, 287–288
　　cost, 288
　　effectiveness, 287
　recovery, advanced, 302–303
　relapse prevention, 302
　self-help group, 298
　stages of, 299–303
　therapy, pharmacological, 299

Parent
　alcohol abuse, 115–116, 152, 164, 191

Parent (*cont.*)
  and drugs, 138
  loss of, 147
Patient, dis-ease as disease, 109
PCP: *see* Phencyclidine
Peer influence, 116–118, 180
  and alcohol abuse, 116–118, 180–181
  and drug abuse, 131, 139
Pentazocine, 14, 33
Pentobarbital, 8–9, 13–16, 33
Period of high risk and drug abuse, 140
Personality
  addictive, 187
  alcohol abuse, 118–119
  causality, 187, 190
  predisposition, 188
  vulnerability, 187
Peyote, 246–248
  and Huichoi Indians of Mexico, 247
Phencyclidine, 13, 20–23, 27, 249
  self-administration, 9–11
Pilocarpine, 308
Polydipsia in rat, schedule-induced, 7–8
Polydrug abuse, 26–27, 89–91, 145–171, 182–
      184, 245, 273–283
  and dependence, 89–91
  popular during the 1980s, 290
  preventing relapse, 291
  treatment issues, 277–281, 290
  treatment techniques, 291–294
  use in United States in 1985, 274–275
Post-traumatic stress disorder, 91–94
Pregnancy and drug use, 133, 138
Problems of alcohol abuse, listed, 175
Problem behavior theory, 186
  predictors, 186–187
Prohibition (United States), 249
Psychiatry, descriptive, 100
Psychopathology
  and alcoholism, 188
  and drug addiction, 257

Rat, 5–33, 66
  breeding selectively, 17–18
    inbreeding, 17–18
  withdrawal symptoms, 28–29
Reinforcement: *see* Alcohol abuse,
      reinforcement
Reinforcer of behavior, defined, 5
Religion and alcoholism, 114
Religiosity and alcoholism, 118–119
Renard Diagnostic Interview, 72
Response, conditioned, 49
Rhesus monkey, 8–9, 12–16
  self-administration of ethanol, 8–9, 12

RO 15-4513, 238
Role playing as therapy, 316
Rum fits, 28

SCID: *see* Structured clinical interview
Scoline, 309
Secobarbital, 266
Sedative–hypnotic drug
  alcohol: *see* Alcohol
  alprazolam, 266
  barbiturate, 266
  benzodiazepine, 266
  glutethimide, 266
  secobarbital, 266
Self-administration by animal, 8–9, 12–16; *see
      also* Rat; Rhesus monkey
  route, 13–14
Self-care, 262
  deficit in alcohol addict, 262
    in cocaine addict, 262
    in opiate addict, 262
Self-control, behavioral, training, 308–311
  and driving-while-intoxicated (DWI), 311
Self-esteem, 261, 267–268
  and alcoholism, 119, 267–268
  deficit in addict, 261
Self-medication, 265–266
Self-regulation
  and distress, human, 258–259
  need, human, for, 256–257
Sensitization, covert, as treatment, 309–310
  and hypnosis, 310
  and valeric acid, 310
Serotonin, 25
Simplex model of drug use initiation, 183
Social skill training, 308
  role playing, 316
Solvent sniffing, 250
Species and alcohol, 15
Status, socioeconomic, and alcoholism, 114–
      115
Stimulant: *see* Cocaine
Stress, *see also* Tension-reduction hypothesis
  and coping, 192–193
  defined, 316
  disorder, post-traumatic, 91–94
  management training, 308, 316–318
    and group counseling, 317
  and stressors, 192–193
  term confusing, 192
  types of, 192–193
  and vulnerability, 192–194
Structured clinical interview (SCID), 51, 57,
      69–83

Substance
  and neuroadaptation syndrome, 54
  psychoactive, 71
    alcohol, 71
    drugs, 71
    tobacco, 71
Superego, part of the mind soluble in alcohol, 266
System, multiaxial, 97–101
Temperance Movement, 99, 249
Tension-reduction hypothesis, 192; *see also* Stress
  of alcoholism, 179
Tobacco, 71, 73, 205–219, 246; *see also* Cigarette smoking; Nicotine; Alcohol abuse
Tolerance, 48, 64, 210
Torpedo californica, 224–227
Tranquilizer
  major, 255
  minor, 255
Treatment, residential, inpatient, for 28 days, 287; *see also separate substances*
Tremor, 28, 29
Triazolam, 236–237
Tryptophan, 25

Unemployment and drug abuse, 134
Unidimensionality, 64–65
  of alcohol, 60
  of cocaine, 60
  of opiate, 60

Urine as drink, 249

Valeric acid, 310
Values, personal, and alcoholism, 118–119
V-code, 100
Vulnerability and alcoholism
  and family, 190–191
  and gender, 189–190
  and personality, 187
  and stress, 192–194

Well-being, 261
  deficit in addict, 261
Wine, 249
Withdrawal syndrome, 48–50, 56–60
  animal models, 29
  autonomic symptoms, 29
  behavioral signs, 29
  convulsion, 29
  gastrointestinal signs, 29
  hyperexcitability, 29
  motor symptoms, 29
  from opiate, 59–60
  performance measures, 31–33
  severity, 30–31
  seizure, 29
Woman alcoholic, 189–190
Work role and drug abuse, 131–135

Zimelidine, 25
Zuckerman's sensation-seeking scale for opiate addicts, 54